The Pediatric Cardiac Anesthesia Handbook

The Pediatric Cardiac Anesthesia Handbook

Second Edition

Viviane G. Nasr, M.D., MPH, FASA

Associate Professor of Anaesthesia
Harvard Medical School
Chief, Division of Cardiac Anesthesia
Francis X. McGowan, Jr. M.D. Chair in Cardiac Anesthesia
Boston Children's Hospital
Boston, MA, USA

James A. DiNardo, M.D., FAAP, FASA

Professor of Anaesthesia
Harvard Medical School
Senior Associate in Cardiac Anesthesia
Boston Children's Hospital
Boston, MA, USA

Library of Congress Cataloging-in-Publication Data
Names: Nasr, Viviane G, author.
Title: The pediatric cardiac anesthesia handbook / Viviane G Nasr.
Description: Second edition. | Hoboken, NJ : Wiley-Blackwell, 2025. |
    Includes bibliographical references and index.
Identifiers: LCCN 2024023168 (print) | LCCN 2024023169 (ebook) |
ISBN 9781119835394 (paperback) | ISBN 9781119835400 (adobe pdf) |
ISBN 9781119835417 (epub)
Subjects: MESH: Heart Defects, Congenital–surgery | Infant | Cardiac
    Surgical Procedures–methods | Anesthesia–methods | Child
Classification: LCC RJ426.C64 (print) | LCC RJ426.C64 (ebook) | NLM WS
    295 | DDC 618.92/12043–dc23/eng/20240701
LC record available at https://lccn.loc.gov/2024023168
LC ebook record available at https://lccn.loc.gov/2024023169

Cover Design: Wiley
Cover Image: © Godong/Alamy Stock Photo

Set in 10/12pt WarnockPro by Straive, Pondicherry, India
Printed in Singapore
M118595_120924

Contents

Preface to the Second Edition   *xix*

Part I   The Basics   *1*

1   Cardiovascular Development   *3*
Embryology   *3*
Cardiovascular Physiology   *3*
    Fetal Circulation   *3*
    Closure of the Ductus Arteriosus   *5*
    Closure of the Foramen Ovale   *6*
    Closure of the Ductus Venosus   *6*
    Pulmonary Vascular Changes   *6*
Myocardial Performance in the Neonate   *7*
    Hemodynamic Changes at Birth   *7*
References and Further Reading   *8*

2   Important Concepts in Congenital Heart Disease   *9*
Pathophysiology of CHD   *9*
Concepts of Shunting, Single-Ventricle Physiology, and Intercirculatory Mixing   *9*
    Shunting   *9*
        Effective Blood Flow   *10*
        Total Pulmonary Blood Flow/Total Systemic Blood Flow   *10*
    Single-Ventricle Physiology   *10*
    Intercirculatory Mixing   *13*
    Classification of Anatomic Shunts   *15*
        Simple Shunts   *15*
        Complex Shunts   *17*
Pulmonary Vascular Pathophysiology   *18*
    Causes of Precapillary PH in CHD   *18*
    Causes of Postcapillary PH in CHD   *18*
Control of Pulmonary Vascular Resistance   *19*
    PaO_2 *19*
    $PaCO_2$ *19*
    pH   *19*
    Variation in Lung Volumes   *19*
    Vasodilator Agents   *20*
    Sympathetic Nervous System Stimulation   *20*
    Anesthetic Agents   *21*
    Vasoactive Agents   *21*

Myocardial Ischemia *21*
  Aortic Diastolic Pressure *21*
  Subendocardial Pressure *22*
  Heart Rate *22*
  Anatomic Coronary Artery Lesions *22*
References and Further Reading *22*

3 Preoperative Evaluation *23*
Clinical History *23*
Physical Examination *23*
Associated Congenital Abnormalities *24*
Laboratory Data *24*
Pregnancy *27*
Psychological Considerations *27*
Preoperative Preparation *27*
  Preoperative Fluid Therapy *28*
  Preoperative Medications *28*
References and Further Reading *31*

4 Intraoperative Management *33*
Intraoperative Monitoring *33*
  ECG and Blood Pressure *33*
  Systemic Oxygen Saturation *34*
  End-tidal CO_2 *34*
  Central Venous Pressure *34*
  Temperature *35*
  Near-infra-red Spectroscopy *36*
  Transcranial Doppler *36*
  Transesophageal Echocardiography (TEE) *38*
Airway Management *38*
Anesthesia Induction and Maintenance *39*
  Induction of Anesthesia *39*
    Mask Induction *39*
    Intravenous Induction *39*
  Maintenance of Anesthesia *40*
References and Further Reading *40*

5 Developmental Hemostasis and Patient Blood Management *41*
Current Concept of Hemostasis (Coagulation, Anticoagulation, and Fibrinolysis) *41*
  Initiation *44*
  Amplification *44*
  Propagation *44*
  Stabilization *44*
  Inhibition of Coagulation *44*
  Fibrinolysis *45*
  Special Considerations in Neonates and Infants *46*
  Cyanosis *46*
Patient Blood Management *46*
References and Further Reading *47*

6   Interpretation of Cardiac Catheterization Data   *49*
    Right-Heart Catheterization   *49*
        Right Atrial Pressure (RAP) Waveform   *49*
        Right Ventricular Pressure (RVP) Waveform   *49*
        Pulmonary Artery Pressure (PAP) Waveform   *50*
    Left-Heart Catheterization   *50*
        Left Atrial Pressure (LAP) Waveform   *51*
        Left Ventricular Pressure (LVP) Waveform   *51*
        Aortic Pressure Waveform   *51*
    Left Ventriculography   *51*
    Coronary Angiography   *53*
        Coronary Anatomy   *53*
        Anatomic Coronary Lesions   *54*
        Coronary Collaterals   *55*
    Cardiac Output Determination   *55*
        Thermodilution Technique   *55*
        Fick Determination   *55*
    Evaluation of Cardiac Shunts   *56*
        Shunt Location   *56*
        Shunt Quantification   *56*
    Saturation Data   *58*
    Resistances   *58*
    Assessment of Pulmonary Vascular Anatomy   *58*
        Evaluation of the Pulmonary Vasculature   *58*
        Pulmonary Artery Wedge Angiogram   *59*
        Pulmonary Vein Wedge Angiogram   *59*
        Assessment of Pulmonary Hypertension (PH)   *59*
    Assessment of Valve Lesions   *60*
        Stenotic Lesions   *60*
        Regurgitant Lesions   *61*
    References and Further Reading   *61*

7   Management of Cardiopulmonary Bypass   *63*
    The Cardiopulmonary Bypass Circuit   *63*
    Differences Between Adult and Pediatric CPB   *65*
        CPB Flow Rates   *65*
        Circuit Size and Component Selection   *65*
        Anesthesia During CPB   *66*
        Monitoring During CPB   *66*
        Hemodilution   *66*
        Priming Solution   *66*
        Ultrafiltration   *68*
            Conventional Ultrafiltration   *69*
            Modified Ultrafiltration   *69*
    Blood Gas Management   *69*
    Deep Hypothermic Circulatory Arrest and Antegrade Cerebral Perfusion Techniques   *71*
        Deep Hypothermic Circulatory Arrest (DHCA)   *71*
            Hypothermia   *71*
            Acid–base Management   *71*
        Antegrade Cerebral Perfusion (ACP)   *72*

Anticoagulation   *73*
Protamine Reversal of Heparin   *74*
Post-CPB Hemostasis   *77*
    Platelet Repletion   *77*
    Fibrinogen Repletion   *79*
    Prothrombin Complex Concentrates (PCC), rVIIA, Desmopressin
    Administration   *79*
    Red Cell Repletion   *81*
    Antifibrinolytics   *83*
References and Further Reading   *84*

8   Echocardiography   *85*
Transthoracic Echocardiography   *85*
Transesophageal Echocardiography   *85*
    Epicardial Echocardiography   *95*
Goals of a Comprehensive Echocardiographic Exam   *96*
    Atrial Identity and Location   *98*
    Ventricular Size and Identity   *98*
    Atrioventricular Relationship   *99*
    Great Vessel Orientation and Identity   *99*
    Ventriculoarterial Relationship   *99*
    Presence of Intracardiac Shunts and Obstructive Lesions   *99*
    Evaluation of the Surgical Repair   *100*
        Patch Leaks   *100*
        Baffle Obstruction   *100*
        Stenotic Valves   *100*
        Regurgitant Valves   *100*
        Stenotic Anastomoses   *100*
        Ventricular Function Assessment   *101*
        Patency of Aortopulmonary Shunts   *101*
        Patency of Cavopulmonary Shunts   *101*
References and Further Reading   *101*

9   Risk Scoring Systems in Patients with Congenital Heart Disease   *103*
Cardiac Surgery   *103*
    Catheterization   *103*
Noncardiac Procedures   *106*
References and Further Reading   *108*

10   Mechanical Circulatory Support   *109*
Extracorporeal Membrane Oxygenation   *109*
    Indications   *109*
    Relative Contraindications   *109*
    Modes of ECMO Support   *109*
        Venovenous (VV) ECMO   *109*
        Venoarterial (VA) ECMO   *110*
    Device and Patient Complications   *110*
    Common Terminology Used During an ECMO Run   *111*
    Intraoperative Considerations for Patients on ECMO   *111*
Ventricular Assist Devices   *113*
    Indications   *113*

Relative Contraindications   113
Current VAD and TAH Technologies   113
Pneumatic Pulsatile Flow Devices   113
Axial Continuous Flow Devices   115
Centrifugal Continuous Flow Devices   118
Complications   119
Anesthetic Considerations for Patients Receiving VAD   119
Induction of Anesthesia and Pre-bypass Management   120
Post-VAD Placement Management   120
BiVAD Insertion   123
References and Further Reading   124

11   Postoperative Cardiac Intensive Care Unit Care   127
Structured Hand-off from OR to CICU Team   127
Sedation/Analgesia Medications   127
Benzodiazepines   129
Opioids   129
Propofol   130
Dexmedetomidine   130
Ketamine   131
Management of Sedation/Analgesia   131
Detection and Treatment of Low Cardiac Output Syndrome   131
Mechanical Ventilation   136
Enhanced Recovery after Surgery and Early Tracheal Extubation   138
Extended CICU Care   139
References and Further Reading   141

Part II   Specific Lesions   143

12   Patent Ductus Arteriosus   145
Introduction   145
Anatomy   145
Physiology   145
Surgical Therapy   145
Catheterization Laboratory Intervention   146
Anesthetic Management   146
Induction and Maintenance   146
Postligation Cardiac Syndrome   147
Noncardiac Surgery   147
References and Further Reading   147

13   Aortopulmonary Window   149
Introduction   149
Anatomy   149
Physiology   149
Surgical Management   149
Catheterization Laboratory Intervention   150
Anesthetic Management   150
Noncardiac Surgery   151
References and Further Reading   151

14 Coarctation of the Aorta *153*
Introduction   *153*
Anatomy   *153*
Physiology   *153*
Surgical Therapy   *157*
Catheterization Laboratory Intervention   *157*
Anesthetic Management   *157*
   Induction and Maintenance   *158*
   Management after Cross-clamp Removal   *158*
Noncardiac Surgery   *159*
References and Further Reading   *159*

15 Atrial Septal Defect *161*
Introduction   *161*
Anatomy   *161*
   Ostium Secundum ASD   *161*
   Ostium Primum ASD   *161*
   Sinus Venosus Defects   *162*
   Coronary Sinus Defect   *163*
Physiology   *163*
Surgical Therapy   *164*
Catheterization Laboratory Intervention   *164*
Anesthetic Management   *164*
   Induction and Maintenance   *165*
Post-CPB Management   *165*
Noncardiac Surgery   *165*
References and Further Reading   *165*

16 Ventricular Septal Defect *167*
Introduction   *167*
Anatomy   *167*
   Subpulmonary or Supracristal Defects   *167*
   Membranous or Perimembranous Defects   *167*
   Conoventricular Defects   *167*
   Inlet or Canal-type Defects   *167*
   Muscular Defects   *167*
Physiology   *167*
Surgical Therapy   *169*
Catheterization Laboratory Intervention   *169*
Anesthetic Management   *169*
   Induction and Maintenance   *169*
Post-CPB Management   *170*
Noncardiac Surgery   *170*
References and Further Reading   *170*

17 Atrioventricular Canal Defects *171*
Introduction   *171*
Anatomy   *171*
   Partial AVC   *171*
   Transitional AVC   *171*

Intermediate AVC   *171*
Complete AVC (CAVC)   *171*
Unbalanced AVC   *173*
Physiology   *173*
Surgical Therapy   *174*
Anesthetic Management   *174*
Induction and Maintenance   *174*
Post-CPB Management   *175*
Noncardiac Surgery   *175*
References and Further Reading   *175*

18   Double Outlet Right Ventricle   *177*
Introduction   *177*
Anatomy   *177*
Physiology   *179*
Surgical Therapy   *180*
Anesthetic Management   *181*
Induction and Maintenance   *181*
Post-CPB Management   *181*
References and Further Reading   *181*

19   Truncus Arteriosus   *183*
Introduction   *183*
Anatomy   *183*
Physiology   *185*
Surgical Therapy   *185*
Catheterization Laboratory Intervention   *185*
Anesthetic Management   *185*
Goals   *185*
Induction and Maintenance   *186*
Post-CPB Management   *186*
Goals   *186*
References and Further Reading   *186*

20   Total Anomalous Pulmonary Venous Return   *187*
Introduction   *187*
Anatomy   *187*
Physiology   *188*
Surgical Therapy   *189*
Anesthetic Management   *189*
Goals   *189*
Induction and Maintenance   *190*
Post-CPB Management   *190*
Goals   *190*
Long-term Outcomes   *191*
References and Further Reading   *192*

21   Left Ventricular Outflow Tract Obstruction   *193*
Introduction   *193*
Anatomy   *193*

Physiology   *195*
  Williams–Beurin and nonsyndromic SVAS   *195*
Surgical Therapy   *195*
Catheterization Laboratory Intervention   *196*
Anesthetic Management   *196*
  Goals   *196*
  Induction and Maintenance   *197*
Post-CPB Management   *198*
References and Further Reading   *198*

22 Mitral Valve   *199*
Mitral Valve Stenosis   *199*
Introduction   *199*
Anatomy   *199*
Physiology   *200*
Surgical Therapy   *200*
Catheterization Laboratory Intervention   *200*
Anesthetic Management   *201*
  Goals   *201*
  Pre-induction   *202*
  Induction and Maintenance   *202*
Post-CPB Management   *202*
Mitral Valve Regurgitation   *203*
Introduction   *203*
Anatomy   *203*
Physiology   *203*
Surgical Management   *204*
Catheterization Laboratory Intervention   *204*
Anesthetic Management   *204*
  Goals   *204*
  Premedication   *205*
  Induction and Maintenance   *205*
Post-CPB Management   *205*
References and Further Reading   *205*

23 Pulmonary Atresia/Intact Ventricular Septum   *207*
Introduction   *207*
Anatomy   *207*
Physiology   *207*
Surgical and Catheter-based Therapy   *209*
Anesthetic Management   *211*
  Goals   *211*
Post-CPB Management   *211*
References and Further Reading   *211*

24 Tetralogy of Fallot   *213*
Introduction   *213*
Anatomy   *213*
Physiology   *213*

Hypoxic or Hypercyanotic Episodes ("Tet Spells")   *216*
Surgical Therapy   *217*
    Palliative Shunts   *217*
    Definitive Repair   *218*
Catheterization Laboratory Intervention   *219*
    PDA stenting   *219*
    RVOT stenting   *219*
    Adult TOF Patients   *219*
Anesthetic Management   *220*
    Goals   *220*
    Induction and Maintenance   *220*
Post-CPB Management   *221*
    Goals   *221*
    Postoperative Junctional Ectopic Tachycardia   *222*
Noncardiac Surgery   *223*
References and Further Reading   *223*

25   Tetralogy of Fallot with Pulmonary Atresia   *225*
Anatomy   *225*
Physiology   *225*
Surgical Therapy   *225*
Anesthetic Management   *227*
Post-CPB Management   *227*
References and Further Reading   *228*

26   Tetralogy of Fallot with Absent Pulmonary Valve   *229*
Anatomy   *229*
Physiology   *229*
Surgical Therapy   *229*
Anesthetic Management   *230*
Post-CPB Management   *230*
References and Further Reading   *230*

27   Transposition of the Great Arteries   *233*
Introduction   *233*
Anatomy   *233*
Physiology   *234*
Surgical Therapy   *237*
    Anatomic Repair or the Arterial (Jatene) Switch Procedure   *237*
    Intraatrial Physiologic Repair: Mustard and Senning Procedures   *239*
    Rastelli, Lecompte, and Nikaidoh Procedures   *240*
Anesthetic Management   *241*
    Goals   *241*
    Induction and Maintenance   *241*
Post-CPB Management   *241*
    Goals   *241*
Noncardiac Surgery   *243*
Congenitally Corrected Transposition of the Great Vessels   *243*
    Introduction   *243*
    Anatomy   *243*

Physiology   *244*
Surgical Management   *244*
Traditional Repair for C-TGV   *244*
Double Switch Procedure and Atrial Switch-Rastelli Procedures   *244*
References and Further Reading   *246*

28   Single-ventricle Lesions   *247*
Introduction   *247*
Physiology and Initial Procedures   *247*
Initial Procedures to Optimize Pulmonary Arterial Blood Flow   *247*
Initial Procedures to Optimize Pulmonary Venous Blood Flow   *249*
Initial Procedures to Optimize Systemic Blood Flow   *250*
Management of Single-ventricle Physiology   *250*
Anesthetic Management, Preinitial Repair   *251*
Goals   *251*
Induction and Maintenance   *253*
Post-CPB Management, Postinitial Repair   *254*
Goals   *254*
Single-ventricle Pathway, Superior Cavopulmonary Shunt or
Bidirectional Glenn   *254*
Anesthetic Management, Presuperior Cavopulmonary Shunt   *259*
Goals   *259*
Induction and Maintenance   *259*
Post-CPB Management, Postsuperior Cavopulmonary Shunt   *259*
Goals   *259*
Definitive Repair: The Fontan Procedure or Total Cavopulmonary Connection   *260*
Fontan Physiology   *260*
Fenestrated Fontan   *264*
Anesthetic Management, Pre-Fontan   *264*
Goals   *264*
Induction and Maintenance   *265*
Post-CPB Management, Post-Fontan Procedure   *265*
Goals   *265*
Noncardiac Surgery   *267*
References and Further Reading   *268*

29   Hypoplastic Left Heart Syndrome   *269*
Introduction   *269*
Anatomy   *269*
Physiology   *269*
Surgical Therapy   *271*
Anesthetic Management   *271*
Goals   *271*
Post-CPB Management   *272*
Biventricular Repair   *272*
The "Borderline" Left Heart   *272*
The Left Heart Rehabilitation   *272*
Staged Left Ventricular Recruitment   *272*
Biventricular Conversion   *273*

Noncardiac Surgery   *273*
References and Further Reading   *273*

30   Interrupted Aortic Arch   *275*
Introduction   *275*
Anatomy   *275*
Physiology   *275*
Surgical Management   *276*
Catheterization Laboratory Intervention   *278*
Anesthetic Management   *278*
 Goals   *278*
 Induction and Maintenance   *279*
Post-CPB Management   *279*
 Goals   *279*
References and Further Reading   *279*

31   Vascular Rings   *281*
Introduction   *281*
Anatomy   *281*
Physiology   *281*
Surgical Management   *281*
Catheterization Laboratory Intervention   *283*
Anesthetic Management   *283*
References and Further Reading   *284*

32   Tricuspid Atresia   *285*
Introduction   *285*
Anatomy   *285*
Physiology   *285*
Surgical Therapy   *287*
Anesthetic Management   *287*
 Goals   *287*
References and Further Reading   *288*

33   Heart Transplantation   *289*
The Donor   *289*
Anesthetic Management of the Recipient   *292*
 Preoperative Evaluation   *292*
 Physical Examination   *292*
 Premedication   *292*
 Preinduction   *292*
 Induction and Maintenance   *293*
Operative Procedure   *295*
Post-CPB Management   *297*
 Goals   *297*
 Preparation for Termination of CPB   *297*
  Impaired Systolic Function   *297*
  Right Ventricular Afterload Mismatch   *298*
  Sinus and Atrioventricular Node Dysfunction   *298*

Impaired Diastolic Function   *298*
Termination of CPB   *299*
Noncardiac Surgery in the Postcardiac Transplant Patient   *300*
Physiology of the Transplanted Heart   *300*
Autonomic Nervous System   *300*
Heart Rate   *301*
Left Ventricular Systolic Function   *301*
Right Ventricular Systolic Function   *301*
Atrial Function   *301*
Diastolic Function   *301*
Issues Unique to Heart Transplant Patients   *302*
Cardiac Allograft Vasculopathy (CAV)   *302*
Hypertension   *302*
Atrial and Ventricular Arrhythmias   *303*
Subacute Bacterial Endocarditis (SBE) Prophylaxis   *303*
Rejection   *303*
Response to Drugs   *304*
Anesthetic Considerations for Noncardiac Surgery in Patients Post Heart
Transplantation   *305*
References and Further Reading   *306*

34   Heart–Lung and Lung Transplantation   *307*
Introduction   *307*
Single-lung Transplantation   *307*
Double-lung Transplantation   *308*
Living Donor Lobar Lung Transplant   *308*
The Donor   *308*
Operative Procedure and Patient Positioning   *309*
Use of CPB   *309*
HLT and *En Bloc* DLT   *309*
SLT and BSSLT   *310*
Anesthetic Management   *310*
Goals   *310*
Preoperative Evaluation   *310*
Premedication   *310*
Preinduction   *311*
Management of One-lung Ventilation   *311*
Endobronchial Intubation   *311*
Single-lumen Endotracheal Tube Plus a Bronchial Blocker   *311*
Single-lumen Endotracheal Tube Plus an E-Z Bronchial Blocker   *313*
Univent™ Tube   *313*
Double-lumen Endotracheal Tube   *313*
Induction and Maintenance   *313*
Special Considerations for SLT and BSSLT   *315*
One-lung Ventilation   *315*
Clamping of the PA   *315*
Allograft Implantation   *315*
Indications for CPB   *316*
Post-CPB Management   *316*

Postoperative Care   *316*
Noncardiac Surgery in Lung Transplant Patients   *317*
  Anesthetic Considerations for Noncardiac Surgery in Patients Post Lung
  Transplantation   *318*
References and Further Reading   *319*

**35 Anomalous Origin of the Left Coronary Artery from the Pulmonary Artery
    and Anomalous Aortic Origin of a Coronary Artery** *321*
Anomalous Origin of the Left Coronary Artery (ALCAPA)   *321*
Introduction   *321*
Anatomy   *321*
Physiology   *321*
Surgical Treatment   *321*
Anesthetic Management   *322*
Anomalous Aortic Origin of a Coronary Artery (AAOCA)   *323*
Introduction   *323*
Anatomy   *323*
Physiology   *323*
Surgical Treatment   *324*
Anesthetic Management   *325*
References and Further Reading   *326*

36 Heterotaxy *327*
Introduction   *327*
Anatomy   *327*
  Position of the Heart in the Chest   *327*
Atrial Anatomy   *327*
Venoatrial Connections   *327*
Ventricular Anatomy   *328*
  Atrioventricular Junction   *330*
Ventriculoarterial Connections   *330*
Tracheobronchial Anatomy   *330*
General Characterizations   *330*
Surgical Therapy   *331*
References and Further Reading   *332*

37 Ebstein Anomaly *333*
Introduction   *333*
Anatomy   *333*
Physiology   *333*
Medical Management   *334*
Surgical Treatment   *336*
Anesthetic Management in Ebstein Anomaly   *337*
  Goals   *337*
Post-CPB Management   *338*
References and Further Reading   *338*

Index *339*

Preface to the Second Edition

The Pediatric Cardiac Anesthesia Handbook, 2nd edition, is intended to provide practical recommendations for the anesthetic management of patients with congenital heart disease. It is written and organized to function as a comprehensive review book and clinical manual. It can be used by both cardiac and non-cardiac anesthesiologists involved in the care of the growing population of patients with congenital heart disease. The first part provides an overview of cardiovascular physiology, basic perioperative assessment, interpretation of hemodynamics, echocardiography, the use of mechanical support devices, and postoperative care. The second part is divided into chapters devoted to individual cardiac lesions. Each chapter provides a summary of lesion anatomy, pathophysiology, preoperative assessment, surgical/interventional management, and postoperative care.

It is our hope that this book will be useful to you in the care of your patients.

Part I

The Basics

1

Cardiovascular Development

The incidence of congenital heart disease (CHD) is approximately 7–10 per 1000 live births. Most congenital heart defects are the result of an interaction of genetic predisposition and environmental factors. Environmental factors such as drugs, viral infection, maternal diabetes, or maternal alcohol abuse may account for specific lesions. Knowledge of cardiac development is a must to understand congenital heart lesions. This chapter reviews the embryology and cardiovascular physiology at birth.

Embryology

It is essential to understand the basic embryology and origin of the cardiac structures in order to appreciate the specific lesions described in the next section of the Handbook. It is beyond the scope of this Handbook to discuss the details of cardiac development, including: (i) cardiac sidedness or asymmetry; (ii) cardiac looping; (iii) formation of outflow tracts; and (iv) septation. The embryologic structures and their corresponding adult structures are listed in Table 1.1.

Cardiovascular Physiology

Circulatory changes occur at birth and continue over the first few days and the first months of life, and are considerable. They need to be appreciated in order to understand their profound effects on neonatal cardiovascular physiology. It is not coincidental that 50% of neonates born with CHD will become ill enough during the first days or weeks of life to require medical or surgical intervention. Optimal perioperative and anesthetic management of the neonate with CHD must be based on a firm understanding of these developmental changes.

Fetal Circulation

Fetal circulatory channels shunt blood away from the lung such that both ventricles, in parallel, contribute to systemic oxygen delivery by pumping blood to the systemic arterial system. This parallel circulation permits normal fetal growth and development even in fetuses with cardiac malformations.

Oxygenated blood from the placenta returns to the fetus via the umbilical vein, which enters the portal venous system. The ductus venosus connects the left portal vein to the left hepatic vein at its junction with the inferior vena cava (IVC). This allows approximately 50% of umbilical venous blood to bypass the hepatic sinuses. The remainder of the umbilical venous flow passes through the liver and enters the IVC via the hepatic veins. Fetal IVC blood is a combination of blood from the lower fetal body, umbilical vein, and hepatic veins. The stream of blood from the ductus venosus has a higher velocity in the IVC than the stream from the lower body and hepatic veins. This higher velocity facilitates delivery of this higher-oxygen content

The Pediatric Cardiac Anesthesia Handbook, Second Edition. Viviane G. Nasr and James A. DiNardo.
© 2025 John Wiley & Sons Ltd. Published 2025 by John Wiley & Sons Ltd.

Table 1.1 Cardiovascular embryologic structure and the corresponding structures in adults.

Embryologic structure	Adult structure
Truncus arteriosus	Aorta Pulmonary trunk
Bulbus cordis	Smooth part of right ventricle (conus arteriosus) Smooth part of left ventricle (aortic vestibule)
Primitive ventricle	Trabeculated part of right ventricle Trabeculated part of left ventricle
Primitive atrium	Trabeculated part of right atrium Trabeculated part of left atrium
Sinus venosus	Smooth part of right atrium (sinus venarum) Coronary sinus Oblique vein of left atrium
Aortic arches	
1	*
2	*
3	Common carotid arteries Internal carotid arteries (proximal part)
4	Right subclavian artery (proximal part) Part of the aortic arch
5	Regresses in the human
6	Pulmonary arteries (proximal part) Ductus arteriosus

blood across the foramen ovale (FO) into the left atrium (LA) (Figure 1.1).

The IVC blood enters the right atrium (RA) and, due to the position of the Eustachian valve, Chiari network, and FO, enters the LA during 80% of the cardiac cycle. During the other 20% (atrial systole), IVC blood crosses the tricuspid valve and enters the right ventricle (RV). The overwhelming majority of superior vena cava (SVC) blood crosses the tricuspid valve and also enters the RV. Blood from the RV is ejected into the pulmonary artery (PA). Approximately 10–15% of blood from the PA passes through the lungs to reach the LA, and the rest is shunted to the distal aorta via the ductus arteriosus (DA). As a result, two-thirds of the total fetal cardiac output is provided by the RV, with the remaining one-third provided via the LV.

The dynamics of shunting at the level of the ductus venosus, FO, and DA result in a preferential delivery of the most highly oxygenated blood to the coronary and cerebral circulations. Obviously, this preferential delivery of oxygenated blood may be compromised *in utero* by cardiac lesions that prevent or reduce left ventricular output. At birth, a series circulation is established in which each ventricle pumps into a specific vascular bed (RV to pulmonary artery, LV to aorta). The removal of the placenta and the initiation of alveolar ventilation at birth have the immediate effect of establishing this series circulation. To maintain the adult series circulation, the fetal channels must be closed (Table 1.2). Complex neurochemical and hormonal influences affect the closing of these fetal shunts. Acidosis, sepsis, hypothermia, hypoxia, and hypercarbia may cause a reopening of the shunts and persistence of the fetal circulation (PFC). Most neonates who are critically ill from CHD have one or more of these inciting factors at the time of presentation. In some instances, the persistence of fetal circulatory

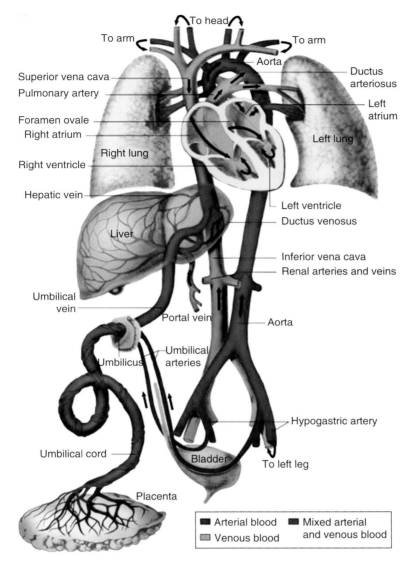

To head

To arm

To arm

Aorta

Superior vena cava

Pulmonary artery

Foramen ovale

Right atrium

Right lung

Right ventricle

Hepatic vein

Liver

Umbilical vein

Portal vein

Umbilicus

Umbilical arteries

Umbilical cord

Placenta

Bladder

Ductus arteriosus

Left atrium

Left lung

Left ventricle

Ductus venosus

Inferior vena cava

Renal arteries and veins

Aorta

Hypogastric artery

To left leg

■ Arterial blood ■ Mixed arterial
□ Venous blood   and venous blood

Figure 1.1 Course of the fetal circulation in late gestation. Note the selective blood flow patterns across the foramen ovale and the ductus arteriosus. *Source:* Reproduced from Greeley et al. (2010)/with permission of Elsevier.

channels may be beneficial or even mandatory for survival.

Closure of the Ductus Arteriosus

In the fetus, patency of the ductus arteriosus is maintained by high levels of prostaglandins (PGI$_2$ and PGE$_1$). There are two stages of ductal closure in the newborn: functional closure and permanent anatomic closure.

Functional closure occurs by contraction of the smooth muscle of the ductal wall and usually occurs within the first day of life. An increase in PO$_2$ and a decrease in prostaglandin levels contribute to functional closure. Oxygen is a dose-dependent ductal constrictor that acts by increasing the rate of oxidative phosphorylation within smooth muscle cells. In addition, the response to

Table 1.2 Fetal structures and their corresponding structure in adults.

Fetal structure	Adult structure
Foramen ovale	Fossa ovalis
Umbilical vein	Ligamentum teres
Ductus venosus	Ligamentum venosum
Umbilical arteries	Medial umbilical ligaments, superior vesicular artery
Ductus arteriosus	Ligamentum arteriosum

oxygen may be age related; full-term neonates have a more dramatic response to oxygen than immature newborns. Norepinephrine and epinephrine, by changing pulmonary and systemic vascular resistances, may secondarily contribute to ductal closure. Acetylcholine has a direct constrictor effect on ductal tissue. Permanent anatomic closure of the duct usually is accomplished by 2–3 weeks of life in the normal full-term neonate. The lumen is sealed by fibrous connective tissue, leaving the vestigial structure, known as the ligamentum arteriosum.

The survival of some neonates with congenital cardiac lesions is dependent on ductal patency. Because functional closure is a reversible event, the use of PGE_1 infusions (0.01–0.05 $\mu g\,kg^{-1}\,min^{-1}$) has been one of the major medical advances in the stabilization of neonates with ductal-dependent heart lesions. Preterm neonates are at risk of delayed ductal closure. This may be due to a decreased degradation of PGE_1, an increased production of PGE_1, or a diminished sensitivity to the ductal-constricting effects of oxygen. In instances in which delayed ductal closure is disadvantageous, prostaglandin inhibitors such as indomethacin (0.1–0.3 $mg\,kg^{-1}$ PO or IV) have been used successfully to promote ductal closure and establish normal patterns of pulmonary blood flow.

Closure of the Foramen Ovale

In utero, the right atrial pressure is higher than the left atrial pressure. IVC blood flows in such a manner as to keep the FO open.

The cessation of umbilical vein flow causes a significant decrease in venous return to the right heart, leading to a decrease in right atrial pressure. In addition, ventilation causes a marked increase in pulmonary arterial and venous blood flows, resulting in an increase in left atrial pressure. This elevation of left atrial pressure relative to right atrial pressure causes the flap-like valve of the FO to functionally close. In instances in which right atrial pressure remains elevated, right-to-left shunting may persist. Functional closure usually progresses to anatomic closure. However, probe patency of the FO may persist in 30% of normal adults and in 50% of children younger than five years of age.

Closure of the Ductus Venosus

The umbilical vessels constrict strongly after mechanical stimulation, and a high oxygen tension facilitates this process. The resultant decrease in umbilical venous blood flow causes passive closure of the ductus venosus. The latter does not appear to be as sensitive as the ductus arteriosus to PaO_2, $PaCO_2$, or pH. The ductus venosus is functionally closed by one week of life and is anatomically closed by three months. The remaining structure is the ligamentum venosum. In addition to the establishment of the adult series circulation, dramatic alterations in pulmonary circulation, cardiac output and distribution, myocardial performance, myocardial cell growth, and hypertrophy continue to occur during the first weeks, months, and even years of life. In the presence of CHD, these changes may be pathologically affected.

Pulmonary Vascular Changes

The fetus has a low pulmonary blood flow secondary to a high pulmonary vascular resistance. The minimal blood flow that reaches the pulmonary bed has a very low PaO_2, which may cause hypoxic pulmonary vasoconstriction and contributes to the elevated pulmonary resistance seen in the fetus. Morphologic examinations of the small arteries of the fetal and newborn lung show a thick medial smooth muscle layer. The fetal pulmonary vasculature is reactive to a number of stimulants. Vasoconstriction is induced by decreases in PaO_2, pH, and leukotrienes. Acetylcholine, histamine, bradykinin, PGE_1, PGE_2, PGI_2 (prostacyclin), and prostaglandin D_2 and beta-adrenergic catecholamines are patent vasodilators of fetal pulmonary vessels.

At birth, alveolar ventilation commences. This reduces the mechanical compression of small pulmonary vessels and increases PaO_2, the result being a dramatic reduction in pulmonary vascular resistance (PVR). During the following weeks and months, remodeling of the pulmonary vessels occurs; the most notable change is a thinning of the medial smooth muscle layer. By six months of life, this process results in a reduction of the PVR to near-normal adult levels. The normal process of postnatal pulmonary maturation may be altered significantly by pathologic conditions, such as those associated with CHD.

Myocardial Performance in the Neonate

In utero, the RV has a cardiac output of approximately 330 ml kg^{-1} min^{-1} compared to the left ventricular output of 170 ml kg^{-1} min^{-1}. At birth, both the RV and LV eject an output of approximately 350 ml kg^{-1} min^{-1}. This requires a minimal stroke volume increase for the RV but a considerable increase in stroke volume for the LV. The high-output state of the newborn effectively limits further increases in cardiac output. This high-output state decreases to about 150 ml kg^{-1} min^{-1} by 8–10 weeks of life.

Hemodynamic Changes at Birth

Myocardial morphology and performance are notably different in the neonate. These differences are summarized as follows and are listed in Table 1.3.

Table 1.3 Neonatal myocardial performance compared to the adult.

- Afterload mismatch
- Limited preload reserve
- Reduced contractile capacity
- Reduced ventricular compliance
- Increased intraventricular dependence
- Incomplete autonomic sympathetic innervation and dominance of parasympathetic
- Immature myocardial metabolism

- *Afterload mismatch*: the neonatal heart is more susceptible to afterload mismatch, and therefore the stroke volume is poorly maintained in the face of increasing outflow resistance (see Chapter 5).
- *Limited preload reserve*: the neonatal heart has a limited preload reserve. Augmentation of stroke volume via the Frank–Starling mechanism is limited compared with an adult.
- *Reduced contractile capacity*: neonatal cardiac cells contain more water and fewer contractile elements than mature myocardium. In addition, there are fewer mitochondria and sarcoplasmic reticulum (SR) and poorly formed T tubules that make the myocardium more dependent on extracellular calcium. Development of the SR, T-tubular system and calcium-handling proteins appears to be rapid, and it has been suggested that they are relatively mature by three weeks in the neonatal heart.
- *Reduced ventricular compliance*: the compliance of the neonatal myocardium is reduced because a deficiency of elastic elements parallels the deficiency of contractile elements.
- *Increased intraventricular dependence*: changes in ventricular pressure are transmitted to the opposite ventricle via the ventricular septum more readily in the immature myocardium. Left ventricular diastolic filling is disproportionately impaired in the neonate by a high right ventricular end-diastolic pressure. This is due to a leftward shift of the intraventricular

septum and a reduction in left ventricular distensibility. Right ventricular diastolic filling is impaired to an equal extent by high left ventricular end-diastolic pressures in neonates. This enhanced ventricular inter-action is caused by reduced ventricular compliance and because, at birth, the LV and RV are of equal mass. The increased volume and pressure load experienced by the LV after birth produce relative left ventricular hypertrophy (LVH). The normal adult LV to RV mass ratio of 2:1 is not seen until several months after birth.

- *Incomplete autonomic innervations*: sympathetic innervation, which is responsible for increasing the heart rate and contractility, is incompletely developed at birth. As a result, the local myocardial release of norepinephrine contributes less to increases in contractility than do increases in circulating catecholamine levels. For this reason, inotropic agents such as dopamine – the effects of which are partially mediated through release of norepinephrine from myocardial nerve endings – may have to be used at higher doses to be effective in younger patients.

On the other hand, the parasympathetic system, which reflexly slows the heart, is fully functional at birth.

- *Immature myocardial metabolism*: the neonatal myocardium is more dependent on anaerobic metabolism than the adult heart, which uses carbohydrates and lactate as primary energy sources. This may have a somewhat protective effect, making the neonatal myocardium more tolerant to the effects of hypoxia.

References and Further Reading

Greeley, W.J., Berkowitz, D.H. & Nathan, A.T. Anesthesia for pediatric cardiac surgery. In: Miller, R.D. (ed.) *Anesthesia*, 7th edn. Churchill Livingstone, Philadelphia (2010).

Jones, C.B. & Crossland, D.S. The interplay between pressure, flow, and resistance in neonatal pulmonary hypertension. *Semin Fetal Neonatal Med* **27**, 101371 (2022).

Kiserud, T. Physiology of the fetal circulation. *Semin Fetal Neonatal Med* **10**, 493–503 (2005).

2

Important Concepts in Congenital Heart Disease

The prevalence of congenital heart disease (CHD) continues to increase. In 2000, it was 11.89 per 1000 children and 4.09 per 1000 adults, whereas in 2010 it was 13.11 per 1000 children and 6.12 per 1000 adults.

The anesthesiologist who cares for patients with CHD faces myriad challenges in the perioperative management of these complex individuals. In major pediatric cardiac centers, almost every lesion is amenable to surgical intervention. The pathophysiology of a wide variety of congenital heart defects can be best understood by applying certain basic principles to each patient. This chapter outlines those principles. The anesthesiologist who understands the cardiovascular physiology, the dynamics of each cardiac lesion, and the planned surgical cardiac or noncardiac intervention will be able to conduct an appropriate anesthetic. Although younger, smaller, and sicker patients are presenting for more complex, innovative surgical and interventional treatment, it is encouraging and impressive that there has been a concomitant decrease in surgical and anesthetic morbidity and mortality.

Pathophysiology of CHD

While some congenital heart defects involve purely obstructive or regurgitant valvular lesions, the presence of shunts (both physiologic and anatomic) is the hallmark of CHD. Anesthetic management of the patient with CHD is dependent on a clear understanding of:

- the concepts of shunting (both physiologic and anatomic), single-ventricle physiology, and intercirculatory mixing
- the types of anatomic shunts and the dynamics of the anatomic shunting process
- the effects of congenital lesions on the development of the pulmonary vascular system
- the factors that influence pulmonary and systemic vascular resistance
- the factors responsible for producing myocardial ischemia.

Concepts of Shunting, Single-Ventricle Physiology, and Intercirculatory Mixing

Shunting

Shunting is the process whereby venous return into one circulatory system is recirculated through the arterial outflow of the same circulatory system. Flow of blood from the systemic venous atrium or right atrium (RA) to the aorta produces a recirculation of systemic venous blood. A flow of blood from the pulmonary venous atrium or left atrium (LA) to the pulmonary artery (PA) produces a recirculation of pulmonary venous blood. Recirculation of blood produces a physiologic shunt. The recirculation of pulmonary venous blood produces a physiologic left-to-right (L-R) shunt, whereas the recirculation of

Figure 2.1 Depiction of blood flows in a normal cardiac physiology without shunting.

$Q_p:Q_s = 1:1$

$Q_{peff} = 2l.min^{-1}.m^{-2}$
No Shunt
$Q_p = 2l.min^{-1}.m^{-2}$

$Q_{seff} = 2l.min^{-1}.m^{-2}$
No Shunt
$Q_s = 2l.min^{-1}.m^{-2}$

systemic venous blood produces a physiologic right-to-left (R-L) shunt. A physiologic R-L or L-R shunt commonly is the result of an anatomic R-L or L-R shunt. In an anatomic shunt, blood moves from one circulatory system to the other via a communication at the level of the cardiac chambers (atrial or ventricular) or great vessels. Physiologic shunts can exist in the absence of an anatomic shunt. Transposition physiology is the primary example of this process.

Effective Blood Flow

Effective blood flow is the quantity of venous blood from one circulatory system reaching the arterial system of the other circulatory system. Effective pulmonary blood flow is the volume of systemic venous blood reaching the pulmonary circulation, whereas effective systemic blood flow is the volume of pulmonary venous blood reaching the systemic circulation. Effective pulmonary blood flow and effective systemic blood flows are the flows necessary to maintain life. Effective pulmonary blood flow and effective systemic blood flow are always equal, no matter how complex the lesions are. Effective blood flow usually is the result of a normal pathway through the heart, but it may occur as the result of an anatomic R-L or L-R shunt.

Total Pulmonary Blood Flow/Total Systemic Blood Flow

Total pulmonary blood flow (Q_p) is the sum of effective pulmonary blood flow and recirculated pulmonary blood flow. Total systemic blood flow (Q_s) is the sum of effective systemic blood flow and recirculated systemic blood flow. Total pulmonary blood flow and total systemic blood flow do not have to be equal. Therefore, it is best to think of recirculated flow (physiologic shunt flow) as the extra, noneffective flow superimposed on the nutritive effective blood flow. These concepts are illustrated in Figures 2.1 and 2.2.

Single-Ventricle Physiology

Single-ventricle physiology is used to describe the circulation wherein complete mixing of pulmonary venous and systemic venous blood occurs at the atrial or ventricular level and the ventricle(s) then distribute output to both the systemic and pulmonary beds. As a result of this physiology, the following factors pertain.

- The ventricular output is the sum of pulmonary blood flow (Q_p) and systemic blood flow (Q_s).
- The distribution of systemic and pulmonary blood flows is dependent on the relative resistances to flow (both intracardiac and extracardiac) into the two parallel circuits.
- Oxygen saturations are the same in the aorta and the pulmonary artery.
- This physiology can exist in patients with one well-developed ventricle and one hypoplastic ventricle, as well as in patients with two well-formed ventricles.

Figure 2.2 Depiction of blood flows and saturations in atrial septal defect (ASD) and transposition of the great arteries (TGA). Effective systemic and effective pulmonary blood flows are equal and are shown as solid lines in both lesions. The shunted flows are shown as dotted lines.

- In the case of a single anatomic ventricle, there is always disruption of the normal pathway of pulmonary venous blood delivery to the aorta or of systemic venous blood delivery to the pulmonary artery as the result of complete or near-complete obstruction to inflow and/or outflow from the hypoplastic ventricle. In this circumstance there must be an alternate, unobstructed pathway to assure postnatal survival. In some instances of a single anatomic ventricle, a direct connection between the aorta and the pulmonary artery via a patent ductus arteriosus (PDA) is the sole source of systemic blood flow (hypoplastic left heart syndrome; HLHS) or of pulmonary blood flow (pulmonary atresia with intact ventricular septum; PA/IVS). This is known as ductal-dependent circulation. In other instances of a single anatomic ventricle, intracardiac pathways provide both systemic and pulmonary blood flow without the necessity of a PDA. This is the case in tricuspid atresia with normally related great vessels, a nonrestrictive ventricular septal defect (VSD) and minimal or absent pulmonary stenosis.

Single-ventricle physiology can exist in the presence of two well-formed anatomic ventricles when there is complete or near-complete obstruction to outflow from one of the ventricles.

- Tetralogy of Fallot (TOF) with pulmonary atresia (PA) where pulmonary blood flow is supplied via a PDA or multiple aortopulmonary collateral arteries (MAPCA).
- Truncus arteriosus.
- Severe neonatal aortic stenosis and interrupted aortic arch; in both lesions a

substantial portion of systemic blood flow is supplied via a PDA.

- Heterotaxy syndrome, where there are components of systemic venous (SVC, IVC, hepatic veins, azygous veins) and pulmonary venous return to both right-sided and left-sided atria. In addition, the atrial morphology can be ambiguous.

Despite the fact that patients with totally anomalous pulmonary venous return (TAPVR) have complete mixing of pulmonary and systemic venous blood at the atrial level, they do not manifest the other features necessary to create single-ventricle physiology. This also holds true for lesions in which a common atrial or ventricular chamber exists due to bidirectional (both L-R and R-L) anatomic shunting across a large defect (atrial septal or ventricular septal) and where there is no obstruction to ventricular outflow. A number of single-ventricle physiology lesions are listed in Table 2.1.

All patients with single-ventricle physiology who have severe hypoplasia of one ventricle will ultimately be staged down the single ventricle pathway to Fontan physiology (this will be discussed in detail later). Patients with single-ventricle physiology and two well-formed ventricles may be able to undergo a two-ventricle (biventricular) repair.

With single-ventricle physiology, the arterial saturation (SaO_2) will be determined by the relative volumes and saturations of pulmonary venous and systemic venous blood flows that have mixed and reached the aorta. This is summarized in the following equation:

$$Aortic\ saturation = \frac{\left[\begin{array}{l}(systemic\ venous\ saturation)(total\ systemic\ venous\ blood\ flow) + \\ (pulmonary\ venous\ saturation)(total\ pulmonary\ venous\ blood\ flow)\end{array}\right]}{[total\ systemic\ venous\ blood\ flow + total\ pulmonary\ venous\ blood\ flow]}$$

This is illustrated in Figure 2.3, where: $SaO_2 = [(65)(1) + (98)(0.85)]/(1.85) = 80\%$.

From this equation, it is apparent that with single-ventricle physiology, three variables will determine arterial saturation: $Q_p:Q_s$; systemic venous saturation; and pulmonary venous saturation.

1) *The ratio of total pulmonary to total systemic blood flow ($Q_p:Q_s$)*: a greater proportion of the mixed blood will consist of saturated blood (pulmonary venous blood) than desaturated blood (systemic venous blood) when $Q_p:Q_s$ is high. Figure 2.4 demonstrates the increase in arterial saturation that occurs with increases in pulmonary blood flow relative to systemic blood flow.

2) *Systemic venous saturation*: for a given $Q_p:Q_s$ and pulmonary venous saturation, a decrease in systemic venous saturation will result in decreased arterial saturation. Decreases in systemic venous saturation occur as the result of decreases in systemic oxygen delivery or increases in systemic oxygen consumption. Systemic oxygen delivery is the product of systemic blood flow and arterial oxygen content. Arterial oxygen content is dependent on the hemoglobin concentration and the arterial saturation.

3) *Pulmonary venous saturation*: in the absence of large intrapulmonary shunts and/or V/Q mismatch, pulmonary venous saturation should be close to 100% breathing room air. In the presence of pulmonary parenchymal disease, pulmonary venous saturation may be reduced. The V/Q mismatch component of pulmonary venous desaturation will be largely eliminated with a FiO_2 of 1.0, while the intrapulmonary shunt contribution will not be eliminated. For any given systemic venous saturation and $Q_p:Q_s$ a reduction in pulmonary venous saturation will result in a decreased arterial saturation.

Table 2.1 Anatomic subtypes of single-ventricle physiology.

	Aortic blood flow from	Pulmonary artery blood flow from
HLHS	PDA	RV
Severe neonate aortic stenosis	PDA	RV
IAA	LV (proximal) PDA (distal)	RV
PA/IVS	LV	PDA
Tetralogy of Fallot with pulmonary atresia	LV	PDA, MAPCAs
Tricuspid atresia, NRGA, with pulmonary atresia (type 1A)	LV	PDA, MAPCAs
Tricuspid atresia, NRGA, with restrictive VSD and pulmonary stenosis (type 1B)	LV	LV through VSD to RV
Tricuspid atresia, NRGA, with nonrestrictive VSD and no pulmonary stenosis (type 1C)	LV	LV through VSD to RV
Tricuspid atresia, D-TGA with nonrestrictive VSD and pulmonary atresia (type 2A)	LV through VSD to RV	PDA, MAPCAs
Tricuspid atresia, D-TGA, with nonrestrictive VSD and pulmonary stenosis (type 2B)	LV through VSD to RV	LV
Tricuspid atresia, D-TGA, with nonrestrictive VSD and no pulmonary stenosis (type 2C)	LV through VSD to RV	LV
Tricuspid atresia, D-loop ventricles, L-TGA, subpulmonic stenosis (type 3A)	LV	LV through VSD to RV
Tricuspid atresia, L-loop ventricles, L-TGA, subaortic stenosis (type 3B)	LV through VSD to RV	LV
Truncus arteriosus	LV and RV	Aorta
DILV, NRGA	LV	LV via BVF
DILV, L-loop ventricles, L-TGA, restrictive BVF DORV, severe PS or PA	LV via BVF, PDA	LV
	LV via VSD	PDA
Ebstein anomaly, functional PA (due to severe TR and high PVR)	LV	PDA

BVF, bulboventricular foramen; D, dextro; DILV, double-inlet left ventricle; HLHS, hypoplastic left heart syndrome; IAA, interrupted aortic arch; L, levo; LV, left ventricle; MAPCAs, multiple aortopulmonary collateral arteries; NRGA, normally related great arteries; PA/IVS, pulmonary atresia with intact ventricular septum; PDA, patent ductus arteriosus; PS, pulmonary stenosis; PA, pulmonary atresia; RV, right ventricle; TGA, transposition of the great arteries; VSD, ventricular septal defect.
Source: Reproduced from DiNardo and Zvara (2008)/with permission of John Wiley & Sons.

Intercirculatory Mixing

Intercirculatory mixing is the unique situation that exists in transposition of the great vessels (TGA) (see Figure 2.2). In TGA, two parallel circulations exist due to the existence of atrioventricular concordance (RA-RV, LA-LV) and ventriculoarterial discordance (RV-Ao, LV-PA). This produces a parallel rather than a normal series circulation. In this arrangement, blood flow will consist of a parallel recirculation of pulmonary venous blood in the pulmonary circuit and systemic venous blood in the systemic circuit. Therefore, the physiologic shunt or the percentage of venous blood from one system that recirculates in the arterial outflow of the same system is 100% for both circuits. Unless there are one or more communications (atrial septal defect,

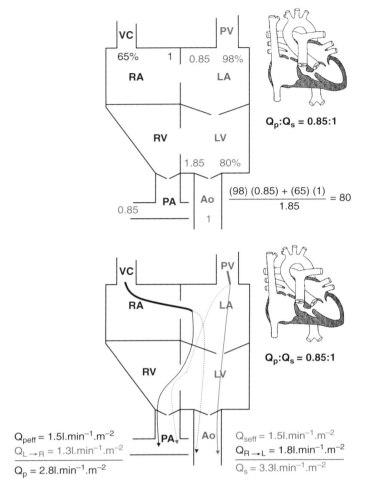

$$\frac{(98)\,(0.85)+(65)\,(1)}{1.85}=80$$

$Q_p:Q_s = 0.85:1$

$Q_{peff} = 1.5 \text{l.min}^{-1}.\text{m}^{-2}$
$Q_{L\rightarrow R} = 1.3 \text{l.min}^{-1}.\text{m}^{-2}$
$\overline{Q_p = 2.8 \text{l.min}^{-1}.\text{m}^{-2}}$

$Q_{seff} = 1.5 \text{l.min}^{-1}.\text{m}^{-2}$
$Q_{R\rightarrow L} = 1.8 \text{l.min}^{-1}.\text{m}^{-2}$
$\overline{Q_s = 3.3 \text{l.min}^{-1}.\text{m}^{-2}}$

Figure 2.3 Blood flows and saturations in tricuspid atresia (single-ventricle physiology). Effective pulmonary and systemic blood flows shown as solid lines. Shunted pulmonary and systemic blood flows shown as dotted lines.

ASD; patent foramen ovale, PFO; VSD; PDA) between the parallel circuits to allow intercirculatory mixing, this lesion is incompatible with life.

An anatomic R-L shunt is necessary to provide effective pulmonary blood flow, whereas an anatomic L-R shunt is necessary to provide effective systemic blood flow. Effective pulmonary blood flow, effective systemic blood flow, and the volume of intercirculatory mixing must always be equal. Total systemic blood flow is the sum of recirculated systemic venous blood plus effective systemic blood flow. Likewise, total pulmonary blood flow is the sum of recirculated pulmonary venous blood plus effective pulmonary blood flow. Recirculated blood makes up the largest portion of total pulmonary and total systemic blood flows, with effective blood flows contributing only a small portion of the total flows. This is particularly true in the pulmonary circuit where the total pulmonary blood flow (Q_p) and the volume of the pulmonary circuit (LA-LV-PA) are two- to three-fold larger than the total systemic blood flow (Q_s) and the volume of the systemic circuit (RA-RV-Ao). The net result is transposition physiology, wherein the pulmonary artery oxygen saturation is greater than the aortic oxygen saturation.

Figure 2.4 Graph of systemic SaO$_2$ versus Q$_p$:Q$_s$ for two different ventricular outputs (300 ml kg^{-1} min^{-1} and 450 ml kg^{-1} min^{-1}) in single-ventricle physiology. In this example, oxygen consumption is assumed to be 9 ml kg^{-1} min^{-1} and SpvO$_2$ = 95%. It is clear that SaO$_2$ peaks at or near a Q$_p$:Q$_s$ of 1:1. Further increases in Q$_p$:Q$_s$ produce minimal to no increases in SaO$_2$.

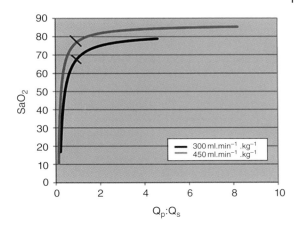

Arterial saturation (SaO$_2$) will be determined by the relative volumes and saturations of the recirculated systemic and effective systemic venous blood flows reaching the aorta. This is summarized in the following equation:

$$Aortic\ saturation = \frac{\left[\begin{array}{l}(systemic\ venous\ sat)(recirculated\ systemic\ venous\ blood\ flow)+\\(pulmonary\ venous\ sat)(effective\ pulmonary\ venous\ blood\ flow)\end{array}\right]}{\left[total\ systemic\ venous\ blood\ flow\right]}$$

where sat = saturation. This is illustrated in Figure 2.2, where SaO$_2$ = [(50)(1) + (99)(1)]/2 = 74.5%.

Obviously, the greater the effective systemic blood flow (intercirculatory mixing) relative to the recirculated systemic blood flow, the greater the aortic saturation. For a given amount of intercirculatory mixing and total systemic blood flow, a decrease in systemic venous or pulmonary venous saturation will result in a decrease in arterial saturation.

Classification of Anatomic Shunts

Anatomic shunts can be characterized as either simple or complex.

Simple Shunts

In an anatomic shunt, a communication (orifice) exists between pulmonary and arterial vessels or heart chambers (Table 2.2). In a simple shunt, there is no fixed obstruction to outflow from the vessels or chambers involved in the shunt. When the shunt orifice is small (restrictive shunt), a large pressure gradient exists across the orifice, and variations in outflow resistance (pulmonary vascular resistance, PVR; systemic vascular resistance, SVR) have little effect on shunt magnitude and direction. In this instance, the magnitude of the shunt is affected by the size of the shunt orifice. However, when the shunt orifice is large, the shunt becomes nonrestrictive and outflow resistance becomes the primary determinant of the magnitude and direction of shunting. These shunts, in which the ratio of PVR to SVR determines the magnitude of shunting, are known as *dependent* shunts. When the communication is very large, no pressure gradient exists between the vessels or chambers involved. In this instance, *bidirectional* shunting occurs, resulting in complete mixing and a functionally common chamber. Net systemic and pulmonary blood flow is then determined by the ratio of systemic to pulmonary vascular resistance (Figure 2.5).

Table 2.2 Simple and complex shunts.

Simple No fixed obstruction to outflow		Complex Obstruction to outflow	
Restrictive (small communication)	**Nonrestrictive (large communication)**	**Partial obstruction**	**Complete obstruction**
Large pressure gradient	Small shunt gradient	Shunt magnitude and direction are largely fixed due to obstruction	Shunt magnitude and direction are totally fixed
Direction and magnitude of shunt are relatively independent of PVR:SVR	Direction and magnitude of shunt are largely dependent on PVR:SVR	Shunt dependence on PVR:SVR is inversely related to the severity of the obstructive lesion	Flow through the shunt is independent of PVR:SVR
Shunt is less subject to control by ventilator or pharmacologic interventions	Shunt is subject to control by ventilator or pharmacologic interventions	Shunt pressure gradient is determined by both the shunt orifice and the obstructive lesion	Shunt pressure gradient is determined only by the shunt orifice
Examples: small VSD, small PDA, small ASD, modified Blalock–Thomas–Taussig shunt	Examples: large VSD, large PDA, CAVC	Examples: TOF, VSD and PS, VSD with coarctation	Examples: tricuspid atresia, mitral atresia, pulmonary atresia, aortic atresia.

ASD, atrial septal defect; VSD, ventricular septal defect; PDA, patent ductus arteriosus; CAVC, common atrioventricular canal; PVR, pulmonary vascular resistance; SVR, systemic vascular resistance; TOF, tetralogy of Fallot; PS, pulmonary stenosis.

Figure 2.5 Influence of orifice size and the pulmonary vascular resistance:systemic vascular resistance (PVR:SVR) ratio on the magnitude and direction of a dependent shunt. (a) PVR and SVR are balanced, resulting in equal pulmonary and systemic blood flows. (b) PVR is reduced relative to SVR, resulting in an increase in pulmonary blood flow and a decrease in systemic blood flow. (c) PVR is elevated relative to SVR, resulting in a decrease in pulmonary blood flow and an increase in systemic blood flow.

Complex Shunts

In complex anatomic shunt lesions, there is obstruction to outflow in addition to a shunt orifice (Table 2.2). The obstruction may be at the valvular, subvalvular, or supravalvular level. The obstruction may be fixed (as with valvular or infundibular stenosis) or variable (as with dynamic infundibular obstruction). In complex shunts, outflow resistance is a combination of the resistance across the obstructive lesions and the resistance across the pulmonary or systemic vascular bed (Figure 2.6). When an obstruction is severe, the SVR or PVR distal to the obstruction will have little effect on shunt magnitude or direction.

Tetralogy of Fallot is a good example of a complex shunt in which there is a partial obstruction to outflow. There is a fixed component of right ventricular outflow obstruction in tetralogy of Fallot secondary to infundibular, valvular, and possibly supravalvular obstruction. A dynamic component of right ventricular obstruction is produced by changes in the caliber of the right ventricular infundibulum. These two components of right ventricular outflow obstruction can produce a R-L shunt. Because right ventricular outflow obstruction is incomplete, increases in PVR will also increase the total right ventricular outflow resistance and increase R-L shunting. Similarly,

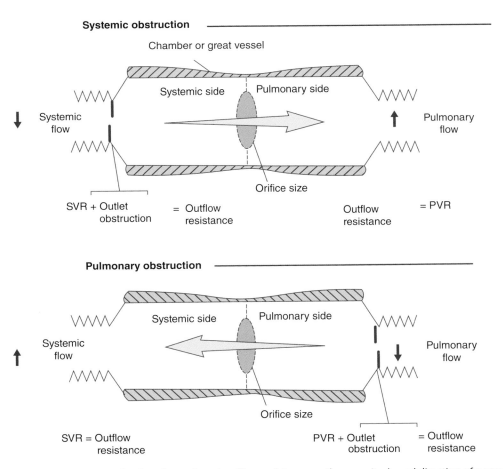

Figure 2.6 Influence of orifice size and total outflow resistance on the magnitude and direction of a complex shunt. Total outflow resistance will be a combination of pulmonary vascular resistance (PVR) or systemic vascular resistance (SVR) and the resistance offered by the obstructive lesion.

a decrease in SVR relative to PVR will increase R-L shunting without any increase in right ventricular outflow resistance.

Another form of complex shunt is present in patients who have single-ventricle physiology. In these lesions, changes in SVR or PVR play no role in determining shunt magnitude or direction. The entire shunt flow is fixed and obligatory across the communication, and complete mixing results. In order for flow of this mixed blood to reach the obstructed circuit, an additional downstream shunt, such as a VSD or PDA, must be present. The downstream shunt may be simple or complex, and is dependent on the ratio of PVR to SVR.

These concepts are critical to a clear understanding of the pathophysiology involved in patients with CHD. Describing a lesion as cyanotic or acyanotic may be misleading and simplistic. For example, in a patient with tetralogy of Fallot, there may be minimal valvular or infundibular obstruction to pulmonary blood flow at baseline, and the patient may not be cyanotic. In fact, this type of patient ('pink Tet') may have a large L-R shunt through the VSD, with increased pulmonary blood flow. During anesthesia, hypercarbia and hypoxemia may develop and result in an increase in both PVR and the dynamic component of infundibular obstruction. This will produce a net R-L shunt and cyanosis ("Tet spell"). Similarly, a cyanotic episode (a net R-L shunt) may be precipitated in the same patient by the SVR reduction that accompanies a febrile illness.

Pulmonary Vascular Pathophysiology

Pulmonary hypertension (PH) may occur as the result of congenital heart lesions. PH is defined as a mean pulmonary artery pressure (mPAP) $\geq$20 mmHg at rest. The stimulus for the development of PH in CHD is exposure of the pulmonary vascular system (both *in utero* and after birth) to abnormal pressure and flow patterns.

Pulmonary hypertension can be considered to have a precapillary cause, a postcapillary

cause (pulmonary venous hypertension), or a combination of both. Precapillary PH is also known as pulmonary arterial hypertension (PAH), and is defined as mPAP $\geq$20 mmHg at rest, pulmonary artery wedge pressure (PAWP) $\leq$15 mmHg, and a pulmonary vascular resistance index (PVRI) >3 Wood units m^{-2} for biventricular circulations. Following cavopulmonary anastomosis (Fontan procedure), the definition is a PVRI >3 Wood units m^{-2} or a transpulmonary gradient >6 mmHg, even in the presence of mPAP $\leq$20 mmHg. Postcapillary PH is most commonly due to left heart disease and is defined as mPAP $\geq$20 mmHg at rest in conjunction with PAWP $\geq$15 mmHg. Postcapillary causes are characteristically associated with interstitial pulmonary edema. Children with longstanding postcapillary PH develop a component of precapillary PH (PAH) due to reactive pulmonary artery vasoconstriction.

Causes of Precapillary PH in CHD

1) Exposure of the pulmonary vascular circuit to systemic arterial pressures and high pulmonary blood flows. Patients for whom the pulmonary vasculature is exposed to high flows and systemic arterial pressures typically have very early development of PAH. This classically occurs in the presence of a large (nonrestrictive) VSD.

2) Exposure of the pulmonary vascular circuit to high pulmonary blood flow in the absence of high pulmonary artery pressures. This type of lesion is associated with a slow progression of PAH. A large ASD or a small (restrictive) PDA are examples of this type of lesion.

Causes of Postcapillary PH in CHD

1) Obstruction of pulmonary venous drainage. Pulmonary venous obstruction may result from stenotic pulmonary veins, which can exist as a primary disease entity or in conjunction with anomalous pulmonary venous return. Cor triatriatum can cause the obstruction of pulmonary venous drainage into the left atrium.

2) The presence of high pressure in the atrial chamber into which there is pulmonary venous drainage. This is generally the left atrium (congenital mitral stenosis, congenital aortic stenosis, severe coarctation of the aorta, severe left ventricular systolic or diastolic function), but may also be the right atrium (totally anomalous pulmonary venous return, heterotaxy syndrome). PH seen in adult patients with acquired heart disease is almost always related to elevated left atrial pressure from left-heart diseases.

The morphologic changes associated with PAH in CHD have three components: (i) an increased muscularity of small pulmonary arteries; (ii) small artery intimal hyperplasia; and (iii) scarring and thrombosis and reduced numbers of intraacinar arteries. These changes produce progressive obstruction to pulmonary blood flow and result in progressive and irreversible elevations of PVR and pulmonary artery pressure. These changes may be graded morphologically using lung biopsy, or angiographically using the pulmonary artery angiogram. Ultimately, these changes elevate PVR and reduce pulmonary blood flow. In addition, the increased muscularity of the small pulmonary arteries enhances the response of the pulmonary vasculature to pulmonary vasoconstrictors.

Control of Pulmonary Vascular Resistance

Alterations in PVR are an important determinant of shunt magnitude and direction in some shunt lesions. Furthermore, the patient with CHD is likely to have an enhanced response of the pulmonary vasculature to vasoconstricting substances. It is therefore necessary to be familiar with the interventions that will alter PVR in the CHD patient. In patients with PH due to a precapillary cause, the following interventions are useful. In patients with a postcapillary cause, use of these interventions (particularly the use of inhaled pulmonary vasodilators) may result in the development of or worsening of interstitial pulmonary edema, with little or no effect on PAP due to the presence of downstream obstruction.

PaO$_2$

Both alveolar hypoxia and arterial hypoxemia induce pulmonary vasoconstriction. A PaO$_2$ lower than 50 mmHg increases PVR over a wide range of arterial pH; however, this effect is enhanced when pH is lower than 7.40. Conversely, high levels of inspired O$_2$ can reduce an elevated PVR.

PaCO$_2$

Hypercarbia increases PVR, independent of changes in arterial pH. Hypocarbia, on the other hand, reduces PVR only through the production of an alkalosis. In fact, reliable reductions in PVR and increases in pulmonary blood flow and PaO$_2$ are seen in children with R-L shunts when hyperventilation to a PaCO$_2$ near 20 mmHg and a pH near 7.60 is obtained. Similarly, post-cardiopulmonary bypass (CPB) hyperventilation to a PaCO$_2$ of 20–33 mmHg and a pH of 7.50–7.56 in patients with preoperative PH results in a reduction in PVR when compared with ventilation that produces normocarbia or hypercarbia.

pH

Both respiratory and metabolic alkalosis reduce PVR, whereas both respiratory and metabolic acidosis increase PVR.

Variation in Lung Volumes

At small lung volumes, atelectasis results in the compression of extraalveolar vessels, whereas at high lung volumes hyperinflation of alveoli results in the compression of intraalveolar vessels. Therefore, PVR is normally lowest at lung volumes at or near the functional residual capacity. Positive end-expiratory pressure (PEEP) may cause an increase in PVR by increasing alveolar pressure through hyperinflation. However, in situations in which PEEP works to recruit atelectatic alveoli and increase arterial PaO$_2$, a decrease in PVR generally is seen.

Vasodilator Agents

There is no intravenous drug that selectively acts as a pulmonary vasodilator. Pulmonary vasodilators (PGE_1, nitroglycerin, milrinone, sodium nitroprusside, and tolazoline) also induce systemic vasodilation.

A number of inhaled agents (of which nitric oxide, NO, is the prototype) capable of providing selective pulmonary vasodilation are now available. NO generated by endothelial NO synthase (eNOS) is an endogenous vasodilator. A wide variety of substances that increase intracellular calcium stimulate the production of NO from L-arginine via eNOS. After it has been formed, NO diffuses from the endothelium to vascular smooth muscle (VSM), where it binds to and activates guanylate cyclase to produce cyclic guanosine monophosphate (cGMP). cGMP acts as a second messenger to catalyze reactions that lead to a reduction of VSM calcium by reduced calcium influx, increased calcium efflux, and a reduced release of intracellular calcium. This produces a relaxation of the VSM and vasodilation. NO is also involved in the modulation of basal VSM tone. This modulation capacity is lost in vessels in which endothelium is removed or damaged.

Inhaled NO selectively reduces pulmonary hypertension and improves ventilation/ perfusion matching in a variety of disease states. Pulmonary selectivity is based on three characteristics of NO.

- Its gaseous state allows delivery to ventilated alveoli by inhalation.
- Its small size and lipophilicity allow ready diffusion into the appropriate cells.
- Its avid binding to and rapid inactivation by hemoglobin prevent systemic vasodilation. NO binds to oxyhemoglobin (Fe^{2+}) to form nitrosylhemoglobin, which is rapidly converted to methemoglobin (Fe^{3+}) and NO_3^-.

Inhaled NO has been used to treat PH in both the pre- and post-CPB period in a variety of congenital heart lesions and in the treatment of persistent PH of the newborn. Generally, approximately 20–40 ppm inhaled NO has been used. Some caution is warranted because both NO dependency and rebound pulmonary hypertension following NO discontinuation have been reported.

An alternative to inhaled NO is aerosolized prostacyclin (PGI_2) and aerosolized PGE_1. PGI_2 and its analogs (iloprost, epoprostenol or Flolan®) and PGE_1 act by binding to prostacyclin receptors and activating cyclic adenosine monophosphate (cAMP). This activates protein kinase A, which leads to a reduction of VSM intracellular calcium, causing vasorelaxation. PGI_2 also stimulates endothelial release of NO. Aerosolized PGI_2 (2–50 ng kg^{-1} min^{-1}) is useful in selectively lowering PVR after congenital cardiac surgery. There is less experience with aerosolized PGE_1 but at doses of 150–300 ng kg^{-1} min^{-1}, it has proved useful in the treatment of neonatal respiratory failure.

Sildenafil is a cGMP-specific phosphodiesterase (PDE_5) inhibitor that also works to increase cGMP levels. Oral, intravenous, and aerosolized forms of sildenafil are effective in reducing PVR.

Sympathetic Nervous System Stimulation

Sympathetic stimulation results in increases in both pulmonary and systemic vascular resistance. In children with pulmonary artery medial hypertrophy, this may result in a hyperactive pulmonary vasoconstrictor response. Blunting of sympathetic outflow associated with hypothermia or pain occurring during a stress response attenuates increases in PVR in children predisposed to PH.

In summary, the control of ventilation by manipulating PaO_2, $PaCO_2$, pH, and lung volumes is the best method for altering PVR independently of SVR. A combination of a high inspired FiO_2, a PaO_2 higher than 60 mmHg, a $PaCO_2$ of 30–35 mmHg, a pH of 7.50–7.60, and low inspiratory pressures without high levels of PEEP will produce reliable reductions in PVR. Attention should be paid to minimizing mean airway pressure as well as giving consideration to an inspiratory:expiratory (I:E) ratio of 1:3 and PEEP titrated to maximize lung compliance.

Conversely, a reduced FiO_2, a PaO_2 of 50–60 mmHg, a $PaCO_2$ of 45–55 mmHg, and the application of PEEP can be used to increase PVR. Inhaled NO and prostacyclin are valuable selective pulmonary vasodilators in some patients.

Anesthetic Agents

Isoflurane, desflurane, and sevoflurane all inhibit hypoxic pulmonary vasoconstriction which may be of some small benefit in preventing an increase in PVR with surgical stimulation. Ketamine does not increase PVR as long as its administration does not result in hypoxemia or hypercarbia. The same holds true for synthetic opioids. Etomidate does not increase PVR but the impaired corticosteroid synthesis associated with its administration is a real concern. Propofol has no direct effect on PVR but causes systemic hypotension due to a combination of reduced SVR, increased venous capacitance, reduced sympathetic output, and myocardial depression. Dexmedetomidine in loading doses of 1 mg kg^{-1} increases peripheral vascular resistance without increasing PVR but at higher doses with plasma levels of 1.9 ng ml^{-1}, parallel increases in both PVR and SVR are seen. Unarousable deep sedation is thought to occur at plasma concentrations above 1.9 ng ml^{-1}.

Vasoactive Agents

Vasopressin has minimal effects on PVR compared with norepinephrine, epinephrine, and phenylephrine, all of which increase SVR but increase PVR as well. Vasopressin also dilates the pulmonary vasculature under hypoxic conditions through a V1 receptor-mediated release of NO. Low-dose vasopressin may be particularly useful as a selective systemic vasoconstrictor in the setting of a pulmonary hypertensive crisis to augment SVR without adverse effects on PVR. High doses of vasopressin (>0.08–0.1 U min^{-1}) should be avoided because of the possible effect on coronary vasoconstriction, which may induce RV ischemia. The benefit of norepinephrine, despite the risk of increasing PVR, is improved RV coronary blood flow and concurrent beta-agonism to support RV contractile function.

The inodilators milrinone and dobutamine reduce both SVR and PVR but milrinone in particular is a weak inotrope. Use of these agents may lead to severe systemic hypotension, requiring the addition of norepinephrine to maintain an adequate blood pressure.

Myocardial Ischemia

Patients with CHD are at higher risk for the development of subendocardial ischemia than is commonly appreciated. In some congenital lesions, there are abnormalities in the coronary circulation predisposing to ischemia, but in many other forms of CHD, ischemia occurs in the presence of normal coronary arteries secondary to myocardial oxygen supply and demand imbalance.

Subendocardial perfusion is largely determined by coronary perfusion pressure (CPP), which is the mean aortic diastolic pressure minus the ventricular end-diastolic pressure. In addition, the time interval available for perfusion (predominantly diastole) is critical. As a result, the relationship between heart rate, diastolic blood pressure, and ventricular end-diastolic pressure will determine whether subendocardial ischemia occurs. These factors as they apply to patients with CHD are considered below.

Aortic Diastolic Pressure

Subendocardial perfusion in a ventricle with systemic pressure occurs predominantly in early diastole. In normal children, some subendocardial perfusion of the pulmonary or right ventricle can occur in systole, as well as in diastole, because the pulmonary ventricular systolic pressure is low. However, in many congenital lesions, systolic pressure in both ventricles is systemic and in some cases the pulmonary ventricle may have suprasystemic pressures. As a result, the perfusion of both ventricles may be dependent on the rapid increase in early diastolic flow.

Aortic diastolic pressure, which is normally low in neonates and infants, is further compromised in single-ventricle physiology lesions because these lesions promote a diastolic run-off of aortic blood into the lower-resistance pulmonary circuit. The subgroup of patients with ductal-dependent systemic blood and patients with truncus arteriosus are particularly at risk for enhanced aortic diastolic run-off. In addition, coronary perfusion is further compromised in patients with hypoplastic left heart syndrome (HLHS) because the coronary ostia are perfused retrogradely down a segment of hypoplastic ascending aorta.

Subendocardial Pressure

Subendocardial pressure is elevated and subendocardial perfusion is compromised in the presence of elevated ventricular end-diastolic pressure. An elevated end-diastolic pressure may be the result of impaired diastolic function (both reduced ventricular compliance and impaired ventricular relaxation), impaired systolic function, increased ventricular end-diastolic volume, or a combination of all three. For example, elevated ventricular end-diastolic pressure occurs as the result of the ventricular volume overload that accompanies single-ventricle lesions, lesions with a high $Q_p:Q_s$, and regurgitant atrioventricular and semilunar valve lesions. The ventricular hypertrophy that accompanies pressure overload lesions is particularly detrimental to subendocardial perfusion. Ventricular hypertrophy reduces ventricular compliance and elevates ventricular end-diastolic pressure. In addition, the extravascular compressive forces that accompany a high external pressure workload further compromise myocardial perfusion by reducing the transmural coronary vascular reserve (CVR). The CVR is the ratio of hyperemic myocardial blood flow to baseline myocardial blood flow.

Heart Rate

The duration of diastole diminishes geometrically as the heart rate increases, while the duration of systole remains relatively constant. As a result, the time available for diastolic coronary artery perfusion falls as the heart rate increases. Consequently, a higher diastolic pressure is necessary to maintain subendocardial perfusion at higher heart rates. Hence, subendocardial perfusion is maintained in the presence of a low diastolic blood pressure if the heart rate is slower. In an infant with HLHS and an aortic diastolic pressure of 25 mmHg, a heart rate of 130–140 bpm may well be tolerated without evidence of subendocardial ischemia, whereas it is unlikely that a heart rate of 170–180 bpm will be tolerated at the same diastolic pressure.

Anatomic Coronary Artery Lesions

Anatomic coronary artery abnormalities complicate the management of patients with a number of congenital cardiac lesions such as pulmonary atresia with intact ventricular septum (PA/IVS), Williams–Beurin syndrome, and anomalous left coronary artery from the pulmonary artery (ALCAPA).

References and Further Reading

Barnea, O., Santamore, W., Rossi, A. *et al.* Estimation of oxygen delivery in newborns with a univentricular circulation. *Circulation* **98**, 1407–1413 (1998).

Diller, G.-P., Uebing, A., Willson, K. *et al.* Analytical identification of ideal pulmonary-systemic flow balance in patients with bidirectional cavopulmonary shunt and univentricular circulation: oxygen delivery or tissue oxygenation? *Circulation* **114**, 1243–1250 (2006).

DiNardo, J.A. & Zvara, D.A. *Anesthesia for Cardiac Surgery*, 3rd edn. Blackwell, Massachusetts (2008).

Santamore, W. P., Barnea, O., Riordan, C.J., Ross, M.P. & Austin, E.H. Theoretical optimization of pulmonary-to-systemic flow ratio after a bidirectional cavopulmonary anastomosis. *Am J Physiol* **274**, H694–700 (1998).

3

Preoperative Evaluation

Clinical History

Clinical history should include medications, allergies, past hospitalizations, and operations, including prior anesthetic experiences, and a thorough review of systems. Performance of age-appropriate activities will aid in the evaluation of cardiac function and reserve. The infant in cardiac failure will manifest symptoms of low cardiac reserve during feeding. A parent might report sweating, tiring, dyspnea, and circumoral cyanosis during feeding. The observation by a parent that the patient cannot keep the same pace as siblings often is a reliable clinical sign that cyanosis or congestive heart failure is worsening. Frequent pulmonary infections may occur as a result of increased pulmonary blood flow in otherwise asymptomatic patients. However, cardiac catheterization data may be several months old by the time the patient presents for surgery, and the newly observed clinical signs may reflect the patient's current cardiac status more accurately.

Physical Examination

An interpretation of vital signs is age specific. The heart rate decreases and blood pressure increases with age. Growth curves also are useful. Congestive heart failure will sequentially inhibit age-appropriate gains in weight, height, and head circumference. It is not unusual for patients with severe congestive heart failure to weigh less at four months of age than at birth. Interestingly, cyanotic children often do not manifest this failure to thrive.

Physical examination may reveal cyanosis, clubbing, or signs of congestive heart failure similar to those seen in adults (hepatomegaly, ascites, edema, or tachypnea). Rales may not be heard in infants and children with congestive heart failure, and the degree of heart failure may be determined more reliably by some of the signs and symptoms outlined above. Cyanosis is visibly detectable when the deoxyhemoglobin concentration is >5 g dl^{-1} and anemia masks the detection of cyanosis. Differentiation between congestive heart failure and an upper respiratory tract infection can be difficult. The physical examination in both conditions may show mild tachypnea, wheezing, and upper airway congestion. Abnormal laboratory findings may help distinguish between the two. The decision to proceed to surgery may be necessary even when the differentiation between worsening congestive heart failure and a respiratory tract infection cannot be made with certainty.

Physical examination should include an evaluation of the limitations to vascular access and monitoring sites. A child may have a diminished pulse or unobtainable blood pressure in the arm in which the subclavian artery has been directly incorporated into a palliative shunt. This obviously has implications for arterial catheter placement, blood pressure monitoring, and use

The Pediatric Cardiac Anesthesia Handbook, Second Edition. Viviane G. Nasr and James A. DiNardo.
© 2025 John Wiley & Sons Ltd. Published 2025 by John Wiley & Sons Ltd.

of pulse oximetry during surgery. More commonly, children requiring shunt procedures will have undergone a modified Blalock–Taussig shunt (tube graft from innominate artery to pulmonary artery). In this circumstance, prior to initiating blood pressure monitoring in the ipsilateral arm, it is necessary to confirm that the blood pressure in that arm accurately reflects blood pressure in the contralateral arm. Finally, the child who has undergone multiple palliative procedures may have poor venous access, which will influence the mode of induction.

Associated Congenital Abnormalities

Approximately 8% of children with congenital heart disease (CHD) have other congenital abnormalities (Table 3.1). Preoperative evaluation must define these defects. For example, conotruncal lesions (tetralogy of Fallot, interrupted aortic arch, truncus arteriosus, ventricular septal defects) are commonly associated with 22q11.2 deletion syndrome. This syndrome has previously been called DiGeorge syndrome, velocardiofacial syndrome, or conotruncal anomaly face syndrome, and is associated with hypocalcemia, immunodeficiency, facial dysmorphia, palate anomalies, velopharyngeal dysfunction, renal anomalies, and speech and feeding disorders. Atrial septal defects, ventricular septal defects, and tetralogy of Fallot are seen in children with VACTERL and CHARGE association. Tracheal stenosis must be considered in patients with VATER association who have undergone tracheoesophageal fistula repair.

The incidence of CHD (primarily atrioventricular canal defects) in patients with trisomy 21 is approximately 50%. As they age, these patients may present with problematic airways due to a large tongue and atlantooccipital instability.

Laboratory Data

A review of pertinent laboratory data and correlation with the clinical findings are necessary. A summary of preoperative evaluation is provided in Table 3.2. The child in congestive heart failure may have mild iron deficiency because of chronically increased metabolic needs. The cyanotic child will be erythrocytotic (not polycythemic) in direct relation to the degree of arterial desaturation. Hematocrit levels higher than 65% are associated with a marked increase in blood viscosity. To avoid possible neurologic sequelae from such extreme viscosity, exchange transfusion should be considered before surgery. This is especially important if the proposed surgery is palliative and cardiopulmonary bypass with hemodilution is not employed. Patients with severe cyanosis and anemia may require transfusion. Cyanosis also affects the coagulation process, and it is not unusual to observe prolongation of prothrombin time (PT), partial thromboplastin time (PTT), and bleeding times. Thrombocytopenia or functional platelet defects also may exist. In the face of reoperation with extensive dissection, the anesthesiologist should plan adequate blood component therapy for each patient.

While preoperative coagulation tests are routinely obtained in most institutions, it should be noted that in the absbence of a congenital coagulation defect, the results of these tests have little or no utility in predicting post-CPB bleeding.

When iron deficiency anemia is diagnosed, treatment with iron supplemental should be initiated. Unfortunately, there is often insufficient time to correct iron deficiency anemia with oral iron supplemention prior to surgery. In this instance, use of the intravenous iron preparations ferumoxytol and ferric iron gluconate allow for rapid iron replacement. Use of recombinant erythropoietin (rEPO) therapy should be reserved for circumstances where use of an asanginous prime is a top priority, as in Jehovah's Witness patients.

Table 3.1 Common syndromes and associated congenital heart diseases.

Syndrome	Associated CHD
CHARGE association (**C**oloboma, congenital **H**eart defects, choanal **A**tresia, **R**enal abnormalities, **G**enital hypoplasia, **E**ar deformities)	65% conotruncal anomalies, aortic arch anomalies
22q11.2 deletion syndrome	Interrupted aortic arch, truncus arteriosus, VSD, PDA, TOF
Duchenne muscular dystrophy	Cardiomyopathy
Ehlers–Danlos syndrome	Aneurysm of aorta and carotids
Ellis–van Creveld syndrome (chondro-ectodermal dysplasia)	50% common atrium
Fetal alcohol syndrome	25–30% VSD, PDA, ASD, TOF
Friedreich ataxia	Cardiomyopathy
Glygogen storage disease II (Pompe)	Cardiomyopathy
Holt–Oram syndrome	ASD, VSD
Leopard syndrome (cardio-cutaneous syndrome)	PS, long PR interval, cardiomyopathy
Long QT syndromes: • Jervell and Lange Nielsen • Romano–Ward	Long QT interval, ventricular tachyarrhythmia
Marfan syndrome	Aortic aneurysm, AR, and/or MR
Mucopolysaccharidosis	AR and/or MR, coronary artery disease, cardiomyopathy
Noonan syndrome	PS (dystrophic valve), LVH, septal hypertrophy
Tuberous sclerosis	Myocardial rhabdomyoma
Shprintzen syndrome (velocardiofacial, 22q deletion)	Conotruncal anomalies, TOF
VACTERL association	VSD, conotruncal anomalies (TOF, truncus arteriosus, etc.)
Williams–Beurin syndrome	Supravalvular AS, PA stenosis
Zellweger syndrome (cerebrohepatorenal syndrome)	PDA, VSD, ASD

AR, aortic regurgitation; AS, aortic stenosis; ASD, atrial septal defect; LVH, left ventricular hypertrophy; MR, mitral regurgitation; PA, pulmonary atresia; PDA, patent ductus arteriosus; PS, pulmonary stenosis; TOF, tetralogy of Fallot; VACTERL, vertebral anomalies, anorectal anomalies, cardiac anomalies, tracheoesophageal fistula or atresia, renal anomalies, limb anomalies; VSD, ventricular septal defect.

Plasma electrolyte concentrations should be screened, especially in patients receiving digitalis and diuretic therapy. Hypocalcemia may be observed in patients with congestive heart failure, as well as those with 22q11.2 deletion syndrome. Severe congestive heart failure may be accompanied by jitteriness and irritability. It is important to rule out hypoglycemia as an alternative cause of these findings.

The chest radiograph serves to confirm other clinical and diagnostic findings, such as cardiomegaly, the quantity of pulmonary blood flow, previous surgical procedures, and the presence of acute pulmonary infections. The electrocardiogram similarly confirms chamber enlargement and the presence of dysrhythmias. Review of the catheterization and echocardiographic data is critical to

Table 3.2 Preoperative evaluation.

History	Signs and symptoms of congestive heart failure (e.g., failure to thrive) Palpitations or syncope Additional congenital anomalies (e.g., airway, genitourinary) Recent and current medications (e.g., diuretics, digoxin, ACE inhibitors) Past surgical and interventional history Last follow-up
Physical examination	Heart murmur, thrill, arrhythmias Tachypnea, increased work of breathing, rales Poor peripheral perfusion, delayed capillary refill, bounding or diminished pulses Cool extremities, mottled skin, sweating Hepatomegaly Edema
Laboratory studies	CBC: erythrocytosis (secondary to cyanosis), anemia (secondary to malnutrition, iron deficiency) Electrolytes: hypokalemia, hyponatremia (secondary to diuretic therapy) Coagulation profile
Additional tests	Echocardiography: function and anatomy ECG: rhythm, signs of atrial or ventricular hypertrophy Chest X-ray: cardiomegaly, pulmonary edema, or infiltrates
Specific studies	Cardiac catheterization: anatomy, pressure gradients, saturations, shunts, resistances Cardiac MRI: anatomy, pulmonary blood flow, RV and LV function

ACE, angiotensin-converting enzyme; CBC, complete blood count; ECG, electrocardiogram; MRI, magnetic resonance imaging; RV, right ventricle; LV, left ventricle.
Source: Modified from Chan and Schure (2011).

a clear understanding of the pathophysiology and surgical plan. The following information should be obtained routinely from a review of the catheterization data.

- Anatomic diagnosis.
- Interpretation of saturation data. Saturation step-ups or step-downs between vessels and chambers are used to detect shunts. Likewise, saturation data are used to calculate the ratio of pulmonary to systemic blood flow (Q_p:Q_s). Saturation data also are used to differentiate intrapulmonary shunting and V/Q mismatch (atelectasis, hypoventilation, pulmonary disease) from intracardiac shunting.
- Interpretation of pressure data. Pressure data are used to compare right and left heart pressures and systemic and pulmonary arterial pressures. In addition, pressure

gradients across valve and shunt orifices are measured. Pressure data can be used to assess ventricular diastolic function (distensibility and compliance).
- Interpretation of angiographic data. Cineangiograms can be used to assess ventricular wall motion (systolic function) and intracardiac and great vessel blood flow patterns.
- Functional status and location of prior surgical interventions. This information will allow intelligent decisions to be made regarding monitor placement and anesthetic management.
- Effect of interventions. Interventions made in the catheterization laboratory to palliate congenital heart lesions (balloon valvuloplasty, balloon septostomy, balloon angioplasty) are common. The effects of these interventions on the underlying

lesion must be assessed. Furthermore, a trial of 100% inspired oxygen or NO may be used to assess the reversible component of pulmonary artery hypertension.

Echocardiography has revolutionized the field of pediatric cardiology in recent years. Unlike adults, who may have limited transthoracic echocardiographic windows, images in pediatric patients are easily obtained. Both transthoracic and transesophageal echocardiography are covered in detail in Chapter 8. Most neonates proceed to surgery without catheterization studies. In rare instances, catheterization is necessary to clearly delineate coronary or aortopulmonary collateral anatomy. Cardiac MRI is increasingly being utilized in the assessment of CHD. MRI provides precise quantification of ventricular volumes, valve regurgitation, and blood flow through the heart. It also provides an assessment of tissue characteristics such as scarring and a better delineation of extracardiac vascular anatomy than echocardiography.

Pregnancy

In teenagers and young females with CHD, conception is a possibility and pregnancy testing is required. The overall risk of CHD occurring in children of parents with CHD is 3–5% compared to 0.8% in the general population.

Psychological Considerations

The anesthesiologist who evaluates the patient with CHD must be aware of the considerable effect that appropriate psychological preparation may have during the preoperative and postoperative periods. The pediatric patient has unique psychological concerns that depend on age and previous surgical and anesthetic experience. In addition, the effect that serious heart disease has on parents and other family members cannot

be minimized and must be addressed sensitively during the preoperative evaluation. Although neonates require no psychological preparation, the perioperative process can overwhelm the parents.

The preoperative psychological preparation must be appropriate to the age of the patient. Fear of separation from parents ("stranger anxiety") can manifest in the infant at 8–12 months with an intense aversion to strangers. Very few toddlers, even if playful and cooperative in the presence of the parent, will leave their parent happily to go to the operating room. Older children have fears of disfigurement or that they will "wake up" or feel pain during and after surgery. Even the withdrawn, seemingly complacent adolescent often is in great turmoil regarding impending surgery. Previous surgery and anesthesia will influence even a young child's ability to cope with the newest operative experience.

Just as excess stress is avoided in the anxious adult patient because of potential alterations in hemodynamics, the pediatric patient requires similar attention. Psychological issues influence not only the conduct of the physical examination but also how much detail is discussed with the parents in the presence of the patient. Obtaining informed consent from the parent in the presence of a school-aged child may create undue stress for the child. On the other hand, weak promises of "no needles" or little discussion about what the child can expect is equally unpleasant and counterproductive. Most experienced pediatric anesthesiologists, aware of the spectrum and unpredictability of children's behavior, prudently plan for alternative approaches to physical examination and, most importantly, how to pleasantly and safely separate the child from the parent for the induction of anesthesia.

Preoperative Preparation

Routine preoperative preparation of the anesthesia equipment is not noticeably different for the pediatric patient. It is important to have various-sized airway equipment so that there can be a quick selection of appropriate airways, masks, and endotracheal tubes. A pediatric circle system with humidification can be used for older children. The resistance to airflow created by the unidirectional valves is not an issue for patients receiving mechanical ventilation. Generally, pressure-limited ventilation is used to avoid inadvertent barotrauma. This mode of ventilation requires vigilance in that changes in chest wall or lung compliance will lead to instantaneous changes in tidal volumes.

Appropriate emergency medications should be available in doses consistent with the patient's weight (Tables 3.3 and 3.4). For critically ill patients and those with marginal reserve, selected infusions should be prepared in anticipation of their use. Careful attention should be paid to dosages because the dose per kg may vary significantly from those used for adults.

Appropriate intravenous (IV) catheters are placed. While the use of air-trap filters in IV lines is commonly recommended, their practical application is limited in that they are easily clogged when blood products are administered, and in that air can be introduced downstream of the filter in many circumstances.

Preoperative Fluid Therapy

Preoperative fluid and nil-per-os (NPO) orders are routinely geared to the age-specific needs of the pediatric patient. Generally speaking, the rule of 2, 4, 6, 8 can be used as the NPO interval for neonates, infants, and children with congenital heart disease.

- 2 hours for clear liquids.
- 4 hours for breast milk.
- 6 hours for formula.
- 8 hours for solid food.

Obviously, in the absence of IV hydration, infants should remain NPO for the shortest possible interval. Because dehydration may have potentially deleterious effects on hemodynamics or on the degree of blood viscosity in the erythrocytotic patient, IV hydration with maintenance fluids before surgery should be considered for certain patients (i.e., cyanotic patients with hematocrit levels of 60% or higher).

Maintenance caloric requirements in the awake neonate and infant are 100 kcal kg^{-1} per day or 4 kcal kg^{-1} h^{-1}. This caloric requirement can be met with glucose 25 g kg^{-1} per day or 1 g kg^{-1} h^{-1}. From a practical point of view, this glucose requirement can be met with 10% dextrose (100 mg ml^{-1}) administered at maintenance volume replacement rate of 4 ml kg^{-1} h^{-1}. Dextrose (10%) administered at half this rate (2 ml kg^{-1} h^{-1}) is usually sufficient to meet the caloric requirements of an anesthetized infant while avoiding both the hyperglycemia and hypoglycemia that can be detrimental to neurologic outcome following deep hypothermic circulatory arrest (DHCA). These dextrose infusions should be discontinued prior to the commencement of cardiopulmonary bypass (CPB), which generally produces mild hyperglycemia. Some patients receive nutritional support as part of their medical stabilization prior to surgery.

High-calorie total parenteral nutrition and intralipid therapy should be discontinued and replaced with a 10% dextrose infusion several hours prior to transport to the operating room. Continued administration of these high-calorie infusions makes intraoperative serum glucose management problematic. In these patients, higher dextrose infusion rates may be necessary pre-CPB to avoid rebound hypoglycemia.

Preoperative Medications

Premedication prior to induction can be used to facilitate a number of objectives. In older children, it can be used to alleviate anxiety prior to an IV or inhalation induction. In younger children, premedication can ease separation of the child from the parents. In infants, judicious premedication alone, or in combination with inhaled

Table 3.3 Commonly used vasoactive drugs and antidysrhythmics.

Drugs	Bolus	Infusion rate	Comments
Adenosine 6 mg in 2 ml (3 mg ml^{-1})	100 µg kg^{-1} rapid IV bolus and flush (max. 6 mg); second dose 200 µg kg^{-1} (max. 12 mg)		Reduce by half for patients who have had a heart transplant. Give as close to IV site as much as possible, followed by a flush
Atropine 8 mg in 20 ml (0.4 mg ml^{-1})	20 µg kg^{-1} IV		Maximum dose 1 mg for child and 3 mg for adolescent
Amiodarone 150 mg in 3 ml (50 mg ml^{-1})	5 mg kg^{-1} IV slowly over 15–30 min	5–15 µg kg^{-1} min^{-1}	Adult max. bolus 300 mg for Vfib and/or VTach
Calcium gluconate 100 mg ml^{-1}	30–60 mg kg^{-1} IV		
Dopamine 400 mg in 10 ml (40 mg ml^{-1})		3–10 µg kg^{-1} min^{-1}	Titrate to effect
Epinephrine 1 mg ml^{-1}	1 µg kg^{-1} to treat hypotension IV; 10 µg kg^{-1} IV for cardiac arrest; repeat every 3–5 min as needed	0.01–0.1 µg kg^{-1} min^{-1}	Titrate to effect
Isoproterenol 1 mg in 5 ml (0.2 mg ml^{-1})		0.01–0.1 µg kg^{-1} min^{-1}	Tachycardia, palpitations, angina, pulmonary edema, hypertension, hypotension, ventricular arrhythmias, tachyarrhythmias
Lidocaine 20 mg in 2 ml (10 mg ml^{-1})	1 mg kg^{-1} IV	20–50 µg kg^{-1} min^{-1}	
Magnesium 50% 1 in 2 ml (0.5 g ml^{-1})	25–50 mg kg^{-1} IV		For torsades de pointes (max. 2 g)
Norepinephrine 4 mg in 4 ml (1 mg ml^{-1})		0.05 µg kg^{-1} min^{-1}	Titrate to effect
Phenylephrine 10 mg ml^{-1} vial	0.5 µg kg^{-1}	0.1 µg kg^{-1} min^{-1}	Titrate to effect
Procainamide 500 mg ml^{-1} 100 mg ml^{-1}	5–15 mg kg^{-1} IV loading dose over 30–60 min	20–80 µg kg^{-1} min^{-1}	ECG monitoring required. Caution: hypotension and prolonged QT, widening of QRS
Vasopressin 20 units ml^{-1}	In children 0.1 unit In adults 1 unit	6–30 mU kg^{-1} h^{-1}	Titrate to effect
Ephedrine 5 mg ml^{-1}	0.05–0.1 mg kg^{-1}		

Table 3.4 Commonly used antihypertensive drugs and beta-blockers.

Drugs	Bolus	Infusion rate	Comments
Esmolol 100 mg in 10 ml ($10\ mg\ ml^{-1}$)	$500\ \mu g\ kg^{-1}$ over 3–5 min	$25–200\ \mu g\ kg^{-1}\ min^{-1}$	Titrate to effect
Hydralazine $20\ mg\ ml^{-1}$	$0.1\ mg\ kg^{-1}$		
Labetalol 100 mg in 20 ml ($5\ mg\ ml^{-1}$)		$0.25\ mg\ kg^{-1}\ h^{-1}$	Titrate to effect
Milrinone 10 mg in 10 ml ($1\ mg\ ml^{-1}$)	$50–100\ \mu g\ kg^{-1}$ loading dose	$0.25\text{-}1\ \mu g\ kg^{-1}\ min^{-1}$	
Nitroprusside 50 mg in 2 ml ($25\ mg\ ml^{-1}$)		$0.5\ \mu g\ kg^{-1}\ min^{-1}$	Titrate to effect; observe for signs of cyanide toxicity
Nitroglycerin 50 mg in 10 ml ($5\ mg\ ml^{-1}$)		$0.5\ \mu g\ kg^{-1}\ min^{-1}$	Titrate to effect
Phentolamine $0.1\ mg\ kg^{-1}$	$0.1\ mg\ kg^{-1}$		If weight above 50 kg, give 5 mg

nitrous oxide, can greatly simplify the placement of an IV catheter. One must always consider how stressful it is for parents to see their child being taken to the operating room crying or upset.

Midazolam 1 mg kg^{-1} (20 mg as a maximum dose) orally in infants and younger children who have not had prior cardiac surgery is useful. In patients who have undergone previous operative procedures, midazolam alone may be insufficient. These patients are remarkably tolerant to midazolam as the result of either heightened anxiety or previous intraoperative and postoperative exposure to benzodiazepines. Oral ketamine (3–5 mg kg^{-1} for infants, 5–10 mg kg^{-1} for children aged more than one year) can be given in conjunction with the midazolam to these patients. In circumstances in which the child will not take oral medication, the intramuscular route can be used. Ketamine 2–3 mg kg^{-1} in combination with midazolam 0.1 mg kg^{-1} is appropriate. Some practitioners add glycopyrrolate (8–10 μg kg^{-1}) as an antisialagogue.

It is worth noting that given the large first-pass metabolism effect (70%) of gastrically administered midazolam and ketamine, a premedication which bypasses oral buccal absorption following direct administration into a gastric tube (G-tube) may have reduced efficacy.

Premedication requires the individualization of dosage to avoid respiratory depression. Lower doses are best used for smaller children and children in congestive heart failure. Premedication should always be administered and assessed in the continuous presence of the anesthesiologist. Older children may opt for placement of an intravenous line (IV).

Digoxin, diuretics, angiotensin-converting enzyme (ACE) inhibitors, and angiotensin II receptor blockers (ARB) are generally withheld on the morning of surgery. ACE inhibitors and ARB can exacerbate hypotension occurring with anesthetic induction. Inotrope and prostaglandin infusions are continued into the operative period for critically ill neonates and children.

References and Further Reading

Chan, D.M. & Schure, A.Y. Congenital heart disease. In: Vacanti, C.A., Sikka, P.K., Urman, R.D., Derswitz, M. & Segal, B.S. (eds) *Essential Clinical Anesthesia*. Cambridge University Press, Cambridge (2011).

Jones, S.E., Jooste, E., Gottlieb, E. *et al.* Preoperative laboratory studies for pediatric cardiac surgery patients: a multi-institutional perspective. *Anesth Analg* **128**, 1051–1054 (2019).

Sullivan, K.E. Chromosome 22q11.2 deletion syndrome and DiGeorge syndrome. *Immunol Rev* **287**, 186–201 (2019).

4

Intraoperative Management

The intraoperative management of patients with congenital heart disease (CHD), including monitoring, invasive line placement (central and arterial), anesthesia induction, and maintenance, is discussed in this chapter. The intraoperative management of each lesion will be discussed in the following chapters.

Intraoperative Monitoring

If the infant or child is awake or minimally sedated, the application of multiple monitors can prevent a smooth induction, even for an initially calm patient. Minimizing stimulation, including distracting discussion in the operating room, will avoid disturbing the child. Ideally, preinduction monitoring should include a noninvasive automated blood pressure cuff, electrocardiogram (ECG), pulse oximeter, and an end-tidal carbon dioxide monitor. In some cases, a pulse oximeter and an ECG may be all that is practical in the early stages of induction. Other monitors are then quickly added as induction progresses.

ECG and Blood Pressure

A five-lead ECG with leads II and V_5 displayed allows rhythm and ischemia monitoring. Intraarterial access is obtained following induction; however, many neonates who have been medically stabilized in the intensive care unit (ICU) preoperatively will have an arterial catheter in place. Generally, percutaneous arterial access can be accomplished in even the smallest neonates, particularly given the wide availability of ultrasound equipment to guide placement. Radial, ulnar, and femoral arteries are the sites most commonly utilized. In many institutions, the axillary artery is preferred over the femoral artery in very small infants as there is better collateral circulation in the axillary artery compared to the femoral artery distribution, reducing the likelihood of end-artery ischemia.

In some institutions, attempts to cannulate the ulnar artery are undertaken after failed attempts to cannulate the radial artery have been made. Posterior tibial and dorsalis pedis arteries may also be used, but these sites often do not reflect central aortic pressure during and immediately following hypothermic cardiopulmonary bypass (CPB) in neonates and infants. Brachial arteries are used in some institutions, but others feel strongly that this site is associated with a high risk of distal limb ischemia. Consideration is given to any previous or proposed surgical procedure which may compromise the reliability of ipsilateral upper extremity intraarterial pressure monitoring such as a Blalock–Thomas–Taussig shunt, modified Blalock–Thomas–Taussig shunt, subclavian artery patch repair of aortic coarctation, or sacrifice of an aberrant subclavian artery. Previous catheterization procedures – particularly those of an interventional nature – may result in femoral or iliac artery occlusion.

The Pediatric Cardiac Anesthesia Handbook, Second Edition. Viviane G. Nasr and James A. DiNardo.
© 2025 John Wiley & Sons Ltd. Published 2025 by John Wiley & Sons Ltd.

Table 4.1 Brief guideline for central and arterial line catheter sizes.

Age/size of child	Central line sizes	Arterial line sizes
Infants <5 kg	4 Fr 5 cm	24 gauge for radial/ulnar 2.5 Fr 2.5 cm for radial/ulnar 2.5 Fr 5 cm for femoral/axillary
Infants/toddlers <10 kg	4 Fr 5 cm 5 Fr 5 cm	22 or 24 gauge for radial/ulnar 2.5 Fr 2.5 cm for radial/ulnar 2.5 Fr 5 cm for femoral/axillary
Preschool children <20–25 kg	5 Fr 8 cm	20 or 22 gauge for radial/ulnar 3 Fr 5 cm for femoral/axillary
Older children	7 Fr adult triple-lumen	20 or 22 gauge for radial/ulnar

Fr, French size.

On occasion, surgical access to a peripheral artery is necessary.

Umbilical artery catheters may be used intraoperatively but are generally replaced with a peripheral arterial catheter and removed postoperatively. Blood pressure monitoring consists of an intraarterial catheter as well as upper and lower extremity noninvasive blood pressure cuffs. This arrangement allows the detection of residual coarctation or aortic arch/isthmus obstruction via a comparison of upper and lower extremity blood pressures. A summary of appropriate arterial and central venous pressure catheters is given in Table 4.1.

Systemic Oxygen Saturation

Oxygen saturation (SaO_2) monitoring is accomplished with pulse oximeter probes on both an upper and a lower extremity; these can be placed in pre- and postductal locations if the physiology warrants.

End-tidal CO$_2$

End-tidal carbon dioxide ($ETCO_2$) monitoring is routinely employed, with the caveat that the difference between $PaCO_2$ and $ETCO_2$ will vary as physiologic dead space varies, and that in some circumstances the difference may be large (>10–15 torr). Any acute reduction in pulmonary blood flow or increase in Zone 1 of the lung (high mean airway pressure, decreased cardiac output, pulmonary embolus, increased intracardiac R-L shunting) will increase this gradient. In patients with single-ventricle physiology (most commonly those with HLHS or truncus arteriosus) with a high Q_P:Q_S prior to the initiation of CPB, the right pulmonary artery may be partially, or completely, occluded by the surgeon to mechanically limit pulmonary blood flow. This maneuver dramatically increases physiologic dead space and $ETCO_2$ will vastly underestimate $PaCO_2$.

Central Venous Pressure

Percutaneous central venous access offers numerous advantages and can be reliably obtained, even in small neonates. The use of real-time ultrasound has helped to improve the successful placement rate to 90–95% in neonates. A brief guideline to central line sizes is provided in Table 4.1. The preoperative use of pulmonary artery catheters for pediatric patients is uncommon. In patients where postoperative assessment of pulmonary artery pressure (PAP) is important, the surgeon may choose to place a transthoracic pulmonary artery catheter.

Central venous access is not without risks, particularly in neonates and infants, and

Table 4.2 Advantages and disadvantages of central venous pressure (CVP) monitoring in neonates and infants.

Advantages	Disadvantages
• Measuring CVP • Infusion site for vasoactive and inotropic agents • Infusion of blood products • Measurement of mixed venous oxygenation saturation to determine CO and Q_p:Q_s • CVP waveform helpful in rhythm analysis • Assessment of SVC drainage during CPB	• Pneumothorax • Hematoma with vascular or tracheal compression/displacement • Thoracic duct injury • Air embolus • Internal jugular or SVC thrombosis • Infection

CO, cardiac output; CPB, cardiopulmonary bypass; CVP, central venous pressure; Q_p:Q_s, pulmonary-systemic shunt ratio; SVC, superior vena cava.

therefore the decision to place a percutaneous central venous catheter must involve consideration of the relative risks and benefits. In particular, the risk of internal jugular or superior vena cava (SVC) thrombosis must be considered, as this complication can be devastating in patients who are to be staged to a superior cavopulmonary connection. The relative risk and benefits of central venous cannulation are outlined in Table 4.2. The risk of thrombosis and infection can be reduced by maintaining a heparin infusion (2 units h^{-1}) through the central line lumens postoperatively, and by removing the lines as soon as possible (typically 1–2 days).

In some institutions, neonates and infants are managed prior to CPB without central venous lines. Transthoracic intracardiac lines (RA, LA, PA) placed by the surgeon prior to the termination of CPB can be used for pressure monitoring, infusion of vasoactive and inotropic agents, and blood product and volume replacement. In older children, particularly those undergoing reoperation with adhesion of the aorta or of the RV to PA conduit to the sternum, large-bore central venous catheters are used in conjunction with a rapid infusion system. In these children, transthoracic intracardiac lines, though suitable for pressure monitoring and infusion of drugs, are insufficient for rapid volume replacement.

Temperature

Rectal, esophageal or nasopharyngeal temperatures are monitored for all CPB cases. Tympanic membrane temperatures are rarely monitored in the current era. Rectal temperature is considered a peripheral temperature site and the equilibration of rectal temperature with tympanic and esophageal temperatures serves as the best index of homogeneous somatic cooling and rewarming. Rectal temperature lags behind esophageal and nasopharyngeal temperatures during both cooling and rewarming.

Both esophageal and nasopharyngeal temperatures are core temperature monitoring sites, and temperature changes at these sites generally mirror brain temperature changes. Even so, esophageal and nasopharyngeal temperatures may either over- or underestimate brain temperature by as much as 5 °C during cooling and rewarming. This observation underscores the importance of providing an adequately long period of core cooling prior to commencement of low-flow CPB or deep hypothermic circulatory arrest (DHCA). The likelihood that the target brain temperature (15–18 °C) will be reached is greatly increased if core cooling is utilized to bring nasopharyngeal or esophageal and rectal temperatures to this target temperature.

Near-infra-red Spectroscopy

Near-infra-red spectroscopy (NIRS) has emerged as a technology that enables continuous monitoring of regional tissue oxygenation. Similar to pulse oximetry, cerebral oximetry uses the fact that oxygenated and deoxygenated hemoglobin absorb near-infrared light to differing degrees. Because the skull is translucent to infra-red light, superficial brain tissue can be accessed using this technology. While initially intended to monitor cerebral oxygenation, NIRS probes placed on the abdominal wall, quadriceps muscle, or on the flank overlying the kidneys are often used to monitor somatic oxygenation.

In the United States, approved cerebral oximetry monitoring systems include Invos^{TM} 5100C and 7100 (Medtronic/Covidien, USA); Fore-Sight Elite® (Casmed/Edwards Lifesciences, USA); Equanox^{TM} three and four-wavelength versions (Nonin Medical, USA); O3® Regional Oximetry (Masimo, USA), and the NIRO-200 NX® system (Hamamatsu Photonics, Japan). All use a light-emitting diode (near-infra-red light 700–1000 nm) and two light sensors placed 3 and 4 cm away from the light source. The diode emits near-infra-red light, which passes through a superficial banana-shaped tissue volume to the detectors. The proximal detector detects light absorbed by extracranial tissues, and this is subtracted from the total signal, allowing the determination of intracranial absorption. The Fore-Sight instrument uses a laser technology. The algorithms used to calculate the cerebral oxygen saturation value are based on the assumption that 25–30% of the intracranial blood is arterial and 70–75% is venous and on the fact that total hemoglobin concentration can be determined because oxy- and deoxyhemoglobin have the same molar absorptivity at 810 nm (isobestic point).

Some monitors display the numerical value rSO_2i, which is the ratio of oxyhemoglobin to total hemoglobin in the light path. The rSO_2i is reported as a percentage on a scale from 15% to 95%. Since this is not an absolute value for tissue oxygenation, clinicians tend to assess trends in rSO_2i relative to an established baseline value such as those obtained prior to induction or commencement of CPB. Newer devices report an absolute value for cerebral oxygenation (StO_2).

Many institutions utilize formal or informal algorithms incorporating the manipulation of FiO_2, $PaCO_2$, acid–base status, CPB flow rate and perfusion pressure, temperature, and hemoglobin concentration to "optimize" NIRS values. Because the normal range of cerebral and somatic NIRS values across the anatomically and physiologically heterogeneous CHD population has not been established, the value of NIRS and the trend in NIRS that requires intervention relies on judgment and experience with the specific monitor. In general, a decrease in a NIRS value of more than 20% requires investigation as to a remediable cause. Figure 4.1 summarizes a comprehensive algorithm to manage intraoperative NIRS data.

Transcranial Doppler

The role of transcranial Doppler (TCD) monitoring in the care of pediatric cardiac surgical patients is evolving. TCD allows the measurement of cerebral blood flow velocity as well as the detection of cerebral microemboli, and is a technology ideally suited for use in neonates and infants. The thin skull of neonates/infants, combined with a low-frequency ultrasonic transducer, allows the transmission of ultrasonic energy into brain tissue with little signal attenuation.

Placement of a 2 MHz pulsed-wave (PW) Doppler probe over the temporal bone allows the ultrasonic signal to be aligned parallel to the proximal (M1) segment of the middle cerebral artery (MCA). The ability of PW Doppler to be gated to a specific depth allows the determination of blood flow velocity in the MCA just distal to the take-off of the anterior cerebral artery. This PW Doppler interrogation yields a velocity spectrum in the MCA for each cardiac cycle. Integration of the area under the velocity spectrum yields the time-velocity integral (TVI) in units of cm per cardiac cycle.

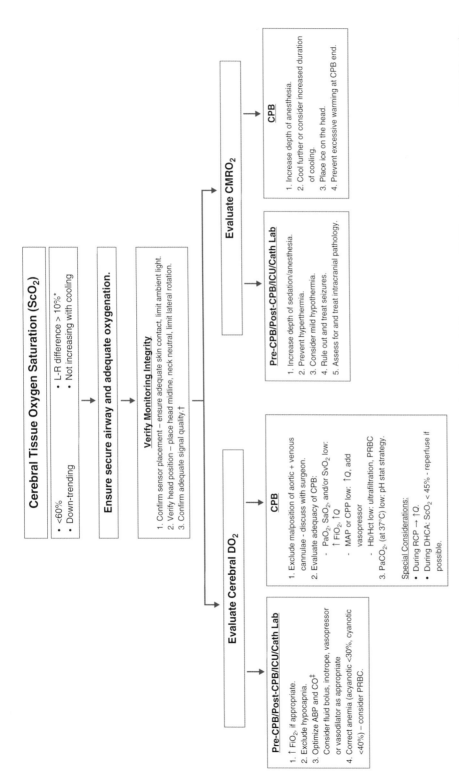

Figure 4.1 A comprehensive algorithm for management of intraoperative NIRS data. ABP, arterial blood pressure; CMRO$_2$, cerebral oxygen consumption; CO, cardiac output; CPB, cardiopulmonary bypass; CPP, cerebral perfusion pressure; DHCA, deep hypothermic circulatory arrest; DO$_2$, oxygen delivery; FiO$_2$, fraction of inspired oxygen; Hb, hemoglobin; Hct, hematocrit; ICU, intensive care unit; L–R, left-right; MAP, mean arterial pressure; PaCO$_2$, partial pressure of carbon dioxide; PaO$_2$, partial pressure of oxygen; PRBC, packed red blood cells; RCP, regional cerebral perfusion (antegrade cerebral perfusion); SaO$_2$, oxygen saturation (by co-oximetry); ScO$_2$, cerebral tissue oxygen saturation; SvO$_2$, mixed venous oxygen saturation; Q, flow (here CPB flow); VE, minute ventilation. *L–R difference may be physiologic, technologic (e.g., geometry, which usually is seen during initial placement) or pathologic. † Indicator specific to each monitor. ‡ Direct measurement of cardiac output by transthoracic echocardiography or pulmonary artery catheter (PAC) (v indirect measures such as mixed venous oxygen saturation, lactate, and acid–base status) infrequent in pediatric congenital heart disease. *Source:* Reproduced from Zaleski and Kussman (2019)/with permission of Elsevier.

The product of vessel TVI and vessel cross-sectional area (units of cm^2) is flow (units of cm^3 per cardiac cycle). If it is assumed that the MCA cross-sectional area remains constant, then there is a linear relationship between TVI and MCA blood flow.

Normal TCD velocity values in various patient subgroups (cyanotic versus noncyanotic, age, following DHCA), and under various CPB conditions (hematocrit, flow, pressure, acid–base status, temperature) have yet to be determined. The TCD determination of cerebral blood flow may prove useful as a continuous surveillance monitor for the detection of inadequate flow or obstructed cerebral venous drainage during CPB.

Cerebral microemboli produce transient increases in reflected Doppler energy compared to the background Doppler spectra. These high-intensity transient signals (HITS) can be counted by the TCD microprocessor and displaced as microembolic events per hour. Due to their higher reflective capacity, gaseous emboli can be detected over a greater distance than particulate emboli, and as a result have a higher sample velocity length (the product of emboli duration and velocity). At present, cerebral emboli detection with TCD requires the constant attention of a skilled observer because TCD technology alone lacks sufficient sensitivity and specificity to distinguish between gaseous brain emboli, particulate brain emboli, and artifacts. TCD emboli detection is being investigated as a tool to refine post-CPB de-airing routines and to reduce the number of cannulation- and perfusion-related iatrogenic embolic events.

Transesophageal Echocardiography (TEE)

This topic is covered in detail in Chapter 8.

Airway Management

Fundamental to the anesthetic care of every patient with CHD is good airway management. The pulmonary vascular resistance (PVR) is altered by changes in ventilatory pattern, PaO_2, $PaCO_2$, and pH. Changes in PVR may dramatically affect shunt magnitude and direction, as well as cardiovascular function and stability. Therefore, prompt control of the airway and of ventilation will allow optimal pulmonary blood flow in each patient.

Children with a high pulmonary blood flow, particularly those with interstitial pulmonary edema, have surprisingly poor lung compliance, necessitating higher than expected airway pressures. Care must be taken not to insufflate the stomach during mask ventilation. The relatively large occiput of infants and small children will cause the head to flex forward; the placement of a small roll under the neck or shoulders will allow the head to remain in the neutral position. Placement of an oral airway in neonates and infants will greatly facilitate mask ventilation by pulling the large tongue away from the pharyngeal wall. In children aged <2–3 years, nasal endotracheal tubes are generally utilized as they provide better stability intraoperatively and postoperatively. This is particularly important in patients undergoing intraoperative TEE examinations. Denitrogenation of the lungs is recommended prior to induction in all patients, including those in whom high inspired O_2 concentrations might temporarily reduce PVR and compromise systemic perfusion.

In patients with high venous pressure and cyanosis, such as those with a bidirectional Glenn shunt or Fontan, nasal endotracheal tubes must be passed cautiously as substantial nasal bleeding can be initiated. Cuffed endotracheal tubes with a leak at or near 20 cmH_2O are generally used in children. The use of a cuffed endotracheal tube will allow higher airway pressures to be utilized as needed in patients where poor pulmonary compliance secondary to lung water, chest wall edema, or abdominal distention are anticipated to compromise minute ventilation.

Anesthesia Induction and Maintenance

Induction of Anesthesia

A variety of induction techniques provide hemodynamic stability and improved arterial oxygen saturation in patients with cyanotic heart disease. Sevoflurane, halothane, isoflurane, and fentanyl/midazolam do not change $Q_P{:}Q_S$ in children with atrial septal defects (ASDs) and ventricular septal defects (VSDs) when cautiously administered with 100% oxygen. Sevoflurane (1 MAC) and fentanyl/midazolam have no significant effect on myocardial function in patients with a single ventricle.

No one anesthetic induction technique is suitable for all patients with CHD. The patient's age, cardiopulmonary function, degree of cyanosis, and emotional state all play a role in the selection of an anesthetic technique. The intravenous administration of induction agents clearly affords the greatest flexibility in terms of drug selection and drug titration, and allows prompt control of the airway. Intravenous induction is the preferred technique in patients with severely impaired ventricular systolic function and those with systemic or suprasystemic pulmonary artery pressures.

Mask Induction

Mask induction of anesthesia can be accomplished safely in the subset of children without severe cardiorespiratory compromise. However, reduced pulmonary blood flow in cyanotic patients will prolong the length of induction and the interval during which the airway is only partially controlled. In addition, in these patients even short intervals of airway obstruction or hypoventilation may result in hypoxemia.

Sevoflurane is the inhalation induction agent of choice. Isoflurane, and particularly desflurane, are unsuitable agents as their pungency causes copious secretions, airway irritation, and laryngospasm. Following administration of a "heavy" premedication such as PO ketamine 5–7 mg kg^{-1} and midazolam 1 mg kg^{-1} or IM ketamine 2–3 mg kg^{-1} and midazolam 0.1 mg kg^{-1}, an inhalation induction with sevoflurane not to exceed 4% inspired concentration (<1.5 MAC) can be performed in children with limited cardiovascular reserve to obtain intravenous access.

Intravenous Induction

Historically, high-dose synthetic opioids (fentanyl 30–50 µg kg^{-1}) in combination with pancuronium (0.1 mg kg^{-1}) were used for intravenous induction in neonates and infants. The vagolytic and sympathomimetic effects of pancuronium counteract the vagotonic effect of synthetic opioids. In current practice, rocuronium (0.6 mg kg^{-1}), vecuronium (0.1 mg kg^{-1}), and cis-atracurium (0.2 mg kg^{-1}) in conjunction with lower dose synthetic opioids (fentanyl 10–30 µg kg^{-1}) are used even in patients with a low aortic diastolic blood pressure and a high baseline heart rate. In older children with mild to moderately depressed systolic function, even lower doses of a synthetic opioid can be used in conjunction with etomidate (0.1–0.3 mg kg^{-1}) or ketamine (1–2 mg kg^{-1}). For patients with both normal and elevated baseline PVR, ketamine causes minimal increases in PAP as long as the airway and ventilation are supported.

The myocardial depressive and vasodilatory effects of propofol and thiopental make them unsuitable as induction agents, except in patients with simple shunt lesions in whom cardiovascular function is preserved.

An alternative to intravenous induction in patients with difficult peripheral intravenous access is intramuscular induction with ketamine (3–5 mg kg^{-1}), succinylcholine (2–5 mg kg^{-1}), and glycopyrrolate (8–10 µg kg^{-1}). Glycopyrrolate is recommended to reduce the airway secretions associated with ketamine administration and prevent the bradycardia that may accompany succinylcholine administration. The dose of succinylcholine per kilogram body weight is highest in infants. This technique provides prompt induction and immediate control of the airway with tracheal intubation. It is useful in circumstances where it is anticipated that initial intravenous access will have to be obtained via the internal or external jugular vein or femoral vein. This technique is hampered by the fact that the short duration of action of succinylcholine limits the period of patient immobility.

An alternative technique combines intramuscular ketamine (3–5 mg kg^{-1}) and rocuronium (1.0 mg kg^{-1}). This technique is hampered by the slightly longer time interval until attainment of adequate intubating conditions and the longer duration of action of rocuronium compared to succinylcholine.

Maintenance of Anesthesia

Anesthesia is generally maintained using a synthetic opioid (fentanyl or sufentanil)- based technique. These opioids may be used in high doses (fentanyl 25–100 µg kg^{-1} or sufentanil 2.5–10 µg kg^{-1}) or in low to moderate doses (fentanyl 5–25 µg kg^{-1} or sufentanil 0.5–2.5 µg kg^{-1}). In either instance, these opioids are used in combination with an inhalation agent (generally isoflurane 0.5–1.0% or sevoflurane 1.0–2.0%), a benzodiazepine (generally midazolam 0.05–0.1 mg kg^{-1}), or dexmedetomidine (0.5–1.0 mg kg^{-1} h^{-1}). Caution must be exercised because the combination of opioids and benzodiazepines is synergistic in reducing systemic vascular resistance.

The high-dose technique is particularly useful in neonates and infants. Patients in this age group presenting for surgery often have significant ventricular pressure and/or volume overload. In addition, many have tenuous subendocardial and systemic perfusion secondary to run-off into the pulmonary circulation and the associated low aortic diastolic blood pressure. Given the limited contractile reserve available in the immature myocardium, it is not surprising that the myocardial depressive and systemic vasodilatory effects of inhalation agents and the synergistic vasodilatory effects of benzodiazepines and opioids may be poorly tolerated in this patient group.

There are unique considerations for the maintenance of anesthesia during CPB. Light anesthesia, particularly during cooling and rewarming, may lead to an elevated SVR, requiring a reduction in pump flow rate, which compromises both somatic perfusion and the efficiency of CPB cooling and rewarming. Subclinical shivering due to inadequate neuromuscular blockade and light anesthesia is an avoidable cause of increased systemic oxygen consumption. Increased systemic oxygen consumption during CPB will manifest as a lower than acceptable venous saturation (<65%) at what should be an adequate CPB flow rate for the patient. Furthermore, for a membrane oxygenator operating at or near its maximum flow capacity, a low venous saturation may result in a lower than acceptable arterial saturation on CPB.

Lower doses of opioids in conjunction with an inhalation agent, benzodiazepine, or dexmedetomidine are suitable for older patients with better cardiovascular reserve. In fact, carefully selected patients (aged >1 year, no pulmonary hypertension, benign past medical history) undergoing simple ASD or VSD closure are candidates for immediate tracheal extubation in the operating room or in the ICU within 2–3 hours. Increasingly, in many institutions immediate or early tracheal extubation is being undertaken in selected infants and older children undergoing more complex repairs.

References and Further Reading

Gleich, S.J., Wong, A.V., Handlogten, K.S., Thum, D.E. & Nemergut, M.E. Major short-term complications of arterial cannulation for monitoring in children. *Anesthesiology* **134**, 26–34 (2020).

Zaleski, K.L. & Kussman, B.D. Near-infrared spectroscopy in pediatric congenital heart disease. *J Cardiothorac Vasc Anesth* **34**, 489–500 (2019).

5

Developmental Hemostasis and Patient Blood Management

Current Concept of Hemostasis (Coagulation, Anticoagulation, and Fibrinolysis)

The classic cascade or waterfall coagulation model (Figure 5.1) is composed of redundant intrinsic (contact activation) and extrinsic (tissue factor, TF) pathways with convergence on factor (F) X activation. This model does not explain several key clinical observations.

- Severe deficiencies of FXII (Hageman factor), high molecular weight kininogen (HMK) and prekallikrein (PK) are not associated with abnormal bleeding. Furthermore, patients with severe FXII deficiency can generate as much thrombin as normal patients during CPB. In addition, the lack of an increase in FXIIa levels during CPB at a time when thrombin generation is increasing suggests that a mechanism other than or in addition to FXII-induced contact phase activation is at work.
- Severe FXI deficiency is associated with bleeding tendencies only when high levels of fibrin are needed, or when surgery takes place in locations with high local fibrinolytic activity, such as the urinary tract or oral cavity.
- FVIII deficiency (hemophilia A) and factor FIX deficiency (hemophilia B) are associated with severe bleeding tendencies. In the presence of both intrinsic and extrinsic pathways, severe deficiencies of FVIII and FIX should not result in clinical bleeding because activation of FX by the TF or FVIIa pathway should be adequate. Clearly, this is not the case.
- Bleeding tendencies similar to those seen with hemophilia A and B occur in patients with severe FVII and are not explained by the classic model in which the intrinsic system plays a major role in initiating coagulation.
- The *in vitro* coagulation tests aPTT and PT only assess the initiation phase of coagulation and are poor predictors of postoperative bleeding.

Current understanding of coagulation is based on the concepts of primary and secondary hemostasis and the cell-based model in which cell-based TF, FVII, and the surface of activated platelets are key components (Figure 5.2). Following vascular injury, primary hemostasis is initiated in conjunction with vasoconstriction. Platelets adhere to exposed subendothelial collagen via the platelet glycoprotein (GP) VI receptor, or to collagen-bound von Willebrand factor (vWF) via the GPIb receptor. Platelet adherence triggers activation via cytosolic signaling that results in stimulation of arachidonic acid metabolism and the release of granular contents. FVIII is brought to the site of the injury bound to multimeric vWF. In addition, when platelets are activated, negatively charged phospholipids move from the inner to the outer leaflet of the membrane bilayer. This surface provides binding sites for enzymes and cofactors of the coagulation system,

The Pediatric Cardiac Anesthesia Handbook, Second Edition. Viviane G. Nasr and James A. DiNardo.
© 2025 John Wiley & Sons Ltd. Published 2025 by John Wiley & Sons Ltd.

Figure 5.1 The classic waterfall model of coagulation with separate, redundant intrinsic and extrinsic pathways.

resulting in the formation of a clot; this is referred to as secondary hemostasis.

Simultaneously, at the site of endothelial disruption, TF-bearing cells are exposed

to blood. TF, also known as tissue thromboplastin or FIII, is abundant and expressed on cells in organs where bleeding can be catastrophic, such as the brain, kidney,

Adhesion and activation

Figure 5.2 Primary platelet plug hemostasis and secondary hemostasis via cell-based coagulation. Also depicted are anticoagulant factors. See text for details. ADP, adenosine diphosphate; APC, activated protein C; AT, antithrombin III; GP, glycoprotein; PS, protein S; TF, tissue factor; TFPI, TF pathway inhibitor; TXA2, thromboxane A2; vWF, von Willebrand factor. *Source:* Negrier et al. (2019)/with permission of Elsevier.

gut, skin, lung, placenta, and in the adventitial cells of blood vessels. TF provides a protective "hemostatic envelope" if the integrity of the vessels or tissue is interrupted. TF may also be expressed by monocytes, endothelial cells, macrophages, and fibroblasts in response to certain pathologic stimuli. Expression of TF by monocytes and macrophages is an important consequence of exposure of blood to artificial biologic surfaces such as those present in CPB and ECMO circuits, and is likely a more important cause of thrombin generation than classic contact activation via the intrinsic pathway.

The process of secondary hemostasis or clot formation and stabilization following primary hemostasis comprises four continuous stages: initiation, amplification, propagation, and stabilization.

Initiation

Once bound to TF, zymogen FVII is rapidly converted to FVIIa and the TF/FVIIa complex is capable of rapidly activating FX and FIX. In the presence of unactivated FV, FXa is capable of catalyzing the conversion of prothrombin (FII) to thrombin (FIIa) in picomolar quantities. Thrombin generation through this reaction is not robust due to the rapid inhibition of FXa and the TF/FVIIa complex by the inhibitor TF pathway inhibitor (TFPI), as well as the rapid inhibition of free FXa by antithrombin III (ATIII). The small amount of thrombin formed is the catalyst for continued thrombin generation because the generated thrombin is capable of activating factors V and VIII, and of inducing further platelet aggregation. In contrast, the FIXa activated by FVIIa/TF does not act on the TF-bearing cell and does not play a significant role in the initiation phase of coagulation. However, FIXa is not inhibited by TFPI and can diffuse to the surface of nearby activated platelets and bind to a specific platelet surface receptor, interact with its cofactor, FVIIIa, and activate FX directly on the platelet surface.

Thrombin and polyphosphate (PolyP) released from activated platelets catalyze formation of FXIa, which in turn catalyzes formation of FIXa on the platelet surface. This drives further FIXa/FVIIIa complex formation and enhances platelet surface FXa and thrombin generation. This is the link between classic extrinsic and intrinsic pathways. While *in vitro* triggering of the intrinsic pathway via contact activation leads to thrombin generation, it does not play a significant *in vivo* role in physiologic hemostasis but may play a critical role in the pathogenesis of thrombosis.

Amplification

Thrombin is a potent platelet activator and further platelet activation occurs. The formation of FVIIIa and FVa allows formation of two platelet phospholipid-bound enzyme complexes which greatly enhance the ability of FXa and FIXa formed by the TF/FVIIa complex to produce thrombin. The FIXa/FVIIIa complex is known as the intrinsic Xase or tenase complex. The FXa/FVa complex is known as the IIase or prothrombinase complex. This phase is characterized by explosive prothrombin activation.

Propagation

The accumulated enzyme complexes (tenase complex and prothrombinase complex) on the platelet surface support robust amounts of thrombin generation and platelet activation. This ensures continuous generation of thrombin and subsequently conversion of fibrinogen to fibrin in order to form a sufficiently large clot.

Stabilization

Thrombin generation leads to activation of FXIII (fibrin stabilizing factor) which covalently links fibrin polymers and provides strength and stability to fibrin incorporated in the platelet plug. In addition, potent antifibrinolytic mechanisms are activated at this stage and are discussed in detail below.

Inhibition of Coagulation

The coagulation process is balanced by the presence of inhibitors of the coagulation process and by the regulated breakdown of fibrin clots (fibrinolysis) to prevent thrombosis. Protein C (PC) and protein S (PS) are vitamin K-dependent proteins. The activated form of PC (APC) has antithrombotic, profibrinolytic, antiinflammatory, and antiapoptotic activities. PS is a required cofactor for APC antithrombotic activities and may have antithrombotic activities independent of PC. PC is converted to its active form APC when thrombin binds to thrombomodulin (TM), a vascular endothelial protein with high concentrations in the microcirculation. Conversion of PC to APC is further enhanced by the endothelial protein C receptor (EPCR). APC in association with PS rapidly inactivates FVa and FVIIIa, the cofactors in the prothrombinase and tenase catalytic complexes respectively. The role of the coagulation inhibitor TFPI has been discussed previously. AT-III inactivates its physiologic target enzymes, thrombin, FXa, and FIXa with relatively low rate constants but this reaction is accelerated 2000–4000-fold in the presence of heparin.

Fibrinolysis

A summary of the fibrinolytic process is illustrated in Figure 5.3. Fibrinolysis is initiated when plasminogen is converted to plasmin. Plasmin is an endopeptidase that cleaves both fibrinogen and fibrin, degrading the fibrin meshwork into soluble fibrin degradation products (FDP) and exposing new carboxy-terminal (C-terminal) lysines at the fibrin surface. FDP do not have the ability to form clots. Plasminogen contains lysine-binding domains which allow it to bind to the lysine residues on fibrin. Fibrin-bound plasminogen is subsequently cleaved to plasmin by tissue plasminogen activator (tPA) and urokinase plasminogen activator (uPA). The endothelium produces tPA, and monocytes, macrophages, and fibroblasts produce uPA in response to fibrin formation. tPA also contains lysine-binding domains which allows binding to fibrin. Free tPA is

capable of converting fibrin-bound plasminogen to plasmin but tPA bound to fibrin lysine residues stimulates activation of plasminogen to plasmin by two orders of magnitude. APC promotes fibrinolysis by binding to and inhibiting the activity of plasminogen activator inhibitor 1 (PAI-1). Conversion of plasminogen to plasmin is also stimulated during contact activation via FXIIa and kallikrein. Plasmin in turn is a potent stimulator of multiple inflammation pathways.

To prevent hyperfibrinolysis, the formation and action of plasmin are negatively modulated. Fibrinolysis is inhibited by plasminogen activator inhibitors PAI-1 (released from activated platelets) and PAI-2 (released from monocytes and macrophages). PAI-1 and PAI-2 inhibit tPA uPA. Once activated via thrombin interaction with TM and directly by plasmin, thrombin-activatable fibrinolysis inhibitor (TAFI) cleaves carboxy terminal lysine residues from fibrin, thus rendering it incapable of binding to either plasminogen or tPA. Recall that the antifibrinolytic agents tranexamic acid (TXA) and epsilon-aminocaproic acid (Amicar®) are lysine analogs which competitively inhibit the binding of tPA and plasminogen to the lysine residues on fibrin. Finally, plasmin and thus fibrinolysis are directly inhibited by

Figure 5.3 The fibrinolytic pathway with activators of fibrinolysis indicated with blue arrows and inhibitors with red arrows. See text for details.

Table 5.1 Comparison of hemostatic factor concentrations and activities between neonates and adults.

	Procoagulant factors	Anticoagulant factors
Increased relative to adult	• Ultra-large WJF multimers • Plasminogen activator inhibitor (PAI)	• Alpha-2-macroglobulin
Decreased relative to adult	• Factors II, VII, IX, X • Platelet reactivity	• Proteins C and S • Antithrombin III (AT III) • Plasminogen • Plasminogen responsiveness • Tissue plasminogen activator (tPA) • Tissue factor pathway inhibitor (TFPI)

alpha-2-antiplasmin and alpha-2-macroglobulin. Alpha-2-antiplasmin is cross-linked into the fibrin network by FXIII and alpha-2-macroglobulin is a ubiquitous serine protease.

Special Considerations in Neonates and Infants

The hemostatic system of neonates and infants in the first six months of life is functionally balanced despite substantial differences in platelet function, fibrinogen and fibrin structure, and pro- and anticoagulant factor concentrations and activities compared to children and adults. These differences are summarized in Table 5.1. In addition, clots formed from adult fibrinogen display high fiber density, a large amount of fiber branching, and a three-dimensional structure. In contrast, clots formed from neonatal fibrinogen display predominantly aligned fibers with increased porosity and a sheet-like, two-dimensional structure. This structure renders neonatal fibrinogen more sensitive to fibrinolysis. Finally, neonatal platelets are hypo-reactive with a diminished aggregative response to all agonists compared to those of children and adults.

Cyanosis

Cyanosis and the accompanying secondary erythrocytosis are associated with poorly defined coagulation abnormalities, including reduced coagulation factor levels due to reduced plasma volume, thrombocytopenia, platelet aggregation abnormalities, and enhanced fibrinolysis.

Patient Blood Management

Patient blood management is rigorously defined as "a patient-centered, systematic, evidence-based approach to improve patient outcomes by managing and preserving a patient's own blood, while promoting patient safety and empowerment." The important components of blood management for pediatric cardiac surgery can be summarized as follows.

- Treatment of preoperative anemia and optimization of hemoglobin (Chapter 3).
- Preoperative screening for coagulation abnormalities in children with a bleeding history (Chapter 3).
- Optimization of CPB circuit size, use of ultrafiltration, optimization of circuit prime composition, acute normovolemic hemodilution (ANH) (Chapter 7).
- Anticoagulation monitoring and reversal (Chapter 7).
- Point-of-care (POC) hemostatic assays and post-CPB transfusion algorithms (Chapter 7).
  - Platelet and fibrinogen repletion.

- – Red cell repletion.
  - o CPB circuit red cell salvage.
  - o Red cell transfusion triggers
- – Rescue therapy for microvascular bleeding: recombinant FVIIa (rFVIIA) and 3 and 4 factor prothrombin complex concentrates (PCC), desmopressin.
- Use of antifibrinolytics (Chapter 7).

References and Further Reading

Negrier, C., Shima, M. & Hoffman, M. The central role of thrombin in bleeding disorders. *Blood Rev* **38**, 100582 (2019).

O'Donnell, J.S., O'Sullivan, J.M. & Preston, R.J.S. Advances in understanding the molecular mechanisms that maintain normal haemostasis. *Br J Haematol* **186**, 24–36 (2019).

6

Interpretation of Cardiac Catheterization Data

The ability to interpret cardiac catheterization data is essential to the cardiac anesthesiologist. Catheterization data provide information about congenital lesions, the location and quantification of intracardiac shunts, assessment of systolic and diastolic function, the extent and distribution of coronary artery abnormalities, and the type and extent of valvular lesions. This information contributes to the preoperative evaluation and serves as a predictor of postoperative functional status.

Right-Heart Catheterization

A fluid-filled catheter capable of making high-fidelity pressure measurements in the right atrium, right ventricle, and pulmonary artery is passed antegrade via a large vein under fluoroscopic guidance. In addition, the catheter may have the capability of making thermodilution cardiac output and mixed venous oxygen saturation measurements. Angiography is performed by recording several cardiac cycles on cine film while radiographic contrast material is injected into the right-heart chambers.

For infants and children, the femoral vein is the usual access site; however, right-heart catheterization via the umbilical vein may be possible in the first few days after birth. Internal jugular or subclavian access may also be used. Transhepatic access to the systemic venous circulation may be necessary in circumstances where the presence of thrombus or stenosis precludes cannulation of femoral, subclavian, or jugular veins.

Right Atrial Pressure (RAP) Waveform

The normal mean right atrial pressure is in the range of 3–6 mmHg. The normal waveform consists of 2–3 positive waveforms (A, C, V) and three negative waveforms (X, X′, Y) (Figure 6.1). The A wave reflects the atrial pressure increase seen during atrial systole, commonly called the atrial kick. The C wave reflects movement of the tricuspid or mitral valve annulus into the atrium during the isovolumic phase of ventricular systole and is often not well seen. The V wave represents passive atrial filling while the tricuspid and mitral valves are closed during ventricular systole. The X descent follows the A and C waves and reflects a combination of the downward displacement of the tricuspid and mitral with the onset of ventricular systole and atrial relaxation following atrial systole. The Y descent follows the V wave and reflects rapid atrial emptying after opening of the tricuspid and mitral valves.

Right Ventricular Pressure (RVP) Waveform

This consists of a rapid rise during isovolumic contraction, peak systolic pressure (typically at 20–30 mmHg), followed by a fall to a minimum diastolic pressure (Figure 6.2).

Figure 6.1 Left atrial pressure. Arrow shows the pacer spike. The paper speed is 50 mm/s. Noted are the A, C, and V waves as well as the X and Y descent. *Source:* Reproduced from DiNardo and Zvara (2008)/with permission of John Wiley & Sons.

Figure 6.2 Right ventricular pressure waveform (red) with aortic pressure waveform (blue).

Pulmonary Artery Pressure (PAP) Waveform

The peak systolic pressure is equal to or less than the RVP. The mean pressure is less than 20 mmHg (Figure 6.3).

Left-Heart Catheterization

A fluid-filled catheter capable of making high-fidelity systolic, diastolic, and mean pressure measurements and of allowing angiographic dye injection is used. The catheter may be passed retrograde via the axillary, brachial or femoral artery to the aortic root under fluoroscopic guidance, where pressures are recorded. In infants and children, the femoral artery is the preferred route. The umbilical artery is small and its course is tortuous so it is not useful except for pressure monitoring and angiography of the descending aorta. Left-heart catheterization can be performed antegrade via the right atrium in patients in whom the atrial septum can be crossed via a patent foramen ovale (PFO) or an atrial septal defect (ASD). This is a common approach in infants and children. In patients in whom the retrograde approach

Figure 6.3 Pulmonary arterial pressure waveform.

to the left ventricle is undesirable, and where an atrial or ventricular level communication does not exist, the atrial septum can be intentionally punctured to gain access to the left atrium using a Brockenbrough needle.

Pressures in the aorta, left ventricle, and left atrium are recorded. Aortography may be performed by recording on cine film the injection of radiographic contrast material into the aortic root. This will allow the detection of aortic regurgitation, congenital aortic arch abnormalities such as coarctation or aortic arch interruption, and acquired aortic lesions such as aortic dissection. Left atrial and ventricular angiography allows the detection of congenital anomalies.

Left Atrial Pressure (LAP) Waveform

The LAP is higher than the RAP and is in the range of 6–9 mmHg.

Left Ventricular Pressure (LVP) Waveform

The normal LVP varies with age and is affected by structural and hemodynamic factors. The peak systolic pressure is equal to the ascending aortic pressure. There is a progressive increase in left ventricular end-diastolic pressure (LVEDP) with age (Figure 6.4).

Aortic Pressure Waveform

The aortic pressure waveform includes a systolic rise, peak, and a dicrotic notch on the downstroke. A widened pulse pressure may result from aortic regurgitation, patent ductus arteriosus (PDA), surgical shunts, or aortopulmonary collaterals. An example of aortic pressure and left ventricular pressure waveform in a patient with aortic stenosis is shown in Figure 6.5.

Left Ventriculography

Left ventriculography is performed by recording several cardiac cycles on cine film as radiographic contrast material is injected into the mid left ventricle. The left ventriculogram allows detection of mitral regurgitation as well as a comparison of both regional and global wall motion in systole and diastole. It also allows calculation of the left ventricular end-diastolic volume (LVEDV) and left ventricular end-systolic volume (LVESV) with computer-assisted planimetry. Angiographic stroke volume (SV) is then defined as [LVEDV − LVESV]. The ejection fraction (EF) is defined as [LVEDV − LVESV)/LVEDV], which is [SV/LVEDV].

Figure 6.4 Left ventricular pressure waveform (blue) then moving to aortic pressure waveform.

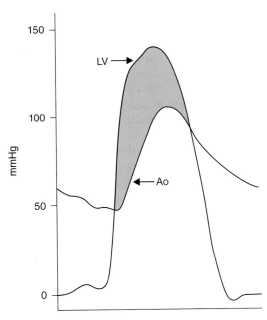

Figure 6.5 Left ventricular and aortic waveform in a patient with aortic stenosis. *Source:* Reproduced from DiNardo and Zvara (2008)/with permission of John Wiley & Sons.

The qualitative analysis of regional wall motion by left ventriculography is another index of systolic function. Left ventriculography is performed in the 30° right anterior oblique (RAO) projection and 60° left anterior oblique (LAO) projection. The ventricle is divided into segments (Figure 6.6) and a visual analysis of regional wall motion is made by comparison of end-diastolic and end-systolic cineangiograms. Five segments are generally analyzed in the RAO projection: anterobasal, anterolateral, apical, diaphragmatic (inferior), and posterobasal. Five segments also may be analyzed in the LAO projection: basal septal, apical septal, apical inferior, posterolateral, and superior lateral. These areas are graded qualitatively for wall motion. Normal areas exhibit a concentric inward movement in systole, while hypokinetic areas exhibit a reduced concentric inward motion in systole. Akinetic areas exhibit no motion with systole. Dyskinetic areas exhibit a paradoxical outward bulging with systole. Aneurysmal areas exhibit characteristic dilation with either hypokinesis or akinesis.

Areas of hypokinesis generally are composed of ischemic myocardium, whereas akinetic areas are composed of infarcted or hibernating myocardium. Improvements in wall motion occur in hypokinetic and akinetic areas when ischemic tissue has been

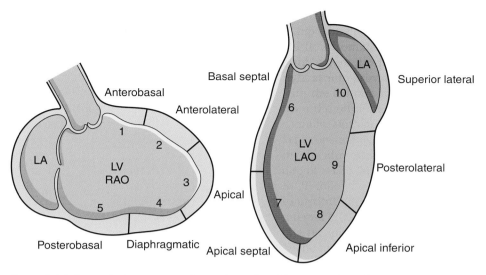

Figure 6.6 Left ventricular segments. *Source:* Reproduced from DiNardo and Zvara (2008)/with permission of John Wiley & Sons.

salvaged by revascularization or by pharmacologic interventions to improve perfusion. The presence of collaterals, the absence of surface ECG Q waves, and the presence of an associated proximal coronary stenosis less than 90% increase the likelihood that medical or surgical intervention will improve the wall motion abnormalities. Dyskinetic and aneurysmal areas, respectively, represent regions with little or no viable myocardium and rarely show improvement in wall motion with surgical or pharmacologic intervention.

Regional wall motion abnormalities are a more sensitive indicator of coronary blood flow insufficiency than is a reduction in a global ejection-phase index of systolic function such as ejection fraction (EF). This is because global systolic function can be maintained in the presence of regional dyssynergy by compensatory increases in wall shortening in areas of normal wall motion, as long as large areas of myocardium are not dyssynergic.

Coronary Angiography

Cine recordings of radiographic contrast material selectively injected into the coronary ostia are made. Special catheters are used for the selective catheterization of the ostia and are advanced under fluoroscopic guidance via the same artery used for left-heart catheterization.

Coronary angiography delineates the normal and pathologic features of the coronary circulation. Normally, angiography is performed in the 60° LAO projection and the 30° RAO projection, with caudal or cranial angulated views if necessary.

Coronary Anatomy

Determination of the areas of myocardium at risk with a particular stenotic or vasospastic lesion requires knowledge of the regional blood supply pattern. The right and left coronary anatomy is illustrated in Figures 6.7 and 6.8. Most patients (85%) have a right dominant system of coronary circulation, where the right coronary artery extends to the crux cordis in the atrioventricular groove and gives rise to the posterior descending branch, left atrial branch, atrioventricular (AV) nodal branch, and one or more posterior left ventricular branches. In a left dominant system (8%), these branches are supplied by the left circumflex artery and the right coronary artery supplies only the right atria

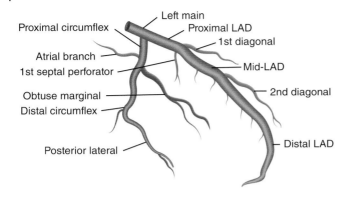

Figure 6.7 Left coronary anatomy. *Source:* Reproduced from DiNardo and Zvara (2008)/with permission of John Wiley & Sons.

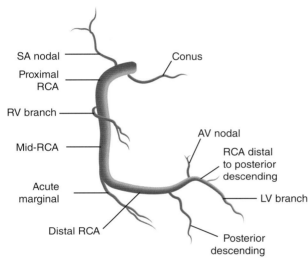

Figure 6.8 Right coronary anatomy. *Source:* Reproduced from DiNardo and Zvara (2008)/with permission of John Wiley & Sons.

and ventricle. In 7% of patients, the system is balanced, with the right coronary artery supplying the posterior descending, left atria, and AV nodal branches, whereas the left circumflex artery supplies the posterior left ventricular branches.

There is variation in the blood supply to various regions of myocardium, but some generalizations can be made (Table 6.1).

Anatomic Coronary Lesions

Coronary stenotic lesions are quantitated visually from moving cineangiograms in several projections. Stenotic areas of the artery are compared with adjacent normal areas, and the percentage reduction in lumen diameter caused by the stenosis is quantified. Thus, a 90% lesion refers to a stenosis that causes a 90% reduction in lumen diameter. It is generally acknowledged that resting coronary blood flow does not decrease until there is an 85% reduction in lumen diameter. This corresponds to a greater than 90% reduction in lumen cross-sectional area. By contrast, a 50% diameter reduction corresponds to a 75% reduction in cross-sectional area. Maximal coronary flow in response to a stimulus for vasodilation is blunted when there is a 30–45% reduction in lumen diameter and is absent when the lumen diameter is reduced by 90%. Interobserver variability exists in the grading of stenotic lesions. In addition, coronary angiography typically underestimates the severity of stenotic lesions and may not accurately predict the physiologic significance of a particular lesion.

Table 6.1 Summary of coronary arterial supply.

1) Anterobasal – LMCA; proximal LAD; 1st diagonal
2) Anterolateral – LMCA; proximal or mid-LAD; 1st diagonal
3) Apical – LMCA; proximal, mid, or distal LAD; 2nd diagonal
4) Diaphragmatic (inferior) – proximal, mid, or distal RCA; PDA
5) Posterobasal – proximal, mid, or distal RCA; PDA
6) Basal septal – LMCA; proximal or mid-LAD, 1st septal
7) Apical septal – LMCA; proximal, mid, or distal LAD
8) Apical inferior – proximal, mid, or distal RCA
9) Posterolateral – LMCA; proximal or distal CIRC marginals
10) Superior lateral – LMCA; proximal CIRC marginals

LMCA, left main coronary artery; LAD, left anterior descending artery; CIRC, circumflex artery; RCA, right coronary artery; PDA, posterior descending artery.

More recently, intravascular ultrasound (IVUS) has been used to assess the function, morphology, and flow of the coronary circulation.

Coronary Collaterals

An extensive network of coronary collaterals is normally present at birth, but these collaterals are not demonstrable by angiography in normal hearts due to their small diameter. It is only when the collateral channels enlarge secondary to regional myocardial oxygen deprivation that they are visible angiographically. The development of collateral pathways in patients with comparable degrees of coronary insufficiency is variable in both extent and time course. The presence of collaterals has been identified as a determinant of reversible wall motion abnormalities. Left ventricular function in the region of an occluded coronary artery is better maintained in the presence of collaterals than in their absence.

Cardiac Output Determination

Two complementary methods are used to determine cardiac output, namely the thermodilution technique and the Fick determination. Both methods measure forward cardiac outputs. Forward cardiac output and total cardiac output are equal only if there are no regurgitant lesions or shunt fractions.

Thermodilution Technique

Thermodilution cardiac output is a modification of the indicator dilution method, in which flow is determined from the following relationship:

$$\frac{Known\ amount\ of\ indicator\ injected}{Measured\ concentration\ of\ indicator} \times time$$

In the thermodilution method, cold water is the indicator.

Fick Determination

The Fick determination is based on the relationship:

$$O_2\ consumption(mlO_2/min)/(arterial - venous\ O_2\ content)(\%mlO_2/dl) \times 10$$

The factor 10 allows conversion of dl to liters since the Hb is measured in g dl^{-1}.

An estimate of VO$_2$ is commonly obtained from LaFarge tables that relate VO$_2$ to body surface area or to heart rate and age. Arterial-venous O$_2$ content difference (A-VO$_2$ difference) is calculated from the difference between the arterial and mixed venous O$_2$ contents where:

$$Content = (O_2\ saturation\ of\ arterial\ or\ mixed\ venous\ blood \times Hb\ concentration \times (1.38)) + (0.003 \times PO_2\ of\ arterial\ or\ mixed\ venous\ blood)$$

This method measures systemic blood flow, which equals forward left heart output. It also can be used to measure pulmonary blood flow or forward right heart output, when O_2 consumption is divided by pulmonary arterial content subtracted from pulmonary venous content. The method is most accurate at low cardiac outputs, where the arterial to venous O_2 difference is great. It is accurate in the presence of intracardiac shunts when the mixed venous O_2 content and pulmonary venous O_2 content are properly determined.

$$Indexed\ systemic\ flow\ (Q_s) = \frac{O_2\ consumption}{systemic\ arterial\ O_2\ content - mixed\ venous\ O_2\ content}$$

$$Indexed\ pulmonary\ flow\ (Q_p) = \frac{O_2\ consumption}{pulmonary\ venous\ O_2\ content - pulmonary\ arterial\ O_2\ content}$$

It is customary to obtain blood samples for baseline calculations while the patient is receiving either room air or minimal supplemental oxygen. This is done both to simplify the calculations and to avoid complicating measurement of PVR in patients who have PVR that may be responsive to supplemental oxygen. The use of room air or minimal supplemental oxygen allows the dissolved oxygen component ($0.003 \times PO_2$ of arterial or mixed venous blood) of the content equation to be ignored. In pediatric patients, O_2 consumption is normally indexed to body surface area (BSA) measured in square meters (m^2).

Evaluation of Cardiac Shunts

A comprehensive discussion of the physiology of shunts is provided in Chapter 2. Oxygen saturation measurements in multiple cardiac chambers and the great vessels are used to localize and quantify cardiac shunts. Additionally, angiography during cardiac catheterization may be used to locate cardiac shunts.

Shunt Location

Shunt localization is usually accomplished using a combination of angiography and measurement of O_2 saturations in the pulmonary veins, superior vena cava (SVC) and inferior vena cava (IVC), right-heart chambers, left-heart chambers, aorta, and pulmonary artery. Oxygen saturation sampling is used to detect O_2 saturation step-up in the right heart in the case of a left-to-right (L-R) shunt or O_2 saturation step-down in the left heart in the case of a right-to-left (R-L) shunt. A step-up is defined as an increase in the O_2 saturation of blood in a particular location that exceeds the normal variability in that location, whereas a step-down is a greater than expected decrease in saturation for a given location.

Shunt Quantification

Shunt quantification is based on comparison of systemic and pulmonary blood flows. Systemic (Q_S) and pulmonary (Q_P) blood flows are calculated by the Fick method previously described:

$$Q_P = VO_2 / (PV\ O_2\ content - PA\ O_2\ content)$$

where PA O_2 content is the pulmonary arterial O_2 content and PV O_2 content is the pulmonary venous O_2 content. Sampling blood from the left atrium (when the pulmonary veins return to the left atrium) will provide a weighted average of the four pulmonary veins' O_2 content. If a R-L atrial level shunt is present, this sampling site will not provide an accurate assessment of pulmonary vein O_2 content. Each of the four pulmonary veins can be entered and sampled separately. When this is done, segmental areas of intrapulmonary shunt and V/Q mismatch can be detected. The PaO_2 or saturation of pulmonary venous blood from a lung segment with V/Q mismatch will improve with an increase in FiO_2, while there will be little or no improvement if an intrapulmonary shunt is present.

$$Q_S = VO_2 / (SVO_2 \ content - MAO_2 \ content)$$

where SA O_2 is the systemic arterial O_2 content and MV O_2 content is the mixed venous O_2 content. True mixed venous blood is a mixture of desaturated blood from the IVC, SVC, and coronary sinus. In a normal heart, a mixed sample of venous blood from these three locations can be obtained from the pulmonary artery. In the presence of an intracardiac L-R shunt, PA O_2 saturation will overestimate true MV O_2 saturation because the pulmonary arterial blood will be a mixture of mixed venous blood and oxygenated pulmonary venous blood from the left heart. In this setting, true mixed venous saturation must be determined from samples taken from the SVC and IVC. If the very low-O_2 content, low-volume blood from the coronary sinus is ignored, then a weighted average of O_2 content of SVC and IVC blood can be used to determine MV O_2 content:

$$(3/4 \times superior \ vena \ cava \ O_2 \ content)$$
$$+(1/4 \times inferior \ vena \ cava \ O_2 \ content)$$

This formula may be used to determine MV O_2 in the catheterization laboratory when L-R shunts exist. More commonly, and particularly in children, the SVC O_2 content is used as a surrogate for MV O_2 content. SVC blood has a lower O_2 content than IVC blood and a higher content than coronary sinus blood; thus, SVC blood provides a very close estimate of the mixture of the three samples. In addition, streaming of blood of varying O_2 contents in the IVC hampers accurate IVC O_2 content sampling.

After Q_P and Q_S have been calculated, shunts can be quantified. For an isolated L-R shunt, the magnitude of the shunt is $[Q_P - Q_S]$. For an isolated R-L shunt, the magnitude of the shunt is $[Q_S - Q_P]$. The ratio $Q_P:Q_S$ is also useful, and can be calculated from content data alone because the VO_2 terms cancel out:

$$Q_P : Q_S = \frac{(SAO_2 \ content - MVO_2 \ content)}{(PVO_2 \ content - PAO_2 \ content)}$$

Furthermore, if the blood is sampled while the patient is receiving either room air or a low FiO_2, the dissolved O_2 portion of the content equation ($PO_2 \times 0.003$) can be ignored. The hemoglobin $\times 1.34$ term cancels out and the equation can be simplified to one using just saturation data from the four sites, as listed above.

A $Q_P:Q_S > 2.0$ constitutes a large shunt, whereas a $Q_P:Q_S < 1.25–1.5$ constitutes a small shunt. Obviously, a $Q_P:Q_S < 1.0$ indicates a net R-L shunt.

For bidirectional shunts, it is necessary to calculate effective pulmonary blood flow (Q_{Peff})

Some important points to remember

1) If no shunts, mixed venous is equal to the PA saturation.
2) If intracardiac shunt, mixed venous saturation is the SVC saturation.
3) In the absence of lung disease, pulmonary venous saturation is 97–100%.

4) The dissolved O_2 is neglected at room air with $FiO_2 = 21\%$ but should be taken into account when supplemental O_2 is provided.

and effective systemic blood flow (Q_{Seff}). Q_{Peff} is the quantity of desaturated systemic venous blood that traverses the pulmonary capillaries to be oxygenated. Q_{Seff} is the quantity of oxygenated pulmonary venous blood that traverses the systemic capillaries to deliver oxygen to tissue. Q_{Seff} and Q_{Peff} are always equal.

$$Q_{Seff} = Q_{Peff} = VO_2 / $$
$$(PVO_2 \; content - MVO_2 \; content)$$

The L-R shunt is defined as $[Q_P - Q_{Peff}]$, while the R-L shunt is defined as $[Q_S - Q_{Seff}]$. The net shunt is the difference between these two calculated shunts.

Saturation Data

The oxygen saturations (%) of blood in the low SVC, the main pulmonary artery, and the aorta are obtained to screen for intracardiac shunts. If an intracardiac shunt is suspected, multiple samples from locations in the great vessels and cardiac chambers are necessary to localize the shunt and determine its magnitude and direction.

Resistances

Systemic and pulmonary vascular resistances are determined using hemodynamic, cardiac output and cardiac index data. Data and formulas are summarized in Table 6.2.

- Systemic vascular resistance (SVR).
- Systemic vascular resistance index (SVRI).
- Pulmonary vascular resistance (PVR)
- Pulmonary vascular resistance index (PVRI)
- Transpulmonary gradient (TPG).
- Mean arterial blood pressure (MAP).
- Mean pulmonary artery pressure (mPAP).
- Pulmonary artery occlusion pressure (PAOP).
- Central venous pressure (CVP).
- Cardiac output (CO).
- Cardiac index (CI).

Assessment of Pulmonary Vascular Anatomy

For infants and children with CHD, special procedures may be necessary to assess the pulmonary vasculature and the extent of pulmonary vascular disease (e.g., oxygen and NO administration).

Evaluation of the Pulmonary Vasculature

Marked increases or decreases in pulmonary blood flow routinely occur in patients with CHD. Pulmonary vascular disease may occur as a consequence of increased pulmonary blood flow in patients with CHD and will

Table 6.2 Formulas and normal values.

$SVR = \dfrac{(MAP - CVP)\,80}{CO}$	700–1600 dynes s cm^{-5} 9–20 Wood units
$PVR = \dfrac{(mPAP - PAOP)\,80}{CO}$	20–130 dynes s cm^{-5} 0.25–1.6 Wood units
TPG = mPAP − PAOP CI = CO/BSA	5–10 mmHg 2.5–4 l min^{-1} m^{-2}
$SVRI = \dfrac{(MAP - CVP)\,80}{CI}$	2000–2400 dynes s cm^{-5} m^{-2} 25–30 Wood units
$PVRI = \dfrac{(mPAP - PAOP)\,80}{CI}$	250–280 dynes s cm^{-5} m^{-2} 3.1–9.5 Wood units

influence the type of corrective or palliative operative procedure performed.

Pulmonary Artery Wedge Angiogram

The pulmonary artery wedge angiogram is recorded on cine film while radiocontrast material is injected into a catheter that is in the pulmonary artery wedge position. Generally, the artery to the posterior basal segment of the right lower lobe is studied. As obstructive pulmonary vascular disease progresses, the wedge angiogram demonstrates progressive increases in the diameter and tortuosity of the pulmonary arteries, a diminution in the blush seen as capillaries fill, and the abrupt termination of dilated, tortuous arteries with a marked decrease in the number of supernumerary arterial branches.

The pulmonary capillary wedge pressure is similar to a left atrial pressure waveform, with a time delay unless there is pulmonary vein stenosis or collaterals.

Pulmonary Vein Wedge Angiogram

In many congenital cardiac lesions with reduced pulmonary blood flow, the pulmonary vasculature may be well visualized with the injection of contrast into collaterals that arise off the aorta. For patients with pulmonary atresia, pulmonary blood flow is markedly diminished and the pulmonary arteries may not be well visualized with contrast injections into collateral vessels. In this instance, the pulmonary vein wedge angiogram may be used to delineate the pulmonary vasculature. Retrograde filling of the parenchymal pulmonary vessels can be seen on cine recordings when contrast is hand-injected into a catheter wedged in a pulmonary vein. When antegrade pulmonary blood flow is severely diminished, retrograde filling of even the main pulmonary artery can occur.

Assessment of Pulmonary Hypertension (PH)

Pulmonary hypertension (PH) may occur as the result of congenital heart lesions. PH is defined as a mean pulmonary artery pressure (mPAP) ≥20 mmHg at rest. The stimulus for the development of PH in CHD is exposure of the pulmonary vascular system (both *in utero* and after birth) to abnormal pressure and flow patterns.

Pulmonary hypertension can be considered to have a precapillary cause, a postcapillary cause (pulmonary venous hypertension), or a combination of both. Precapillary PH is also known as pulmonary arterial hypertension (PAH), and is defined as mPAP ≥20 mmHg at rest, pulmonary artery wedge pressure (PAWP) ≤15 mmHg, and a pulmonary vascular resistance index (PVRI) >3 Wood units m^{-2} for biventricular circulations. Following cavopulmonary anastomosis (Fontan procedure), the definition is a PVRI >3 Wood units m^{-2} or a transpulmonary gradient >6 mmHg, even in the presence of mPAP ≤20 mmHg. Postcapillary PH is most commonly due to left heart disease and is defined as mPAP ≥20 mmHg at rest in conjunction with PAWP ≥15 mmHg. Postcapillary causes are characteristically associated with interstitial pulmonary edema. Children with longstanding postcapillary PH, such as those with pulmonary vein stenosis, develop a component of precapillary PH (PAH) due to reactive pulmonary artery vasoconstriction.

A comprehensive evaluation of PH at the time of cardiac catheterization must include evaluation of the following potential causes.

- *Left atrial hypertension*: an elevated LAP can result from a number of causes (mitral valve disease, LV diastolic dysfunction, LV systolic dysfunction, loss of AV synchrony). This is by far the most common cause of elevated PAP in adults with acquired heart disease.
- *Pulmonary venous obstruction*: this may be the result of obstruction to pulmonary vein entry into the venous circulation, such as total anomalous pulmonary venous return, cor triatriatum, or the result of obstructive disease inherent to the veins themselves.
- *Pulmonary vascular disease*: chronic exposure of the pulmonary arterial bed to high flow and/or pressure leads to extensive

structural changes. There is progressive muscularization of peripheral arteries, medial hypertrophy of muscular arteries, and a gradually reduced arterial number due to occlusive neointimal formation with fibrosis. Chronic left atrial hypertension can lead to the development of a similar process through the chronic elevation of PAP.

- *High Q_P:Q_S*: when a large nonrestrictive intracardiac communication exists, particularly at the ventricular level, the PAP may be systemic or just subsystemic. The question that must be answered is whether the elevated PAP is due to high flow into a low-resistance pulmonary bed (high Q_P:Q_S, normal PVR, large L-R shunt) or normal/low flow into a high-resistance pulmonary bed (normal/low Q_P:Q_S, high PVR, pulmonary vascular disease).

Determination of the etiology of pulmonary hypertension requires measurement of the PAP, LAP, pulmonary artery occlusion pressure (PAOP), transpulmonary gradient (TPG), and pulmonary vascular resistance (PVR), as summarized in Table 6.3.

Nitric oxide (NO) and oxygen trials are conducted after baseline cardiac index,

Q_p:Q_s, and PVR determinations are obtained. After 100% oxygen administration, all measurements are repeated and PVR is calculated. After 10 min of 100% oxygen and NO (20–80 ppm), all measurements are repeated and PVR is recalculated.

Assessment of Valve Lesions

The impressive technologic advances in Doppler echocardiography and magnetic resonance cardiac imaging now allow the noninvasive assessment of valvular pathology. Evaluation via cardiac catheterization, however, provides important information. Analysis of the pressure data from right- and left-heart catheterization, combined with an analysis of ventriculography and aortography data, will delineate the extent and nature of valvular lesions.

Stenotic Lesions

The analysis of stenotic valve lesions is based on obtaining a valve orifice area from flow and pressure-gradient data. Valve areas commonly are normalized for body surface area in infants and children.

Table 6.3 Characteristic findings in pulmonary hypertension from different etiologies.

Etiology	Pressures	LAP	TPG	PVR	Q_P
LA hypertension	PAD ≈ PAOP ≈ LAP (acute)	⇑⇑	⇔	⇔	⇔
	PAD > PAOP ≈ LAP (chronic)	⇑⇑	⇑	⇑	⇔
Pulmonary vein obstruction	PAD ≈ PAOP ≫ LAP	⇔	⇑⇑	⇑⇑	⇔ sl ⇓
Pulmonary vascular disease	PAD ≫ PAOP ≈ LAP	⇔	⇑⇑	⇑⇑	⇔ sl ⇓
Large L-R shunt	PAD ≈ PAOP ≈ LAP	sl⇑	⇔ sl ⇑	⇔ sl ⇑	⇑⇑

LAP, left atrial pressure; PAD, pulmonary artery diastolic pressure; TPG, transpulmonary gradient (mPAP-LAP; normal 5–10 mmHg); PVR, pulmonary vascular resistance (TPG/cardiac output; normal <2 Wood units); PAOP, pulmonary artery occlusion pressure; Q_P, pulmonary blood flow.

Regurgitant Lesions

The quantification of regurgitant lesions with catheterization techniques is more difficult and less accurate than for stenotic lesions. Two approaches are available: one method is qualitative and the other is quantitative. Qualitative analysis is based on assessing the amount of contrast material regurgitated into the left atrium during left ventriculography for mitral regurgitation, or into the left ventricle during aortography for aortic regurgitation.

The degree of regurgitation is graded from mild to severe (1+ to 4+). In mild aortic regurgitation, a small amount of contrast enters the left ventricle during diastole but clears with each systole. In mild mitral regurgitation, a small amount of contrast enters the left atrium during systole but clears in diastole. In severe aortic regurgitation, the left ventricle is filled with contrast after the first diastole and remains opacified for several systoles. In severe mitral regurgitation, the left atrium is filled with contrast after the first systole and becomes progressively opacified with each beat. In addition, contrast is seen refluxing into the pulmonary veins. Similar qualitative analysis is used to grade tricuspid regurgitation.

The quantitative method of assessing regurgitation is based on calculation of the regurgitant fraction:

$$Regurgitant\ fraction = \frac{regurgitant\ stroke\ volume}{total\ stroke\ volume}$$

$$Regurgitant\ stroke\ volume = total\ stroke\ volume - forward\ stroke\ volume$$

References and Further Reading

DiNardo, J.A. & Zvara, D.A. *Anesthesia for Cardiac Surgery*, 3rd edn. Blackwell, Massachusetts (2008).

Joffe, D.C., Shi, M.R. & Welker, C.C. Understanding cardiac shunts. *Paediatr Anaesth* **110**, 799 (2018).

7

Management of Cardiopulmonary Bypass

The Cardiopulmonary Bypass Circuit

The cardiopulmonary bypass (CPB) circuit (Figure 7.1) is intended to isolate the cardiopulmonary system so that optimal surgical exposure can be obtained for operations on the heart and great vessels. In order for this isolation to be effective, the CPB circuit must:

- perform the functions of the intact cardiopulmonary system
- be capable of adding oxygen and removing carbon dioxide from blood
- provide adequate perfusion of all organs with this blood
- fulfill all of these requirements without causing permanent damage to the cardiopulmonary system, the blood, or any of the patient's end organs.

During CPB, blood is drained from the patient via one or more venous cannulas, primarily by gravity and a siphon effect. The effectiveness of gravity drainage is dependent on venous cannula size, the relative height of the patient above the venous reservoir, the length and diameters of the venous tubing, the maintenance of a continuous fluid column, the characteristics of the venous reservoir, and patient volume status. Venous cannulas are typically placed in the superior vena cava (SVC) and inferior vena cava (IVC) (two cannulas) or in the right atrium (single cannula). An active process (vacuum-assisted

venous drainage or kinetic-assisted venous drainage) can be used, recognizing that there may be an increased risk of air entrainment in the venous line.

Despite adequate venous drainage on CPB, blood return to the left ventricle may occur from a number of sources. Thebesian vein blood (veins in the walls of all four heart chambers that drain the myocardium) drains to the left atrium/ventricle. This flow will cease when the aortic cross-clamp terminates coronary blood flow. Bronchial vein blood drains to the pulmonary veins. The bronchial circulation may be very large in patients with cyanotic heart disease.

With extracardiac left-to-right (L-R) shunts, a large portion of pulmonary blood flow may be supplied by anatomic (patent ductus arteriosus [PDA], aortopulmonary collaterals) or surgical systemic-to-pulmonary artery communications (Blalock–Thomas–Taussig, Waterston, Potts, central shunts). If these communications are not ligated or controlled before the institution of CPB, the blood return to the pulmonary artery – and subsequently to the left atrium and left ventricle – may be very large. Flow return to the left ventricle may also result from an incompetent aortic valve. In this instance, retrograde filling of the left ventricle with blood from the aortic cannula will occur until the aortic cross-clamp is applied. To prevent left ventricular distention, which causes myocardial damage and compromises subendocardial blood flow, the left atrium must be

The Pediatric Cardiac Anesthesia Handbook, Second Edition. Viviane G. Nasr and James A. DiNardo.
© 2025 John Wiley & Sons Ltd. Published 2025 by John Wiley & Sons Ltd.

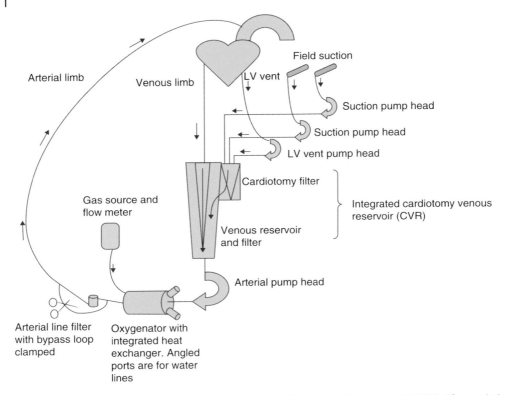

Figure 7.1 A simplified diagram of the CPB circuit. *Source:* Reproduced from Matte (2015)/with permission of John Wiley & Sons.

opened or a left ventricular vent catheter placed. The junction of the left atrium and right superior pulmonary vein provides relatively easy access to the left atrium. The vent can then be easily placed across the mitral valve into the left ventricle.

Cardiotomy suction is used to scavenge blood from the surgical field and improve exposure. Most systems utilize a roller head pump to provide the suction. This is an important source of blood conservation because such blood is returned to the venous reservoir after passing through a screen filter to remove particulate contaminants from the surgical field. In order to avoid clotting the CPB circuit, the patient must be heparinized prior to using cardiotomy suction during cannula placement, before the initiation of CPB.

From the venous reservoir, blood is transported via a pump to the oxygenator and heat exchanger unit. The pump can either be a roller pump or a centrifugal pump. Most pediatric perfusion practices use roller heads for their arterial pumps, since in modern heart-lung machines such pumps have the advantage of very low primes, as it is common for the arterial head to be positioned close to the venous reservoir and oxygenator. The oxygenator serves as the artificial lung and allows gas exchange (oxygen, carbon dioxide) via either a solid or microporous membrane. Only membrane oxygenators, which can be classified as either microporous or true membrane, are currently used in the care of pediatric cardiac surgical patients. Integral to the oxygenator is the heat exchanger, which employs countercurrent heat exchange to cool or warm the blood. The temperature-adjusted, oxygenated blood is then transported through an arterial line filter, the role of which is to reduce the delivery of microemboli into the arterial circulation.

From the arterial filter, the blood reaches the patient's circulation via the arterial cannula. The arterial cannula is typically placed into the ascending aortic arch, but alternative placement sites include the femoral artery and the subclavian artery.

Differences Between Adult and Pediatric CPB

Differences between adult and pediatric CPB systems are outlined in Table 7.1. It is not uncommon for a pediatric perfusion group to utilize 3–5 different-sized oxygenators, along with four or five different custom tubing packs. This array of equipment is required in order to appropriately size major circuit components to a wide range of patients.

CPB Flow Rates

Once proper arterial inflow and venous drainage are assured, the CPB parameters are adjusted to achieve target flow rates, temperature, and acid–base status.

Flow rates during CPB are chosen to provide systemic oxygen delivery. Systemic hypothermia is routinely employed during pediatric CPB, with many operations performed at temperatures of 28–32 °C. Systemic hypothermia reduces whole-body and cerebral oxygen consumption by 5–6% for each 1 °C decrease in body temperature. Flows of $1.8–2.5 \text{ l min}^{-1} \text{ m}^{-2}$ are commonly used for infants, children, and adults during mild to moderate systemic hypothermia. Due to age-related differences in the relationship of weight to body surface area, when these flow rates are expressed in ml $\text{kg}^{-1} \text{ min}^{-1}$ they will be substantially higher in the neonate than in the adult (Table 7.2). Low-flow CPB in neonates and infants is conducted at temperatures of 18–22 °C and flow rates of 50–75 ml $\text{kg}^{-1} \text{ min}^{-1}$ or approximately 0.7–1.2 l min m^{-2} (Table 7.3).

Circuit Size and Component Selection

The selection of the components of a pediatric CPB circuit is a sophisticated process which takes into consideration the size of the patient (generally age and weight specific), the anticipated flow rates for blood and fresh

Table 7.1 Differences between adult and pediatric cardiopulmonary bypass systems.

	Adult	Pediatric
Estimated blood volume	65 ml kg^{-1}	<10 kg: 85 ml kg^{-1}
Dilution effects on blood volume	25–33%	Up to 100–200%
Addition of whole blood or packed red blood cells to prime	Rarely	Usually
Oxygen consumption	2–3 ml $\text{kg}^{-1} \text{ min}^{-1}$	6–8 ml $\text{kg}^{-1} \text{ min}^{-1}$
Full CPB flow at 37 °C	50–75 ml $\text{kg}^{-1} \text{ min}^{-1}$	150–200 ml $\text{kg}^{-1} \text{ min}^{-1}$
Minimum CPB temperature	Rarely <30 °C	Commonly <30 °C
Use of total circulatory arrest or regional cerebral perfusion	Rare	Common for some defects: HLHS, hypoplastic aortic arch
Perfusion pressure	50–80 mmHg	30–50 mmHg
Acid–base management	Primarily alpha-stat	Primarily pH-stat ≤30 °C
Measured PaCO$_2$ differences	30–45 mmHg	20–80 mmHg

HLHS, hypoplastic left heart syndrome.

Table 7.2 Full cardiopulmonary bypass flow rates relative to patient weight.

Patient weight (kg)	Full CPB flow rates (ml kg^{-1} min^{-1})
<3	150–200
3–10	125–175
10–15	120–150
15–30	100–120
30–50	75–100
>50	50–75

Table 7.3 Cardiopulmonary bypass flow rate relative to patient temperature.

Patient temperature (°C)	Flow rate (l min^{-1} m^{-2})
≥35	≥2.5
32	2.2
30	2.0
28	1.8
26	1.6
24	1.4
22	1.2
20	1.0
18	0.7

Source: Reproduced from DiNardo et al. (2015)/with permission of Wolters Kluwer Health.

gas during CPB, and the capacity of the heat exchanger. The final circuit configuration untimately determines the circuit prime volume as discussed below. **Figure 7.2** is a detailed summary of the circuit components utilized to optimally match circuit size to patient size and anticipated flow rates.

Anesthesia During CPB

The perfusionist can be provided with doses of sedatives, analgesics, and muscle relaxants by the anesthesiologist. However, it should be kept in mind that there is substantial absorption of fentanyl and midazolam by the components of the CPB circuit. Some centers deliver volatile anesthetics to the patient during CPB via fresh gas flow to the membrane oxygenator.

Monitoring During CPB

Standard monitors during CPB include:

- standard ASA monitors (ECG, temperature, blood pressure, pulse oximetry, capnography):
  - 12-lead ECG
  - two temperature sites: nasopharyngeal/oropharyngeal or esophageal AND rectal.
- intraarterial catheter (mean arterial pressure; MAP)
- central venous pressure (CVP); an increase in CVP should raise concern for venous cannula malposition
- urine output.

Near-infra-red spectroscopy (NIRS) and/or transcranial Doppler are utilized by many, but not all, centers.

Hemodilution

Due to their small blood volumes and the need for the CPB circuit to be primed, pediatric patients potentially experience more hemodilution than their adult counterparts. For example, a 70 kg adult has an estimated blood volume of 5250 ml (70 kg × 75 ml kg^{-1}). Using a CPB circuit with a 1-liter prime volume results in 20% hemodilution.

In contrast, a 3 kg neonate has an estimated blood volume of 255 ml (85 kg × 3 ml kg^{-1}). Consequently, using a CPB circuit with a 400 ml prime volume will result in 160% hemodilution. Optimal miniaturization of the circuit size as discussed previously is a key component of blood management.

Priming Solution

For adults, a crystalloid prime is typically used. In children, in order to mitigate the anemia caused by hemodilution, red cell

					Pack (AV Loop)	Boot	BSA for 3.0	BSA for 3.6	Prime Volume
FX 05 43ml (75R)	Max Flow per IFU (oxy/CR) 1500/1500	Defoamer = ≥500 ml	ALF 32u VF 47u	HFMO 0.5 m² HE 0.035 m²	Infant 3/16×1/4) Boot to 1200	3/16"	≤0.4	≤0.33	215
Q range	0.1–1.5 LPM MOV=15	**V range**	0.05–5 LPM	5 LPM only for 10s in an emergency	Infant (3/16×1/4) Venous line to 1410	1/4"	0.41–0.47	0.34–0.39	230
D101 87ml (100R)	Max Flow per IFU (oxy/CR) 2500 / NS	Defoamer = entire filter medium	D131 ALF 40u VF 51u 28ml	HFMO 0.61 m² HE 0.06 m²	Child (1/4×3/8) CVR to 2100	1/4"	0.48–0.70	0.40–0.50	400
Q range	Up to 2.5LPM MOV = 30	**V range**	Up to 5 LPM, max 2:1 VQ	Max VQ 4:1 for ≤10 min in an emergency	[Toddler Pack set up on standby]				
FX 15–30 144ml (175R)	Max Flow per IFU (oxy/CR) 5000/4000	Defoamer = ≥2000 ml	ALF 32u VF 47u	HFMO 1.5 m² HE 0.14 m²	Child (1/4×3/8) 1/4 boot to 2100	1/4"	0.48–0.70	0.51–0.58	530
Q range	0.5–5 LPM MOV = 70	**V range**	0.5–15 LPM	15 LPM only for 10s in an emergency	Child (1/4×3/8) 1/4 arterial to 3150	3/8"	0.71–1.05	0.59–0.87 (+/– MUF)	570
					Adult (3/8×1/2) GSD to 3200	3/8"	1.06–1.2	0.87–0.89	660
3.0 C.I. Cases ASD, VSD, AS, PS, TOF, CAVC, BDG, ALCAPA, IAA, AP window, Heart Tx, Lung Tx, Ebstein's, MVR, PVR, TVR, T/PAPVR, PVS, Truncus, D-TGA			**3.6 C.I. Cases** Fontan, APCs, L-TGA, Stage 1, Significant AI, BiV, Anticipated long CPB run		Adult (3/8×1/2) 3/8 boot to 4.4	3/8" KVAD	1.21–1.46	0.90–1.22	730
					Adult (3/8×1/2) HFMO to 5000	1/2" KVAD	1.47–1.66	1.23–1.39	760
FX 25 260ml (250R)	Max Flow per IFU (oxy/CR) 7000/5000	Defoamer = ≥2500 ml	ALF 32u VF 47u	HFMO 2.5 m² HE 0.2 m²	Adult (3/8×1/2)	1/2" KVAD	≥1.67	≥1.4	950
0.48–0.70	0.5–7 LPM MOV = 150	**V range**	0.5–20 LPM	20 LPM only for 10s in an emergency					

Max Flows (ml/min) (max RPM 162)
3/16" boot 1200, arterial 1500
1/4" boot 2100, arterial 3150, venous 1410
3/8" boot 4400, arterial >3150, venous 3750

1/4 LHB 10' = 150 ml, 3/8 LHB 10'= 270 ml

SMUF Circuit Volume = 55/70 ml

Figure 7.2 A comprehensive summary of the various circuit CPB configurations available across patient sizes to accommodate the different CPB flows required for various procedure types (cardiac index of 3.0 or 3.6 liters per minute [LPM]). In the PACK column the first line is the arterial and venous line diameter tubing sizes while the second line indicates which component determines the maximal flow rate, in LPM, of the circuit. This is further clarified in the lower left corner where max RPM 162 is the maximum revolutions per minute (162) for the occlusive roller pump head. Below this, for each of the three sizes (3/16, ¼, 3/8 inches diameter), the limitation to flow in LPM imposed by each component (boot, arterial line, venous line) is summarized. The boot is the portion of the arterial venous loop that resides within the occlusive roller head of the pump. V, sweep gas flow rate; Q, blood flow rate; LPM, liters per minute; MOV, minimal operating volume; IFU, information for use; oxy/CR, oxygenator/cardiotomy reservoir; ALF, arterial line filter pore size; VF, venous filter pore size; BSA, body surface area; C.I., cardiac index; HFMO, hollow fiber membrane oxygenator surface area; HE, heat exchanger surface area; CVR, cardiotomy venous reservoir; KVAD, kinetic venous active drainage; GSD, gravity siphon drainage; MUF, modified ultrafiltration; SMUF, simplified modified ultrafiltration circuit volumes; LHB, left heart bypass tubing volumes for 10 inches of ¼ inch or 3/8 inch tubing.

mass in the form of packed red blood cells or whole blood is often added to the prime solution. Priming volumes vary significantly and depend on the specific equipment (oxygenator, tubing, etc.) used.

To determine the patient's hematocrit (Hct) on CPB when a clear prime (crystalloid/colloid) is employed, the following equation is utilized:

Hct on bypass

$$= [\text{Estimated blood volume} (EBV \times Hct)/(EBV + \text{circuit prime volume})].$$

If the calculated Hct is deemed acceptable, the prime can be buffered and the patient can be placed on bypass with a clear prime. If the calculated Hct is deemed too low (generally the cut-off is 25%), red cell mass may be added to the circuit to reach the desired dilutional Hct once the patient is placed on bypass. The amount of blood required in the circuit prime can be calculated using the equation:

$$\text{Prime blood needed}\,[\text{ml}]$$
$$= (\text{EBV} + \text{circuit volume})$$
$$\times (\text{desired Hct on bypass}) - (\text{EBV} \times \text{Hct})\,/$$
$$(\text{Hct of prime blood})$$

where estimated blood volume (EBV) = patient weight [kg] × blood volume [ml kg^{-1}]; circuit prime volume = calculated from components used; and Hct of prime blood = whole blood (35–40%) versus packed red blood cells (PRBC) (65–75%).

Institutional practice varies with regard to the type of red blood cells used for priming the circuit (red blood cell [RBC] versus whole-blood units) and the lowest acceptable calculated Hct. While most centers use RBC units when required to prime the bypass circuit, there is variable use of whole blood or RBCs reconstituted with fresh frozen plasma (FFP) to prevent the dilution of coagulation factors at the onset of bypass when the prime volume is large relative to the patient's blood volume. In general, even with use of a miniaturized CPB circuit, a prime of whole blood or RBCs reconstituted with FFP is utilized in neonates and infants to mitigate significant dilution of coagulation factors and to reduce the need for factor repletion with FFP in the post-CPB period.

Acute normovolemic hemodilution (ANH) involves the removal of blood, usually shortly after the induction of anesthesia, and its simultaneous replacement by an adequate volume of colloids or crystalloids to maintain normovolemia. As a result of the hemodilution process, blood volume subsequently lost during surgery will contain fewer RBCs, thereby reducing the net RBC mass lost and possibly the need for allogeneic blood transfusion. In addition, the platelets and plasma proteins in the whole-blood withdrawal will be free of the changes induced by CPB. The removed whole can be retransfused following termination of CPB and protamine administration. In general, this is a technique applicable only to adult-sized patients with a high preoperative Hct.

Once the desired Hct on CPB is determined, calculations are done as described above to define the patient Hct necessary to achieve that target, the target Hct$_\text{T}$. The volume of blood to be removed by ANH is then:

$$[\text{EBV} \times (\text{Hct}_\text{S} - \text{Hct}_\text{T})]\,/\,\text{Hct}_\text{A}$$

where Hct$_\text{S}$ is the patient's starting Hct and Hct$_\text{A}$ = (Hct$_\text{S}$ − Hct$_\text{T}$)/2.

A key component of red cell conservation is salvage of red cells from the CPB circuit once it is disconnected from the patient. The technology exists for this process to be used for any size CPB circuit. The advantage of this approach is that unheparinized blood with a relatively high Hct (60–70%) is made available for post-CPB transfusion, obviating the need for transfusion of additional autologous units to increase red cell mass. This blood, however, is devoid of platelets, clotting factors, mediators of fibrinolysis, and inflammatory mediators.

Ultrafiltration

Ultrafiltrators are devices commonly added to the CPB circuit to remove excess fluid and produce hemoconcentration. When used in conjunction with CPB, these devices produce an ultrafiltrate that occurs as the result of a hydrostatic pressure gradient across a semipermeable membrane. These are the same devices that can be used for hemodialysis when they are used in conjunction with a dialysate. When used during CPB, they are commonly called hemoconcentrators as they produce an increase in hematocrit by removing excess fluid.

These devices consist of a core of microporous hollow fibers made of polysulfone, polyamide, or polyacrylonitrile material arranged in a bundle. The pore size generally is 0.30–0.40 microns. Due to the pressure drop across the device, blood inflow must be obtained from the arterial side of the CPB circuit while blood outflow is diverted to the cardiotomy reservoir or venous reservoir. The ultrafiltrate is collected in a container connected to a vacuum source. The ultrafiltrate is discarded and has the composition of glomerular filtrate.

The rate at which ultrafiltrate is produced is dependent on the transmembrane pressure gradient (TMP). TMP is determined by the arterial inlet pressure (Pa), the venous outlet pressure (Pv), the absolute value of applied suction at the outlet (Pn), the oncotic pressure at the inlet (Pi), and the oncotic pressure at the outlet (Po):

$$TMP = \frac{Pa + Pv}{2} + Pn - \frac{Pi + Po}{2}$$

Pn is increased by using the regulated vacuum source connected to the outlet of the device. TMP should not exceed 500 mmHg.

Conventional Ultrafiltration
Conventional ultrafiltration (CUF) is utilized in nearly all pediatric bypass cases, and involves the removal of excess volume in the venous reservoir *during* bypass. An excess venous reservoir volume can be caused by the crystalloid component of cardioplegia, valve testing solution, or simply when a patient has an elevated circulating blood volume. CUF removes excess volume by passing blood, either passively or actively with a roller head, through the ultrafilter.

Modified Ultrafiltration
Modified ultrafiltration (MUF) allows ultrafiltration to continue *after* weaning from CPB. MUF allows the bypass circuit to remain primed while both the patient's blood volume and the bypass circuit volumes are hemoconcentrated. MUF may be performed utilizing either an arteriovenous or venoarterial system. In the arteriovenous system,

inflow to the ultrafilter is drawn with a roller pump directly from the aortic cannula. Outflow from the ultrafilter is directed to the right atrium. In the venoarterial system, the right atrium provides inflow to the ultrafilter with the aid of a roller pump, while outflow from the ultrafilter is returned to the aortic cannula. With both systems, blood volume is kept constant as ultrafiltrate is lost by replacing the ultrafiltrate with blood from the CPB circuit. The endpoint for termination of MUF following CPB varies from institution to institution, and may depend on a set time interval (10–15 min), a set target Hct (40%), or a set volume removed (750 ml m^{-2}).

The major advantage of MUF over CUF is that, by allowing hemoconcentration to continue after CPB, MUF normally allows for a greater degree of hemoconcentration than can be obtained with CUF alone, especially in small children. Some institutions utilize both CUF and MUF, as the techniques are not mutually exclusive. However, when a standardized volume of fluid is removed, there is no difference in clinical outcome or hemoconcentration between CUF and MUF.

Blood Gas Management

Electrochemical neutrality is important in the preservation of cellular protein and enzyme structure and maintenance of the constant transcellular hydrogen (H$^+$) ion gradient necessary for many cellular processes. In addition, optimal functioning of the imidazole buffering system is dependent on maintenance of cellular electrochemical neutrality. The imidazole group of the amino acid histidine is present on many blood and cellular proteins, and is an important buffer.

Electrochemical neutrality occurs when there are equal concentrations of hydroxyl (OH$^-$) and hydrogen (H$^+$) ions. As the temperature decreases, the dissociation constant (pK) of aqueous systems such as those found in cells increases. This process results in a reduction in the concentrations of OH$^-$ and H$^+$ ions as the temperature decreases. If there are equal concentrations of OH^- and H^+, then electrochemical neutrality will be maintained. Thus, in order for electrochemical neutrality to be maintained, the pH must increase as temperature decreases. In an electrochemically neutral cell at 37 °C, the measured pH will be 7.40, whereas in an electrochemically neutral cell at 20 °C, the measured pH will be 7.80. Changes in cellular pH during hypothermia are mediated through $PaCO_2$ homeostasis. As the temperature decreases, the solubility of CO_2 in blood increases. If the total CO_2 content of blood is held constant, this increase in CO_2 solubility will result in a reduction in $PaCO_2$. For example, if the total CO_2 content is held constant and the measured $PaCO_2$ at 37 °C is 40 mmHg, then the measured $PaCO_2$ at 20 °C will be 16 mmHg. This situation causes the pH to increase as the temperature decreases for electrochemical neutrality to be maintained.

pH-stat and alpha-stat regulation are acid–base management methods that directly influence blood flow to the brain and other organs. Although pH-stat and alpha-stat acid–base management is frequently mentioned in association with temperature-corrected and temperature-uncorrected blood gases, it must be emphasized that these are entirely different concepts. The method of blood gas interpretation (corrected or uncorrected) does not dictate the method of acid–base management (pH-stat or alpha-stat). It is important to point out that at a patient temperature of 37 °C, there is no difference between pH-stat and alpha-stat management. However, the difference between the two strategies becomes more marked as patient temperature progressively falls below 37 °C, and is not clinically relevant until patient temperature is below 30 °C.

When a blood gas sample is drawn from a hypothermic patient and sent to the blood gas laboratory, the sample is warmed to 37 °C before measurement. The values obtained at 37 °C are termed "temperature-uncorrected" values, and they are converted to temperature-corrected values using a nomogram. The nomogram accounts for temperature-induced changes in pH, O_2 solubility, and CO_2 solubility in a closed-blood system. When pH and $PaCO_2$ are measured at 37 °C and then corrected to a lower temperature, the electrochemically neutral pH will be higher and the corrected $PaCO_2$ will be lower than the normal values at 37 °C. Therefore, electrochemical neutrality is maintained by keeping pH alkalotic in temperature-corrected blood gases and normal in temperature-uncorrected gases; this is known as alpha-stat regulation. For practical purposes, it is easier to use uncorrected values and keep pH and $PaCO_2$ in the range considered normal at 37 °C. Cerebral blood flow and oxygen consumption are appropriately coupled when alpha-stat regulation is used. An exception to this is that during deep hypothermia, there is loss of cerebral autoregulation such that cerebral blood flow varies directly with arterial pressure.

pH-stat regulation involves maintaining pH and $PaCO_2$ at normal values when temperature-corrected gases are used, and at acidotic values when temperature-uncorrected gases are used. pH stat is achieved by adding CO_2 to the ventilating gas during hypothermic CPB to increase $PaCO_2$ and decrease the pH. In contrast to alpha-stat regulation, in which the total CO_2 content is kept constant, pH-stat regulation results in an increase in total CO_2 content. The cerebral vasculature maintains vasomotor responses to varying $PaCO_2$ during hypothermic CPB. This response is maintained during moderate hypothermia and is attenuated during deep hypothermia, despite the fact that deep hypothermia induces a loss of cerebral blood flow autoregulation. When pH-stat regulation is used with moderate hypothermic CPB, there is an uncoupling of cerebral blood flow and metabolism and a loss of cerebral autoregulation. As a result, cerebral blood flow varies linearly with arterial blood pressure and cerebral hyperperfusion exists, with the cerebral blood flow far in excess of that dictated by the cerebral metabolic rate. This hyperperfusion state is the result of reduced cerebral oxygen consumption induced by hypothermia and cerebral vasodilation resulting from a disproportionately high $PaCO_2$ for the degree of hypothermia present.

Additionally, pH-stat management suppresses the cerebral metabolic rate, which may prolong oxygen availability during periods of circulatory arrest. pH-stat also decreases pulmonary blood flow which can exist even during total bypass due to collateral circulations. This has obvious benefits for preventing the steal of blood from the cerebral circulation, while at the same time improving heat transfer for the cooling and warming phases of bypass. The potential danger of the hyperperfused state is an increased delivery of microemboli into the cerebral circulation.

Alpha-stat management is common in adult cardiac surgery, where patients are more likely to have a particulate embolic load due to calcified plaques in arterial vessels. Children are less likely than adults to suffer from particulate embolic events on bypass due to vascular disease. However, they are more likely to require hypothermic bypass and to suffer from inadequate brain cooling due to collateral circulations stealing from the effective cerebral blood flow. For this reason, pH-stat blood gas management is frequently utilized during pediatric CPB.

Deep Hypothermic Circulatory Arrest and Antegrade Cerebral Perfusion Techniques

Deep Hypothermic Circulatory Arrest (DHCA)

Deep hypothermic circulatory arrest involves cooling a patient on bypass to <20 °C, ceasing the arterial pump flow, and exsanguinating the patient's blood volume into the bypass venous reservoir. It permits a bloodless, uncluttered surgical field, simplified cannulation, and limited blood exposure to foreign surfaces, invoking less inflammation.This technique improves surgical exposure for the surgeon during complex aortic arch repairs,

the correction of anomalous pulmonary venous drainage, or when the patient's size and/or anatomy would prevent adequate venous drainage during surgical repair.

Hypothermia

Hypothermia is arguably the most important component of DHCA. DHCA in children is generally conducted with rectal or bladder and esophageal temperatures ≤18 °C. It may take as long as 20 minutes on CPB to reach this temperature before initiation of DHCA.

Hypothermia-induced reduction in cerebral metabolic rate for oxygen ($CMRO_2$) slows the rate of depletion of high-energy phosphates and the development of intracellular acidosis. This in turn delays or prevents the neuronal energy failure which leads to terminal membrane depolarization and subsequent neuronal injury or death during an ischemic episode. Q_{10} defines the ratio of organ O_2 consumption at a defined temperature to the O_2 consumption at a temperature 10 °C lower. The cerebral Q_{10} is approximately 3.65 in children and 2.3 in adults. Consequently, the cerebral metabolic rate will still be approximately 10–15% of its normothermic baseline at 15 °C. If it is assumed that 3–5 minutes of cerebral ischemia can be tolerated at 37 °C and the Q_{10} is 3.0, 9–15 minutes of ischemia can be tolerated at 27 °C and 27–45 minutes can be tolerated at 17 °C.

In addition to reducing $CMRO_2$, hypothermia also serves to ameliorate some of the sequalae of neuronal ischemia when instituted *prior* to the ischemia insult. Specifically, hypothermia markedly reduces release of the excitatory neurotransmitters glutamate, aspartate, and glycine which accompany cerebral ischemia and subsequent reperfusion.

Acid–base Management

The acid–base strategy (alpha-stat versus pH-stat) utilized before and after DHCA is institution dependent. There are several potential advantges to the use of pH-stat management during cooling prior to DHCA.

- *Suppression of CMRO$_2$*: better suppression of CMRO$_2$ with pH-stat as compared to alpha-stat management. At 17 °C, CMRO$_2$ is decreased 40% over that seen with alpha-stat management.
- *Brain cooling*: during the cooling phase of deep hypothermia, pH-stat management provides faster and more homogeneous brain cooling than does alpha-stat management. This is felt to be a direct consequence of the increased CBF which accompanies pH-stat management.
- *Oxyhemoglobin dissociation curve*: hypothermia induces a leftward shift of the oxyhemoglobin dissociation curve such that during alpha-stat management at 17 °C, the P$_{50}$ of fetal hemoglobin is 5.0 compared to 20.0 at 37 °C. The increased affinity of hemoglobin for O$_2$ reduces the ability of hemoglobin to off-load O$_2$ to tissue. As a result, a substantial portion (56–96%) of the O$_2$ delivered to brain during CPB at 17 °C is obtained from dissolved O$_2$, making a high CBF to CMRO$_2$ ratio necessary. pH-stat management is advantageous in this setting because:
  - it results in increased CBF compared to alpha-stat management
  - the relative acidosis which accompanies pH-stat management induces a rightward shift of the oxyhemoglobin dissociation curve such that the P$_{50}$ of fetal hemoglobin increases to 6.9 at 17 °C, improving off-loading of O$_2$ from hemoglobin to the brain.
- *Aortopulmonary collaterals (APCs)*: the presence of numerous and often large collateral vessels from the arch vessels and thoracic aorta to the pulmonary arterial system is common in neonates, infants, and children with atretic pulmonary arterial systems. The number and size of these vessels increase in proportion to the duration of cyanosis. These vessels are capable of stealing blood from the cerebral circulation to the pulmonary circulation particularly in the setting of alkalosis, which tends to reduce pulmonary vascular resistance while increasing cerebral vascular resistance. pH-stat management during cooling results in better cerebral protection than alpha-stat management when circulatory arrest is induced in the presence of APCs.
- *Cerebral oxygenation*: in animal studies pH-stat management has been demonstrated to increase pre-DHCA cortical O$_2$ saturation (ScO$_2$) and to increase the half-life of arrest ScO$_2$ compared to alpha-stat management. pH-stat management has also been demonstrated to provide better preservation of intracellular pH and cerebral energy stores (high-energy phosphates) and tissue oxygenation.

Most institutions target a Hct minimum of 25% prior to the onset of DHCA and aim to keep the duration of DHCA <40–45 minutes. Longer DHCA durations have been associated with poorer postoperative neurobehavioral outcomes across multiple domains and a higher incidence of white matter injury, stroke, and seizures. The use of adjunct therapies such as allopurinol, erythropoietin, barbiturates, inhalation anesthesic agents, and steroids to mitigate the neuronal damage which accompanies the use of DHCA has not proved clinically fruitful.

Antegrade Cerebral Perfusion (ACP)

Antegrade cerebral perfusion is a bypass strategy that can often limit, or even eliminate, the need for DHCA.

The technique involves diverting pump arterial blood flow, commonly through the innominate artery, solely to the right subclavian and right common carotid arteries. It is commonly employed for aortic arch reconstruction in children with hypoplastic left heard syndrome (HLHS) undergoing the Norwood procedure and in children with aortic hypoplasia or interruption undergoing biventricular repair. This technique is felt to provide both cerebral and some limited somatic (subdiaphragmatic viscera) perfusion. Somatic perfusion is felt to be the result of the extensive network of arterial collaterals in the neonate which link the supra- and subdiaphragmatic viscera such as the internal thoracic and intercostal arteries.

Access to the innominate artery can be obtained via placement of the arterial cannula into the open, distal end of a 3 or 3.5 mm PTFE graft with the proximal end anastomosed to the distal right innominate or proximal right subclavian artery. Obviously, in patients undergoing the Norwood procedure, this graft, when anastomosed distally to the right pulmonary artery, will constitute a modified Blalock–Thomas–Taussig shunt. In patients undergoing biventricular repair, the graft serves as the primary cannulation site. The graft is oversewn at its insertion site once separation from CPB has occurred.

In circumstances where the ascending aorta is of reasonable size the aorta cannula can be advanced up the innominate artery from the right side of the aortic arch during arch reconstruction. Alternatively, the cannula can be left in the ascending aorta with a cross-clamp applied just distal to the innominate artery for reconstruction of distal and descending aortic lesions.

The flow rate, acid–base strategy, and temperature utilized during ACP vary among institutions. ACP flow rates of 20–$40\ ml\ kg^{-1}\ min^{-1}$ are commonly utilized and have been shown to adequately perfuse the cerebral circulation, although some centers utilize higher flow rates (60–$70\ ml\ kg^{-1}\ min^{-1}$). Unilateral or bilateral cerebral NIRS is used by most centers to fine-tune flow rates. Some centers also employ transcranial Doppler (TCD) and somatic NIRS. That said, there is poor correlation between ACP flow rate and both cerebral oxygenation as determined by NIRS and cerebral blood flow velocity as determined by TCD. In addition, there is poor correlation between ACP flow rate and mean arterial blood pressure measured in the radial or brachial artery. Also at issue is whether unilateral assessment of cerebral blood flow by NIRS and TCD is adequate or whether bilateral assessment is necessary given that perfusion of the left side of the brain is dependent on the circle of Willis.

There is no clear evidence to date that use of ACP provides better neurobehavioral outcomes than judicious use of DHCA.

Anticoagulation

Unfractionated heparin (UFH) in conjunction with activated clotting time (ACT) measurement is used to achieve and monitor anticoagulation during CPB. The ACT is a whole-blood coagulation assay which evaluates the intrinsic hemostatic activation system; it is similar to activated partial thromboplastin time (aPTT), a test run on a platelet-poor plasma sample, to which phospholipid activant and a contact activant such as kaolin, silica, ellagic acid, or Celite® has been added. A whole-blood ACT test also uses a contact activator but uses the platelets in the sample as the phospholipid activatant. As such, the ACT factors other than UFH, such as thrombocytopenia, dysfunctional platelets, antiplatelet drugs, and dilution of clotting factors, can prolong the ACT.

Most institutions use an age- or weight-based protocol to administer the initial pre-CPB dose of UFH, and add heparin to the CPB prime as the prime volume would be expected to decrease plasma heparin levels with the initiation of CPB. Typical doses are 300–$400\ units\ kg^{-1}$ to achieve an ACT >480 s pre-CPB. This is quite distinct from the lower ACT targeted during ECMO, an important difference being that the CPB circuit is constantly contaminated with high levels of procoagulant tissue factor released during surgical trauma while the ECMO circuit generally is not. The CPB circuit commonly contains 3 units of heparin for each milliliter of prime volume. Some centers utilize the Hepcon® heparin management system (HMS), wherein the heparin dose–response test (HDR) determines a patient's ACT responsiveness to heparin. An estimate of the patient's blood volume can then be used to determine the heparin dose necessary to reach the target heparin concentration (THC) that will result in an ACT $\geq$480 s.

Heparin resistance or, more accurately, low heparin sensitivity (LHS) is defined as the failure to reach and/or maintain a target ACT (usually 450–480 seconds) after a standard heparin dose (300– 400 IU kg^{-1}). LHS can be managed with additional doses of UFH, administration of FFP which contains antithrombin III (ATIII), or administration of pure ATIII in a dose of 7–10 IU kg^{-1}.

Heparin should always be given via a central venous line from which blood return can be easily demonstrated or, as is common in infants/neonates, directly into the heart (usually the right atrium) by the surgeon. This is necessary to ensure that the heparin dose has reached the central circulation. An ACT can be drawn within minutes of heparin administration as peak arterial ACT prolongation occurs within 30 s and peak venous ACT prolongation within 60 s.

In some circumstances, particularly children with documented heparin-induced thrombocytopenia (HIT) or heparin-induced thrombocytopenia with thrombosis (HITT), an alternative to UFH for anticoagulation for CPB is necessary. Currently, the best alternative is bivalirudin, a bivalent direct thrombin inhibitor (DTI). It binds to both the active and fibrin-binding sites of thrombin and, as opposed to UFH, it has the ability to inhibit clot-bound thrombin. Bivalirudin's activity is independent of cofactors and therefore the anticoagulation response is predictable independent of ATIII levels. Bivalirudin is metabolized via proteolytic cleavage (80%) as well as renal mechanisms (20%) and the estimated average half-life of bivalirudin in the pediatric population is 15–18 minutes. This is important because there is no reversal agent for bivalirudin, and termination of its anticoagulant effect requires sufficient metabolism to allow for thrombin generation and clot formation.

The ACT and aPTT are the most commonly used monitoring tests for bivalirudin. Quantitative, drug-calibrated assays such as the ecarin clotting time (ECT), dilute thrombin time, and chromogenic anti-IIa assay have been shown to be superior to aPTT and ACT testing in terms of monitoring serum bivalirudin concentration, but none are commercially available or FDA approved for clinical use in the United States. A comprehensive protocol for use of bivalirudin for CPB anticoagulation is shown in Figure 7.3.

Protamine Reversal of Heparin

Protamine is normally given after bypass once stable hemodynamics are exhibited and the surgeon is satisfied with the repair. Protamine should not be administered until the likelihood of having to reinstitute CPB is minimal. After protamine neutralization of heparin begins, cardiotomy suction should not be used. This practice ensures the usefulness of the bypass circuit should the reinstitution of bypass be required. The venous cannulas are usually removed before protamine administration. The arterial cannula is left in place until adequate hemostasis is achieved and circuit blood is no longer required.

There are several approaches to the neutralization of heparin with protamine, all with reportedly good clinical results. Some centers use a ratio of 1.0–1.3 mg of protamine for each 100 units of heparin determined to exist at the termination of CPB. This ratio is based on the *in vitro* protamine-to-heparin neutralization ratio of 1.3:1.0. The amount of heparin present is determined by obtaining an ACT when CPB terminates, and using a reverse extrapolation of the patient's heparin dose–response curve to correlate ACT and heparin level. Some centers simply administer a fixed dose of protamine based on the patient's weight (3–4 mg kg^{-1}) regardless of the heparin dose administered. Some centers use heparin assays and then calculate the protamine dose based on the patient's blood volume and a protamine-to-heparin neutralization ratio ranging from 1:1 to 1.3:1.

Regardless of the method utilized, the ACT should be checked after administration of

Table 7.5 ROTEM assays.

ROTEM test	Description and interpretation
INTEM	Contact activation. Reagent contains phospholipid and elllagic acid as activators and provides information similar to that of the aPTT.
EXTEM	Tissue factor activation. Reagent contains tissue factor as an activator and provides information similar to that of the PT.
HEPTEM	Contains yophilized heparinase for neutralizing unfractionated heparin; used in conjunction with INTEM reagent and compared to ITEM analysis to assess heparin effect.
APTEM	Contains aprotinin for inhibiting fibrinolysis; used in conjunction with EXTEM reagent and compared to EXTEM analysis to assess fibrinolysis.
flBTEM	Utilizes cytochalasin D, an actin polymerization inhibitor, to block the pl1 atelet contribution to clot formation. Used in conjunction with EXTEM reagent and when compared to EXTEM analysis allows qualitative anallysis of the fibrinogen contribution to clot strength independent of platelets.
NATEM	Native whole-blood sample analyzed following only recalcification. Impractical for clinical use given long CFT time.

Source: Reproduced from Whiting et.al. (2014)/with permission of John Wiley & Sons.

"standard" platelet dose of 0.1–0.2 units kg^{-1} is expected to increase the platelet count by 50,000 μl^{-1}; however, doses of 0.5–1.0 units kg^{-1} (5–10 ml kg^{-1}) are commonly administered to neonates and infants following complex procedures to target a platelet count >100,000 μl^{-1}.

Fibrinogen Repletion

The minimum fibrinogen content per unit of cryoprecipitate is specified as 50 mg/unit but the actual concentration can vary considerably (300–3000 mg dl^{-1}). The "standard" cryoprecipitate dose of 0.1–0.2 units kg^{-1} is expected to increase fibrinogen levels by 75 mg dl^{-1} but doses of 0.5–1.0 units kg^{-1} (5–10 ml kg^{-1}) are commonly administered to neonates and infants following complex procedures. Fibrinogen concentrate can be used in place of cryoprecipitate at a dose of 70 mg kg^{-1} or using the equation from the package insert: dose = (target level − measured level)/1.7 × weight (kg), to reach a target level. Generally, a target fibrinogen concentration >150–200 mg dl^{-1} is sought. It should

be kept in mind that cryoprecipitate is a non-purified blood product and in addition to fibrinogen, it contains fibronectin and platelet microparticles, and coagulation factors VIII, XIII, and von Willebrand factor.

Prothrombin Complex Concentrates (PCC), rVIIA, Desmopressin Administration

The decision to administer rFVIIa or a PCC for hemostasis should be based on surgeon and anesthesiologist assessment that refractory bleeding despite maximal, standard blood component therapy is present and the recognition that these agents are strongly prothrombotic. Particular caution should be used when administering these agents to patients with structures at risk for thrombosis such as mBTTT shunts or small ascending aortas.

Prothrombin complex concentrates are formulations containing vitamin K-dependent clotting factors. PCCs are classified as four-factor prothrombin complex concentrates (4FPCCs) containing factors II, VII, IX, and X, and three-factor prothrombin complex

Cardiac Surgery Intraoperative Targeted Transfusion Algorithm

- Perform ROTEM/TEG during rewarming phase of bypass
- Optimize Temperature (>36 deg C), pH (>7.2), iCa++ (>1 mmol/L), and Hb (>7.5 g/dL)
- Continue antifibrinolytics and consider ANH, mini circuits, retrograde priming and cell salvage

Figure 7.7 Society of Cardiovascular Anesthesiologists ROTEM/TEG-based cardiac surgery intraoperative transfusion algorithm. ANH indicates acute normovolemic hemodilution; A10, amplitude at 10 minutes; CT, clotting time; DDAVP, 1-deamino-8-d-arginine vasopressin; ECMO, extracorporeal membrane oxygenation; EXTEM, extrinsic pathway thromboelastometry; FIBTEM, fibrinogen-based thromboelastometry; FF, functional fibrinogen; FFP, fresh frozen plasma; Hb, hemoglobin; HEPTEM, heparinase thromboelastometry; HIT, heparin-induced thrombocytopenia; hTEG, heparinase thromboelastography; iCA++, ionized calcium; INTEM, intrinsic pathway thromboelastometry; LY30, clot lysis at 30 min; MA, maximum amplitude; ML, maximum lysis; PCC, prothrombin complex concentrate; R, reaction time; ROTEM, rotational thromboelastometry; TEG, thromboelastograph. *Source:* Reproduced from Raphael et al. (2019)/ with permission of Elsevier.

Figure 7.8 Society of Cardiovascular Anesthesiologists non-ROTEM/TEG-based cardiac surgery intraoperative transfusion algorithm. ACT, activated clotting time; ANH, acute normovolemic hemodilution; CPB, cardiopulmonary bypass; DDAVP, 1-deamino-8-d-arginine vasopressin; FFP, fresh frozen plasma; Hb, hemoglobin; iCA++, ionized calcium; INR, international normalized ratio; PCC, prothrombin complex concentrate; PLT, platelets; RBC, red blood cell; rFVIIa, recombinant activated factor VII; RV, right ventricle; T, temperature. *Source:* Reproduced from Raphael et al. (2019)/with permission of Elsevier.

concentrates (3FPCCs) containing factors II, IX, and X, with negligible amounts of FVII. The 4FPCC available in the US are factor eight-inhibitor bypass activator (FEIBA™; Baxter Healthcare Corporation) and KCentra® (CSL Behring). FEIBA contains activated FVII and protein C while KCentra contains inactivated FVII as well as proteins C and S, AT-III, and heparin. 4FPCC are usually administered as rescue therapy in standardized doses of 10 units (IU) kg^{-1}. Recombinant FVIIa is usually administered as rescue therapy in a standardized dose of 90 µg kg^{-1}.

Desmopressin (DDAVP) is a vasopressin analog that increases circulating levels of coagulation FVIII and von Willebrand factor by stimulating the release of stored von Willebrand factor from the Weibel–Palade bodies in the endothelium. There is little or no evidence to support the use of DDAVP in treatment of post-CPB microvascular bleeding in children.

Red Cell Repletion

This is likely the most controversial decision in post-CPB transfusion management. There is very limited consensus and a great deal of institutional variation as to the optimal post-CPB Hb and there is limited evidence to strongly support any one strategy. That said, Figure 7.9 is an example of a consolidated approach to red cell transfusion based on both Hb thesholds and physiologic data. It

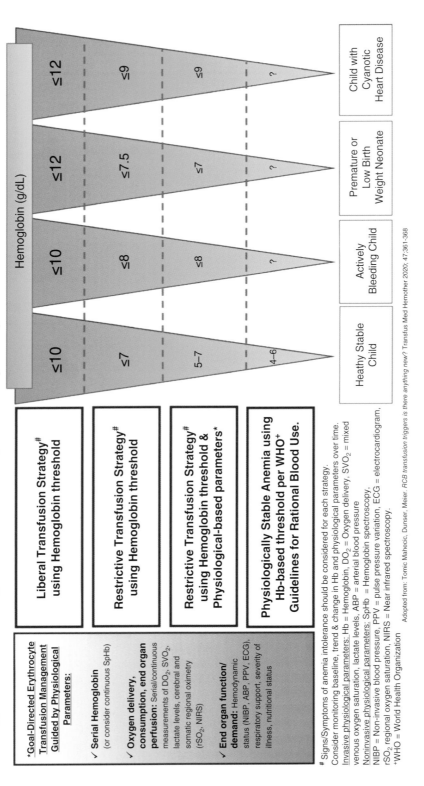

Figure 7.9 A consolidated approach to red cell transfusion based on both Hb thresholds and physiologic data. *Source:* Reproduced from Downey and Goobie (2022)/ with permission of the American Society of Anesthesiologists (ASA).

is important to note that a consolidated approach must be individualized to the patient based on comprehensive assessment of all available physiologic data used to assess DO_2 and VO_2 at the systemic and tissue level. Unfortunately, physiology-based transfusion therapy is hampered by the lack of technology to determine oxygen delivery (DO_2) and oxygen consumption (VO_2) at the level of the microcirculation.

Antifibrinolytics

Because activation of the fibrinolytic pathway plays an important role in the coagulopathy observed during and after cardiac surgery, prophylactic administration of antifibrinolytic agents in neonates and children undergoing cardiac surgery with CPB is relatively routine. Currently available antifibrinolytic agents are the lysine analogs tranexamic acid (TXA) and epsilon-aminocaproic acid (Amicar®) which competitively inhibit the binding of TPA and plasminogen to the lysine residues on fibrin. This inhibits formation of plasmin and thus degradation of fibrin. Plasmin generation after tissue injury also induces thrombin generation, complement activation, and activation of monocytes, neutrophils, and platelets. Thus there are potential advantanges to higher plasma levels of these agents. Unfortunately, there is no consensus on the optimal plasma levels of these agents and hence there is great institutional variation in dosing regimens. There is also concern that high plasma levels of both TXA and Amicar are associated with seizures as a result of enhanced neuronal excitation due to their interactions with gamma-aminobutyric acid (GABA) and glycine receptor-mediated neurotransmission. A summary of the dosing schedules to obtain target plasma levels of TXA and Amicar across various age groups is given in Table 7.6.

Table 7.6 Dosing schedules to obtain target plasma levels of TXA and Amicar across various age groups.

Agent	Population	Targeted concentration	Loading dose	Infusion	CPB dose
Epsilon-aminocaproic acid (AMICAR)	6.8–18.9 kg	260 µg/ml	75 mg/kg	75 mg/kg/h	75 mg/kg
	2.7–3.7 kg	50 µg/ml	40 mg/kg	30 mg/kg	10 mg/l
Tranexamic acid (TXA)	5–40 kg	20 µg/ml	6.4 mg/kg	2.0–3.1 mg/kg/h	**NA**
	0–2 months	20 µg/ml	15 mg/kg	2.5 mg/kg/h	20 mg/l
	2–12 months	20 µg/ml	9 mg/kg	2 mg/kg/h	20 mg/l
	>12 months (max 20 kg)	20 µg/ml	4 mg/kg	2 mg/kg/h	20 mg/l
	0–2 months	60 µg/ml	50 mg/kg	7 mg/kg/h	60 mg/l
	2–12 months	60 µg/ml	26 mg/kg	6 mg/kg/h	60 mg/l
	>12 months (max 20 kg)	60 µg/ml	13 mg/kg	5.5 mg/kg/h	60 mg/l
	0–2 months	150 µg/ml	120 mg/kg	17 mg/kg/h	150 mg/l
	2–12 months	150 µg/ml	65 mg/kg	14 mg/kg/h	150 mg/l
	>12 months (max 20 kg)	150 µg/ml	31 mg/kg	14 mg/kg/h	150 mg/l

References and Further Reading

Bartoszko, J. & Karkouti, K. Managing the coagulopathy associated with cardiopulmonary bypass. *J Thromb Haemost* **19**, 617–632 (2021).

Downey, L.A. & Goobie, S.M. Perioperative pediatric erythrocyte transfusions: incorporating hemoglobin thresholds and physiologic parameters in decision-making. *Anesthesiology* **137**, 604–619 (2022).

Levy, J.H., Ghadimi, K., Kizhakkedathu, J.N. & Iba, T. What's fishy about protamine? Clinical use, adverse reactions, and potential alternatives. *J Thromb Haemost* **21**, 1714–1723 (2023).

Matte, G.S. *Perfusion for Congenital Heart Surgery*. Wiley Blackwell, Chichester, (2015).

Matte, G.S. & DiNardo, J.A. Pediatric cardiopulmonary bypass. In: Gravlee, G.P., Davis, R.F., Hammon, J.W. & Kussman, B.D. (eds) *Cardiopulmonary Bypass and Mechanical Support, Principles and Practice*, 4th edn. Wolters Kluwer, Philadelphia (2015).

Raphael, J., Mazer, C.D., Subramani, S. *et al.* Society of Cardiovascular Anesthesiologists Clinical Practice Improvement Advisory for Management of Perioperative Bleeding and Hemostasis in Cardiac Surgery Patients. *Anesth Analg* **129**, 1209–1221 (2019).

Whiting, D. & DiNardo, J.A. TEG and ROTEM: technology and clinical applications. *Am J Hematol* **89**, 228–232 (2014).

8

Echocardiography

Echocardiography is an indispensable tool in the diagnosis and management of congenital heart disease.

Transthoracic Echocardiography

Transthoracic echocardiography (TTE) is the primary imaging tool in the diagnosis and assessment of congenital and acquired heart disease in neonates, infants, children, and adolescents. A complete TTE exam is noninvasive, can be performed on site anywhere, and provides detailed anatomic, hemodynamic, and physiologic information. It is particularly valuable in neonates, infants, and children, given their smaller size, as a shallower depth of penetration of the ultrasound beam is needed to image the heart, compared to adults.

Image resolution and depth of penetration are inversely related, with higher frequency transducers having higher resolution but less depth of penetration. High-frequency probes (8 or 12 MHz) focus at depths of 4–5 cm, whereas low- or mid-frequency probes (2.5, 3, 5 MHz) focus at depths of 12–16 cm. Consequently, a high-frequency transducer with excellent image resolution can be used in infants and neonates, whereas the depth of penetration necessary to image an adolescent or adult will necessitate use of a lower frequency probe with poorer image resolution.

The imaging widows typically used in a comprehensive TTE exam are shown in Figure 8.1. Figures 8.2–8.9 summarize the images obtained during a comprehensive TTE exam.

Transesophageal Echocardiography

Transesophageal echocardiography (TEE) is a valuable, semiinvasive imaging modality which allows monitoring and diagnostic imaging of the heart before, during, and after cardiac or noncardiac procedures without interruption. The esophageal position of the ultrasonic transducer provides imaging without the constraints imposed by the interposition of the chest wall and lungs between the TTE transducer and the heart. In addition, TEE provides better visualization of posterior cardiac structures such as the left and right atrium and the pulmonary veins given its direct proximity to these structures. Figures 8.10 and 8.11 summarize terminology used to describe manipulation of the TEE probe, the four standard transducer positions within the esophagus and stomach, and the conventions of image display. It should be noted that in some pediatric institutions, the vertex of the displayed image is inverted (vertex at the bottom of the screen rather than the top) compared to what is shown in Figure 8.11. Figures 8.12–8.17 summarize the images obtained during a comprehensive TEE exam.

Multiplane 7.5 MHz probes are available for intraoperative use in neonates, infants,

The Pediatric Cardiac Anesthesia Handbook, Second Edition. Viviane G. Nasr and James A. DiNardo.
© 2025 John Wiley & Sons Ltd. Published 2025 by John Wiley & Sons Ltd.

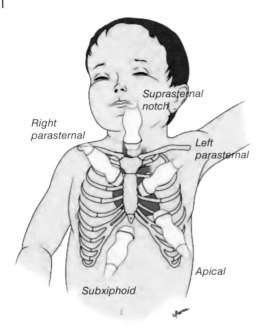

Figure 8.1 Transducer locations for standard transthoracic echocardiogram (TTE) imaging windows. *Source:* Reproduced from Lai and Ko (2016)/with permission of John Wiley & Sons.

Figure 8.2 Subxiphoid long-axis (frontal) sweep; shown are corresponding TTE images. (1) DAo, descending aorta; LA, left atrium; LV, left ventricle; RA, right atrium. (2) Ao arch, aortic arch; AoV, aortic valve; LPA, left pulmonary artery; RPA, right pulmonary artery; TV, tricuspid valve. (3) Ao, aorta; MPA, main pulmonary artery; RSVC, right superior vena cava. (4) LV, left ventricle; RAA, right atrial appendage; RV, right ventricle; RVOT, right ventricular outflow tract. *Source:* Reproduced from Lai and Ko (2016)/with permission of John Wiley & Sons.

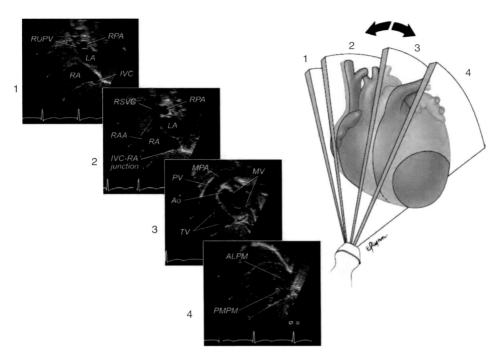

Figure 8.3 Subxiphoid short-axis (sagittal) sweep; shown are corresponding TTE images. (1) IVC, inferior vena cava; LA, left atrium; RA, right atrium; RPA, right pulmonary artery; RUPV, right upper pulmonary vein. (2) IVC–RA junction, inferior vena cava–right atrial junction; LA, left atrium; RA, right atrium; RAA, right atrial appendage; RPA, right pulmonary artery; RSVC, right superior vena cava. (3) Ao, aorta; MPA, main pulmonary artery; MV, mitral valve; PV, pulmonary valve; TV, tricuspid valve. (4) ALPM, anterolateral papillary muscle; PMPM, postero-medial papillary muscle. *Source:* Reproduced from Lai and Ko (2016)/with permission of John Wiley & Sons.

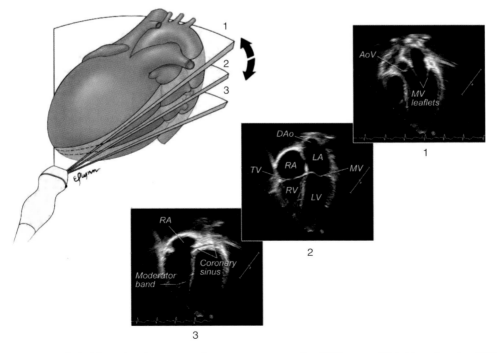

Figure 8.4 Apical four-chamber sweep; shown are corresponding TTE images. (1) AoV, aortic valve; MV leaflets, mitral valve leaflets. (2) DAo, descending thoracic aorta; LA, left atrium; LV, left ventricle; MV, mitral valve; RA, right atrium; RV, right ventricle; TV, tricuspid valve. (3) RA, right atrium. *Source:* Reproduced from Lai and Ko (2016)/with permission of John Wiley & Sons.

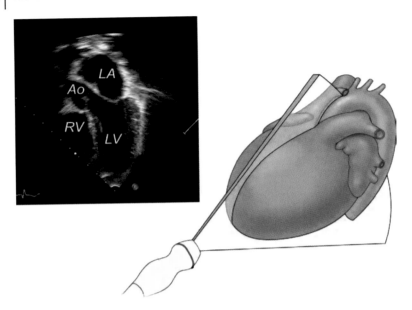

Figure 8.5 Apical long-axis view; shown is corresponding TTE image. Ao, aorta; LA, left atrium; LV, left ventricle; RV, right ventricle. *Source:* Reproduced from Lai and Ko (2016)/with permission of John Wiley & Sons.

Figure 8.6 Parasternal long-axis sweep; shown are corresponding TTE images. (1) LV, left ventricle; RA, right atrium; RV, right ventricle; TV, tricuspid valve; VS, ventricular septum. (2) Ao, aortic valve; CS, coronary sinus; DAo, descending aorta; LA, left atrium; LV, left ventricle; MV, mitral valve, RV, right ventricle. (3) LV, left ventricle; MPA, main pulmonary artery; PV, pulmonary valve; RVOT, right ventricular outflow tract; VS, ventricular septum. *Source:* Reproduced from Lai and Ko (2016)/with permission of John Wiley & Sons.

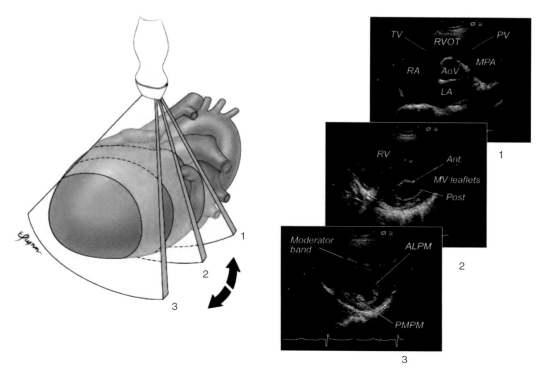

Figure 8.7 Parasternal short-axis sweep; shown are corresponding TTE images. (1) AoV, aortic valve; LA, left atrium; MPA, main pulmonary artery; PV, pulmonary valve; RA, right atrium; RVOT, right ventricular outflow tract; TV, tricuspid valve. (2) Ant. MV, anterior mitral valve; Post. MV, posterior mitral valve; RV, right ventricle. (3) ALPM, anterolateral papillary muscle; PMPM, posteromedial papillary muscle. *Source:* Reproduced from Lai and Ko (2016)/with permission of John Wiley & Sons.

Figure 8.8 Suprasternal notch aortic arch view; shown is corresponding TTE image. LA, left atrium; LCCA, left common carotid artery; LIV, left innominate vein; LSCA, left subclavian artery; RA, right atrium; RIA, right innominate artery; RPA, right pulmonary artery. *Source:* Reproduced from Lai and Ko (2016)/with permission of John Wiley & Sons.

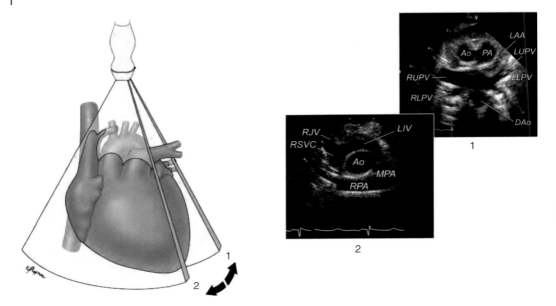

Figure 8.9 Suprasternal view of pulmonary veins; shown are corresponding TTE images. (1) Ao, aorta; DAo, descending aorta; LAA, left atrial appendage; LLPV, left lower pulmonary vein; LUPV, left upper pulmonary vein; PA, pulmonary artery; RLPV, right lower pulmonary vein; RUPV, right upper pulmonary vein. (2) Ao, aorta; LIV, left innominate vein; MPA, main pulmonary artery; RJV, right jugular vein; RPA, right pulmonary artery; RSVC, right superior vena cava. *Source:* Reproduced from Lai and Ko (2016)/with permission of John Wiley & Sons.

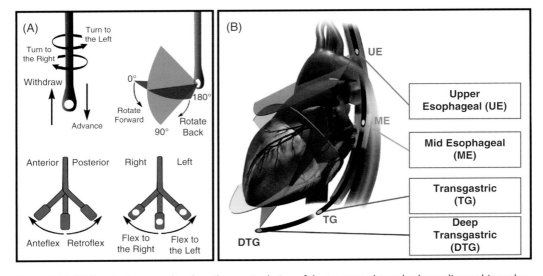

Figure 8.10 (A) Terminology used to describe manipulation of the transesophageal echocardiographic probe. (B) The four standard transducer positions within the esophagus and stomach. The associated imaging planes for each of the defined positions are depicted by the corresponding-colored quadrants. *Source:* Reproduced from Puchalski et al. (2019)/with permission of Elsevier.

A. Multiplane angle 0

B. Multiplane angle 90

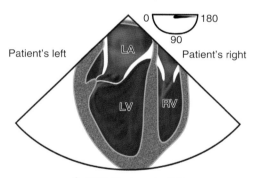

C. Multiplane angle 180

Figure 8.11 Conventional display and orientation of TEE images with transducer location and vertex of the image quadrant at the top of the display. A, B, and C depict image display and orientation at multiplane angles of 0°, 90°, and 180° respectively. *Source:* Reproduced from Puchalski et al. (2019)/with permission of Elsevier.

and children. Two-dimensional TEE probes are available as a micro-multiplane probe for patients >2.5 kg, and a mini-multiplane probe for patients >3.0–3.5 kg. The adult 2D and 3D TEE probes are available for use in patients >25 kg and >30 kg, respectively.

These probes possess two-dimensional, continuous-wave (CW) Doppler, pulsed-wave (PW) Doppler, color flow (CF) Doppler, and M-mode capabilities. Although intraoperative TEE can be performed safely in the smallest patients (2.5–3.5 kg), caution must be exercised as the presence of the probe in the esophagus may cause tracheal and bronchial compression with compromise of ventilation, inadvertent tracheal extubation, right main stem bronchial intubation, esophageal perforation, aortic arch compression with loss of distal perfusion, and compression of the left atrium resulting in left atrial hypertension or compromise of ventricular filling. In particular, ante- or retroflexion of the probe must be performed with caution in small patients.

Absolute contraindications to placement of a TEE probe in a child under anesthesia are:

- unrepaired tracheoesophageal fistula
- esophageal obstruction or stricture
- perforated hollow viscus
- active gastric or esophageal bleeding.

Relative contraindications to placement of a TEE probe in a child under anesthesia are:

- history of esophageal or gastric surgery
- history of esophageal cancer
- esophageal varices or diverticulum
- recent gastrointestinal bleed
- active esophagitis or peptic ulcer disease
- vascular ring or aortic arch anomaly wherein placement of the probe is likely to cause airway or vascular compromise
- oropharyngeal pathology
- severe coagulopathy including significant thrombocytopenia
- cervical spine injury or anomaly
- limited esophageal windows due to previous gastrostomy or fundoplication.

Intraoperative TEE has a major impact on post-CPB decision making (such as return to CPB to repair residual lesions) in approximately 15% of cases when it is used nonselectively. TEE is particularly useful in cases involving the repair of a semilunar or

Imaging plane	3D model	2D TEE image	Acquisition protocol	Structures imaged

Midesophageal views

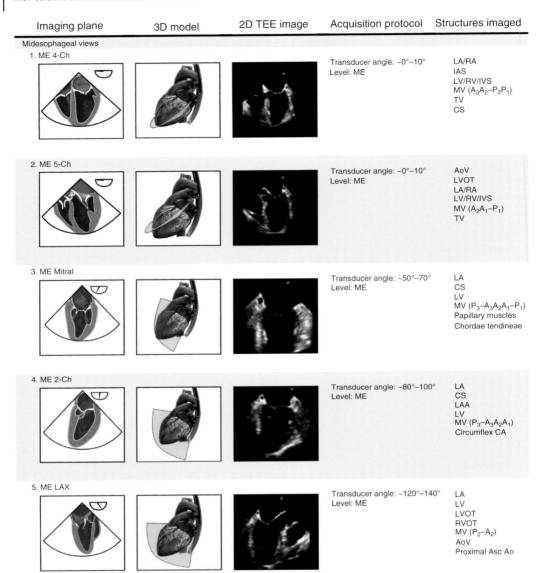

1. ME 4-Ch

Transducer angle: ~0°–10°
Level: ME

LA/RA
IAS
LV/RV/IVS
MV (A_3A_2–P_2P_1)
TV
CS

2. ME 5-Ch

Transducer angle: ~0°–10°
Level: ME

AoV
LVOT
LA/RA
LV/RV/IVS
MV (A_2A_1–P_1)
TV

3. ME Mitral

Transducer angle: ~50°–70°
Level: ME

LA
CS
LV
MV (P_3–$A_3A_2A_1$–P_1)
Papillary muscles
Chordae tendineae

4. ME 2-Ch

Transducer angle: ~80°–100°
Level: ME

LA
CS
LAA
LV
MV (P_3–$A_3A_2A_1$)
Circumflex CA

5. ME LAX

Transducer angle: ~120°–140°
Level: ME

LA
LV
LVOT
RVOT
MV (P_2–A_2)
AoV
Proximal Asc Ao

Figures 8.12–8.17 The 28 views included in a comprehensive TEE exam. Shown from left to right for each view depiction is the imaging plane, a 3D model of probe position and the corresponding image plane, a 2D TEE image, the acquisition protocol, and the structures imaged. 2D, two-dimensional; 3D, three-dimensional; AoV, aortic valve; Asc. Ao, ascending aorta; CA, coronary artery; CHD, congenital heart disease; CS, coronary sinus; DTG, deep transgastric; IAS, interatrial septum; IVC, inferior vena cava; IVS, interventricular septum; LA, left atrium; LAA, left atrial appendage; LAX, long axis; LCA, left coronary artery; LLPV, left lower pulmonary vein; LUPV, left upper pulmonary vein; LV, left ventricle; LVOT, left ventricular outflow tract; ME, midesophageal; MV, mitral valve; PA, pulmonary artery; PV, pulmonary valve; RA, right atrium; RAA, right atrial appendage; RCA, right coronary artery; RLPV, right lower pulmonary vein; RUPV, right upper pulmonary vein; RV, right ventricle; RVOT, right ventricular outflow tract; SAX, short axis; SVC, superior vena cava; TG, transgastric; TTE, transthoracic echocardiography; TEE, transesophageal echocardiography; TV, tricuspid valve; UE, upper esophageal. *Source:* Reproduced from Puchalski et al. (2019)/with permission of Elsevier.

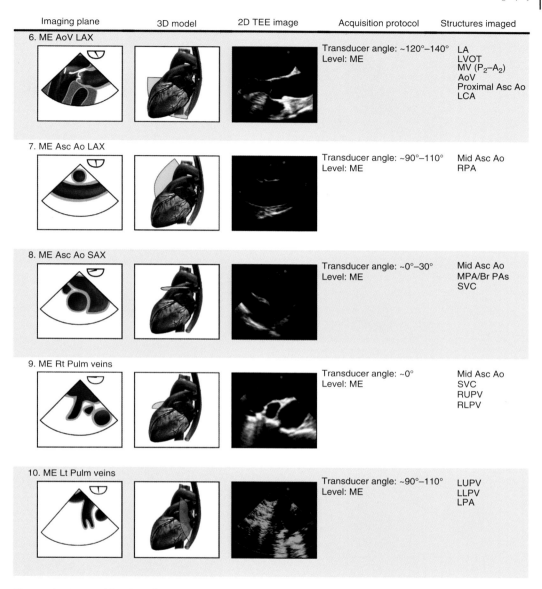

Imaging plane	3D model	2D TEE image	Acquisition protocol	Structures imaged
6. ME AoV LAX			Transducer angle: ~120°–140° Level: ME	LA LVOT MV (P_2–A_2) AoV Proximal Asc Ao LCA
7. ME Asc Ao LAX			Transducer angle: ~90°–110° Level: ME	Mid Asc Ao RPA
8. ME Asc Ao SAX			Transducer angle: ~0°–30° Level: ME	Mid Asc Ao MPA/Br PAs SVC
9. ME Rt Pulm veins			Transducer angle: ~0° Level: ME	Mid Asc Ao SVC RUPV RLPV
10. ME Lt Pulm veins			Transducer angle: ~90°–110° Level: ME	LUPV LLPV LPA

Figures 8.12–8.17 (Continued)

atrioventricular valve, complex ventricular outflow tract reconstructions, and for the delineation of a complicated anatomy that cannot be completely delineated with transthoracic echocardiography (TTE) preoperatively. In the subset of patients undergoing valve repair and outflow tract reconstruction, TEE provides the best immediate assessment of adequacy of the operative procedure and, if necessary, directs its revision. TEE is less helpful in the assessment of residual arch obstruction following aortic arch reconstruction, such as after a Stage 1 procedure, as this area is poorly visualized. While the detection of retained intracardiac air is certainly facilitated using intraoperative TEE, it remains to be determined what role the technology will play in improving cardiac

Imaging plane	3D model	2D TEE image	Acquisition protocol	Structures imaged

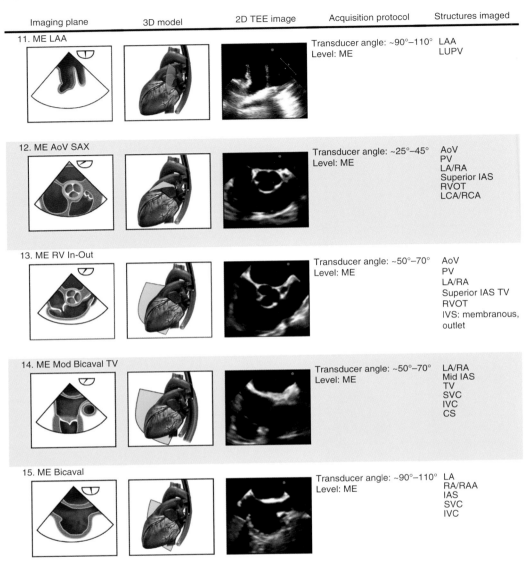

11. ME LAA — Transducer angle: ~90°–110° Level: ME — LAA, LUPV

12. ME AoV SAX — Transducer angle: ~25°–45° Level: ME — AoV, PV, LA/RA, Superior IAS, RVOT, LCA/RCA

13. ME RV In-Out — Transducer angle: ~50°–70° Level: ME — AoV, PV, LA/RA, Superior IAS TV, RVOT, IVS: membranous, outlet

14. ME Mod Bicaval TV — Transducer angle: ~50°–70° Level: ME — LA/RA, Mid IAS, TV, SVC, IVC, CS

15. ME Bicaval — Transducer angle: ~90°–110° Level: ME — LA, RA/RAA, IAS, SVC, IVC

Figures 8.12–8.17 (Continued)

de-airing algorithms, particularly in neonates and infants.

The role of TEE in the detection of residual ventricular septal defects (VSDs) following the repair of both simple and complex defects deserves some discussion. Residual defects <3 mm are detectable by TEE but generally do not require immediate reoperation as they are hemodynamically insignificant. The majority (75%) of these small defects are not present at the time of hospital discharge, as determined by TTE. Residual defects of 3–4 mm detected by TEE require further analysis with intraoperative oximetry to determine the ratio of pulmonary to systemic blood flow (Q_P:Q_S) and hemodynamic data to measure left atrial pressure (LAP) and pulmonary artery pressure (PAP). A residual defect ≥4 mm or a lesion associated with a Q_P:Q_S >1.5:1 likely requires a return to CPB for an additional attempt at closure.

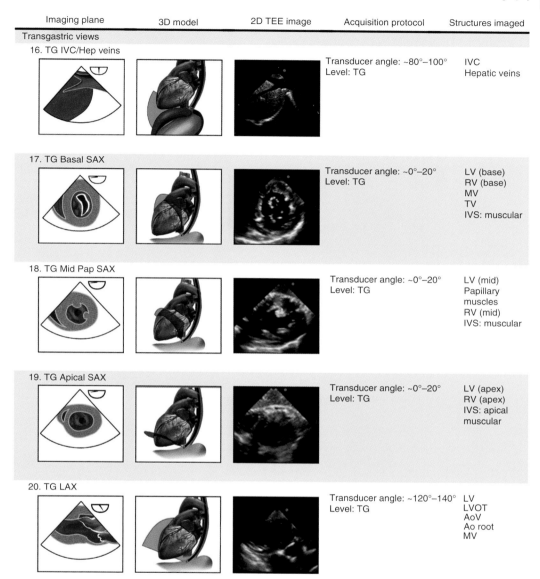

Imaging plane	3D model	2D TEE image	Acquisition protocol	Structures imaged
Transgastric views				
16. TG IVC/Hep veins			Transducer angle: ~80°–100° Level: TG	IVC Hepatic veins
17. TG Basal SAX			Transducer angle: ~0°–20° Level: TG	LV (base) RV (base) MV TV IVS: muscular
18. TG Mid Pap SAX			Transducer angle: ~0°–20° Level: TG	LV (mid) Papillary muscles RV (mid) IVS: muscular
19. TG Apical SAX			Transducer angle: ~0°–20° Level: TG	LV (apex) RV (apex) IVS: apical muscular
20. TG LAX			Transducer angle: ~120°–140° Level: TG	LV LVOT AoV Ao root MV

Figures 8.12–8.17 (Continued)

Epicardial Echocardiography

Transesophageal echocardiography imaging of some cardiac structures, such as the distal ascending aorta, aortic arch, right ventricular outflow tract, and pulmonary artery bifurcation, may be suboptimal due to the interposition of the trachea and main bronchi between the transducer and structures of interest. In addition, it may be difficult to align the Doppler beam parallel to some cardiac structures, resulting in Doppler spectra that will underestimate the true velocity and thus the calculated gradient. Surgeon-performed epicardial imaging can be used as an adjuvant to TEE imaging to overcome these limitations. It provides an unlimited number of imaging

Imaging plane	3D model	2D TEE image	Acquisition protocol	Structures imaged
Deep transgastric views				
21. DTG 5-Ch			Transducer angle: ~0°–20° Level: DTG	LV/RV LVOT AoV Ao root MV IVS
22. DTG RVOT			Transducer angle: ~50°–90° Level: DTG	LV/RV RVOT PV LVOT AoV MV IVS
23. DTG Atr Sept			Transducer angle: ~80°–90° Level: DTG	RA/RAA LA RPA IAS SVC IVC
Upper esophageal views				
24. UE Ao Arch LAX			Transducer angle: ~0°–10° Level: UE	Ao arch Innominate vein
25. UE Ao Arch SAX			Transducer angle: ~70°–90° Level: UE	Ao arch Innominate vein MPA Br PAs PV

Figures 8.12–8.17 (Continued)

planes and allows the surgeon to perform a goal-directed interrogation of the cardiac structures of particular concern. Some institutions have a standardized epicardial echocardiography (e-Echo) protocol for assessment of Stage 1 repairs and determination of a technical performance score.

Goals of a Comprehensive Echocardiographic Exam

Following a comprehensive TEE or TTE exam, segmental anatomy (atria, ventricle, great vessels) should be defined by the three-letter system outlined in Table 8.1.

Imaging plane	3D model	2D TEE image	Acquisition protocol	Structures imaged

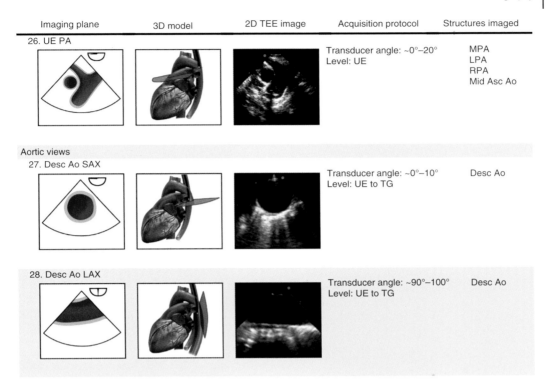

26. UE PA

Transducer angle: ~0°–20°
Level: UE

MPA
LPA
RPA
Mid Asc Ao

Aortic views

27. Desc Ao SAX

Transducer angle: ~0°–10°
Level: UE to TG

Desc Ao

28. Desc Ao LAX

Transducer angle: ~90°–100°
Level: UE to TG

Desc Ao

Figures 8.12–8.17 (Continued)

Table 8.1 Segmental anatomy.

Structure	Location	Nomenclature
Atria	RA rightward LA leftward	S (situs solitus)
	RA leftward LA rightward	I (situs invertus)
	Ambiguous systemic and pulmonary venous connections and ambiguous atrial anatomy	A (situs ambiguous, heterotaxy)
Ventricles	RV anterior and rightward LV posterior and leftward	D (dextro) loop
	RV anterior and leftward LV posterior and rightward	L (levo) loop
Great Vessels	Normal aortic/PA relationship	S
	Aorta anterior and rightward of PA	D transposition
	Aorta anterior and leftward of PA	L transposition

LA, left atrium; LV, left ventricle; PA, pulmonary artery; RA, right atrium; RV, right ventricle.

Thus, a normal heart would have (S,D,S) segmental anatomy while D-transposition would give (S,D,D) segmental anatomy. Whereas most people with normal segmental anatomy do not have congenital heart disease, a patient with segmental anatomy other than (S,D,S) is likely to have significant congenital heart disease. That said, most patients with congenital heart disease (HLHS, TOF, ASD, VSD, CAVC) have normal segmental anatomy.

Atrial Identity and Location

The identity of the atrial chamber can best be determined by examining appendage anatomy. The right atrial appendage (RAA) is best seen in the transverse plane. Flexion of the probe will allow better visualization. The RAA has the following characteristics:

- a broad junction with the right atrium (RA)
- it is short and blunt (Snoopy's nose).

The left atrial appendage is seen in multiple views. It has the following characteristics:

- a narrow junction with the LA
- it is long, narrow, and crenulated (Snoopy's ear).

The SVC and IVC normally return to the RA, as does the coronary sinus when it is not unroofed into the posterior wall of the LA. The pulmonary veins normally return to the LA. The RA will have a Eustachian valve; the LA septal surface has the flap of the fossa ovalis.

In patients with heterotaxy syndrome, both atria have systemic and pulmonary venous connections and the atria themselves may have ambiguous morphology. The entry points of the SVC and pulmonary veins into the atrial chambers can exhibit considerable variability in heterotaxy syndrome. In some of these patients, the IVC is interrupted between the kidneys and liver and the hepatic veins drain directly either to the floor of the right-sided atrium (situs solitus) or the left-sided atrium (situs invertus). The infrahepatic portion of the IVC drains via the azygous or hemiazygous system to a right- or left-sided SVC.

Ventricular Size and Identity

A chamber is considered a ventricle if it receives more than 50% of the ventricular inlet (fibrous ring of an AV valve). The AV valve need not be patent for the chamber to be considered a ventricle, as is the case with tricuspid or mitral atresia. Likewise, the chamber does not need to be large to be considered a ventricle, as is the case with hypoplastic left heart syndrome. In the absence of any AV connection (as in double inlet LV), the chamber is called a bulboventricular foramen (BVF).

The right and left ventricles have different morphologies.

- Right ventricle:
  - has the tricuspid valve (three leaflets) with a chordal attachment to the septum via one of the leaflets; there are three papillary muscles that are located apically
  - the septal leaflet of the tricuspid valve inserts slightly lower on the intraventricular septum than the anterior leaflet of the mitral valve, creating the ventriculoatrial septum (VAS) which separates the RA from the LV. A defect in this area is the source of a Gerbode defect (LV to RA shunt)
  - has a triangular shape and a trabeculated endocardial surface
  - has the moderator band, a band of tissue that stretches from the lower intraventricular septum to the anterior RV wall and is best seen in the four-chamber view with retroflexion of the TEE probe
  - there is conus or an infundibulum in the RV; this creates a lack of fibrous continuity between the tricuspid valve and pulmonary valve.
- Left ventricle:
  - has the mitral valve (two leaflets) with no chordal attachment to the septum; there are two papillary muscles that are located at the junction of the apical and middle two-thirds of the chamber

- has an ellipsoid shape and a smooth endocardial surface
- there is no conus or infundibulum in the LV; as a result, there is fibrous continuity between the mitral valve and aortic valve.

Atrioventricular Relationship

Normally there is atrioventricular concordance (RA to RV, LA to LV) due to the presence of situs solitus and D loop ventricles; atrioventricular concordance can also exist in the presence of situs invertus and L loop ventricles. Atrioventricular discordance (RA to LV, LA to RV) exists in the presence of situs solitus and L loop ventricles or situs invertus and D loop ventricles. It is important to remember that the morphology of the AV valve in both atrioventricular concordance and atrioventricular discordance is determined by the morphology of the corresponding ventricle, *not* the atria.

Great Vessel Orientation and Identity

Normally, the great vessels are oriented at 45° to each other when they leave the heart, with the pulmonary artery (PA) anterior to the aorta. When they are viewed echocardiographically, one vessel will be observed in the short axis and the other will have a sausage shape. When the great vessels are transposed, they are oriented parallel to each other when they leave the heart. When they are viewed echocardiographically, both vessels will be observed in the same axis. The rule of thumb when viewing transposed vessels in the short axis is that the anterior vessel is invariably the aorta. When the vessels are aligned side by side, the determination is more difficult and usually requires finding the arch of the aorta, the coronary arteries, or the branch pulmonary arteries to make the determination.

After the great vessels are identified, their relationship to the ventricles must be delineated. This requires creativity in finding the views that allow this connection to be seen.

Ventriculoarterial Relationship

Normally there is ventriculoarterial concordance (RV to PA, LV to Ao); ventriculoarterial discordance (LV to PA, RV to Ao) is transposition. If the aorta is anterior and rightward of the PA, it is dextro (D); if the aorta is anterior and leftward of the PA, it is levo (L). As a rule, it is the relationship of the great arteries to each other (side by side, anterior/posterior) and to the ventricles that determines the relationship of the great vessels to a VSD rather than the position of the VSD itself. For example, in double outlet RV (DORV), what determines whether a VSD is subpulmonary or subaortic is both the position of the VSD (it is usually conoventricular) and the position of the great vessels relative to the VSD. Another key feature in DORV is the presence of bilateral conus; neither the tricuspid valve nor the mitral valve is in fibrous continuity with the pulmonary valve or the aortic valve.

In tetralogy of Fallot there is aortic override over the RV but the mitral valve is in fibrous continuity with the aortic valve (NOT DORV). In d-transposition of the great arteries (D-TGA), there is fibrous continuity between the mitral valve and pulmonary valve and conus between the tricuspid valve and aortic valve (NOT DORV).

Presence of Intracardiac Shunts and Obstructive Lesions

Color flow (CF) Doppler is indispensable in identifying intracardiac shunts, including those not seen with two-dimensional imaging. Continuous-wave (CW) Doppler is useful in determining velocities and gradients across restrictive communications or valves, whereas pulsed-wave (PW) Doppler can be used to assess less restrictive orifices as well as hepatic and pulmonary venous blood flow. The RVOT must be examined carefully for both dynamic and fixed obstructive lesions. Two-dimensional echocardiography in combination with Doppler will clearly delineate dynamic obstructive lesions. The use of CW Doppler to determine intracardiac pressures is also valuable. Do not forget to look for a PDA.

Evaluation of the Surgical Repair

A comprehensive preoperative TEE study is the foundation of repair assessment. This allows the operator to focus the examination on the repaired lesions. Look for the common things, detailed below.

Patch Leaks

After ventricular septal defect (VSD) and atrial septal defect (ASD) repairs, detection of residual VSD leaks can be more difficult than it sounds, because the VSD patch produces areas of echo attenuation in the RV and RVOT that may mask leaks. Multiplane imaging improves detection but does not completely resolve this problem. It may be difficult to distinguish CFD flow from a perimembranous VSD from a TR jet. CW Doppler, however, can be useful in this scenario. For example, assuming:

Systolic blood pressure = 120 mmHg
RVSP = 39 mmHg
CVP =14 mmHg

If the peak velocity by CW Doppler is 4.5 m/sec, then the gradient is 81 mmHg and the defect is a VSD. If the peak velocity is 2.5 m/sec, then the gradient is 25 mmHg and the defect is TR.

Baffle Obstruction
- Fontan baffle evaluation requires careful examination with CF Doppler, looking for subtle evidence of flow acceleration in what is a low-velocity venous pathway. In addition, the baffle fenestration, if present, must be evaluated for patency, pressure gradient, and direction of flow.
- Senning, Mustard (baffling of systemic and pulmonary venous blood).

Stenotic Valves
After valvuloplasty regarding mitral stenosis, the following grades are generally used.

- Insignificant = pulsed/CW Doppler mean gradient ≤5 mmHg.
- Potentially significant = pulsed/CW Doppler mean gradient of 5–8 mmHg.
- Significant = pulsed/CW Doppler mean gradient of >8 mmHg. A mean mitral valve inflow gradient of more than 5–7 mmHg has been suggested as a cut-off point for consideration of further repair or valve replacement.

Regurgitant Valves
- After valvuloplasty but also after transvalvular approaches to lesions (such as transtricuspid or pulmonary valve approach to a VSD).
- Regarding mitral regurgitation, the following classifications are generally used in conjunction with objective data such as the width of the vena contracta.
  - Insignificant = absent or trivial regurgitation jet width (<2 mm) by color Doppler at the level of the valve leaflets.
  - Potentially significant = regurgitant jet width 2–4 mm by color Doppler at the level of the valve leaflets.
  - Significant = regurgitant jet width >4 mm by color Doppler at the level of the valve leaflets. Return to bypass for further correction or valve replacement is often considered for more than mild MR, due to the increased risk for reoperation.

Stenotic Anastomoses
- Pulmonary vein anastomosis to LA in total or partially anomalous pulmonary venous return.
- SVC to PA in bidirectional cavopulmonary connection and Fontan.
- Residual outflow tract gradients:
  - after tetralogy of Fallot repairs
  - after resection of subaortic membranes or LVOT reconstruction.

- Residual gradients across fenestrated atrial or ventricular septum (TOF repair).
- Residual gradients across ASD or VSD left open in the course of a staged repair (tricuspid atresia, TOF with pulmonary atresia, hypoplastic left heart syndrome).
- Coronary artery imaging and patency: must be evaluated following any procedure involving coronary artery reimplantation or translocation:
  - arterial switch for transposition of the great vessels
  - aortic translocation such as Nikaidoh procedure
  - Ross procedure (transplantation of the pulmonic valve to the aortic valve position and creation of an RV-to-PA conduit)
  - anomalous aortic origin of a coronary artery (AAOCA)
  - anomalous origin of the left or right coronary artery from the pulmonary artery (ALCAPA and ARCAPA).

Ventricular Function Assessment
- After all repairs.
- Particular attention should be paid to (1) patients with reimplanted or translocated coronary arteries and (2) patients who may have had air in the coronary arteries during the de-airing process.

Patency of Aortopulmonary Shunts
Continuous-wave Doppler will detect a high-velocity signal with flow in systole and diastole. CF Doppler will help position the CW Doppler beam.

Patency of Cavopulmonary Shunts
Pulsed-wave Doppler will reveal a phasic venous blood flow pattern that exhibits respiratory variation.

References and Further Reading

Lai, W.W. & Ko, H.H. The normal pediatric echocardiogram. In: Lai, W.W., Mertens, L.L., Cohen, M.S. & Geva, T. (eds) *Echocardiography in Pediatric and Congenital Heart Disease: From Fetus to Adult*, 2nd edn. John Wiley & Sons, Chichester (2016).

Puchalski, M.D., Lui, G., Miller-Hance, W. *et al.* Guidelines for performing a comprehensive transesophageal echocardiographic examination in children and all patients with congenital heart disease: recommendations from the American Society of Echocardiography. *J Am Soc Echocardiogr* **32**, 173–215 (2019).

Stern, K.W.D., Emani, S.M., Peek, G.J., Geva, T. & Kutty, S. Epicardial echocardiography in pediatric and congenital heart surgery. *World J Pediatr Congenit Heart Surg* **10**, 343–350 (2019).

9

Risk Scoring Systems in Patients with Congenital Heart Disease

Risk scores have been developed to predict perioperative morbidity and mortality in children with CHD undergoing cardiac surgery or diagnostic and interventional cardiac catheterization procedures. Scores have also been developed to delineate risk for patients with CHD undergoing noncardiac procedures. Development of a risk assessment tool requires rigorous statistical analysis to derive the components of the score from a representative derivation cohort, followed by validation of the score in a separate validation cohort.

Cardiac Surgery

The Society of Thoracic Surgeons European Association for Thoracic Surgery (STAT) mortality category groups operative procedures into five risk categories, with group 1 having the lowest mortality risk and 5 having the highest (www.sts.org/sites/default/files/CHSD%20Appendix%20C%20-%20STAT%20Categories.pdf).

The Society of Thoracic Surgeons Congenital Heart Surgery Database provides risk-adjusted mortality rates defined by patient age and primary procedure. Other risk scores include Risk Adjustment for Congenital Heart Surgery (RACHS) which groups operative procedures into six categories based on mortality (Table 9.1).

Catheterization

The Congenital Cardiac Catheterization Project on Outcomes (C3PO) includes four procedure-type risk categories with cases classified based on the expected risk of clinically important adverse events (AEs). However, C3PO is not structured to account for advancements in technology and new interventions.

Other procedure risk category methodologies have also been developed by the Congenital Cardiac Interventional Study Consortium (CCISC) and the Improving Pediatric and Adult Congenital Treatment (IMPACT) registries. The CCISC model, Catheterization Risk Score for Pediatrics (CRISP), which was developed in 2015, uses only three categories of procedure risk (Table 9.2). Similar to C3PO, it is not structured to assess the risk of new interventions. In addition, the hemodynamic risk component used in C3PO, CRISP, and IMPACT assigns equal significance to all abnormal hemodynamic variables.

More recently, the Procedural Risk in Congenital Cardiac Catheterization (PREDIC3T) score was created (Table 9.3). Multivariate analysis of the PREDIC3T score, the hemodynamic vulnerability score, and age has been conducted to provide odds ratios for the occurrence of high-severity adverse events (Table 9.4).

Table 9.1 Individual procedures by RACHS category.

RACHS category	Procedure	RACHS category	Procedure
1	PDA >30 d Coarctation >30 d ASD	4	Truncus arterio repair Double switch Hypoplastic arch repair Unifocalization Rastelli ASO/VSD Konno Atrial septectomy
2	VSD TOF Vascular ring Coarctation <30 d AP window	5	TV repositioning Ebstein anomaly <30 d Truncus/IAA
3	ASO TOF/PA Ross ALCAPA DORV repair Coarctation/VSD BTS CAVC	6	Norwood procedure DKS

PDA, patent ductus arteriosus; ASD, atrial septal defect; VSD, ventricular septal defect; TOF, tetralogy of Fallot; AP, aortopulmonary; ASO, arterial switch operation; PA, pulmonary atresia; ALCAPA, anomalous left coronary artery to the pulmonary artery; DORV, double outlet right ventricle; BTS, Blalock–Taussig shunt; CAVC, complete atrioventricular canal; PAB, pulmonary artery band; TV, tricuspid valve; DKS, Damus–Kaye–Stansel.

Table 9.2 Calculation of the risk score for the original 20-point risk score.

Assigned points	0	1	2
Patient status/timing (X_1)	Elective	Emergent/urgent	Postoperative
Age (X_2)	>1 year	30 days–1 year	<30 days
Weight (X_3)	>10 kg	2.5–10 kg	<2.5 kg
Inotropic support (X_4)	None	Yes–stable	Yes–unstable or ECMO
Respiratory status (X_5)	Own airway	Stable on ventilator or known difficult/unusual airway	Respiratory failure on mechanical ventilation
Systemic illness/failure (X_6)	None	Medically controlled or 1 organ system failure	Uncontrolled or >1 organ system failure
ASA score (X_7)	1 or 2	3	4 or 5
Physiologic category (X_8)	Category 1	Category 2	Category 3
Precatheterization diagnosis (X_9)	Category 1	Category 2	Category 3
Procedure risk category (X_{10})	Category 1	Category 2	Category 3

ASA, American Society of Anesthesiologists; ECMO, extracorporeal membrane oxygenator/mechanical cardiopulmonary support.

Table 9.3 PREDIC3T case-type risk categories.

	Risk category 0	Risk category 1	Risk category 2	Risk category 3	Risk category 4	Risk category 5
Diagnostic case		Diagnostic ≥1 y	Diagnostic 1 mo to <1 y	Diagnostic ≤30 d		
Valvuloplasty		Pulmonary valvuloplasty >30 d	Pulmonary valvuloplasty + procedure >30 d	Pulmonary valvuloplasty +/− procedure ≤30 d		Aortic valvuloplasty +/− procedure, ≤30 d Aortic valvuloplasty +/− procedure, >30 d Mitral valvuloplasty Atretic valve perfomation with or without valvuloplasty
Device of coil closure		Fontan fenestration or baffle leak device closure	ASD or PFO closure Venous collateral occlusion PDA closure	Fontan fenestration or baffle leak device closure+ Systematic pulmonary collateral closure +/− procedure	ASD or PFO closure+ procedure	VSD closure
Balloon angioplasty and/ or stent placement				Pulmonary artery (1 vessel) + RVCT conduit dilation/stent Aorta (coarctation) dilation and/or stent	Pulmonary artery (1 vessel) + procedure Pulmonary artery (>2 vessels) Pulmonary vein dilation and/or stent RVOT conduit dilation and/or stent POA dilation and/or stent	Pulmonary artery (≥2 vessels) +RVOT +/− procedure Aorta (coarctation dilation and/or stent procedure
Other	Endomyo-cardial biopsy with coronary angiography			Atrial septostomy		Atrial septostomy + procedure TPV implantation +/− procedure Atrial septum static dilation and/or stent placement

ASD, atrial septal I defect; PDA, patent ductus arteriosus; PFO, patent foramen ovale; RVOT, right ventricular outflow tract; TPV, transcatheter pulmonary valve; VSD, ventricular septal defect.

C-statistic 0.716, 96% bootstrapped CI (0.705–0.732).

Noncardiac Procedures

Using the large ACS NSQIP database (www.facs.org/quality-programs/data-and-registries/acs-nsqip/) and the NSQIP

Table 9.4 Multivariate analysis of predictors for outcome of high-severity (level 3/4/5) adverse events.

	OR (95% CI)	P value
PREDICT case-type risk category		
0		
1		
2		
3		
4		
5		
Hemodynamic vulnerability score		
0	1.00	. . .
1	1.27 (1.07–1.50)	0.006
2	1.89 (1.60–2.23)	<0.001
≥3	2.03 (1.71–2.42)	<0.001
Age		
<1 mo	1.47 (1.21–1.79)	<0.001
1–11 mo	1.18 (1.01–1.39)	0.041
1–18 y	1.00	. . .
≥19 y	1.51 (1.25–1.82)	<0.001

C-statistic 0.74. OR, odds ratio.

definitions of mild, moderate, and severe CHD based on residual lesion burden and functional capacity, a rigorously derived risk assessment model for in-hospital mortality following noncardiac surgical procedures in children with major and severe CHD was developed. A derivation cohort of 4375 (ACS NSQIP years 2012–2013) and a validation cohort of 2869 (ACS NSQIP year 2014) patients were used. Multivariable analysis was utilized to predict mortality and eight preoperative predictors were retained in a final multivariable logistic regression model as summarized in Table 9.5.

These variables were used to create a risk stratification score ranging from 0 to 10 that showed very good calibration and discrimination in the validation cohort (area under the curve: 0.831 [95% CI 0.787–0.875]). Scores ≤3 were associated with low risk of mortality (OR 1.54, 95% CI 0.78–3.04), scores ranging from 4 to 6 were associated with medium risk (OR 4.19, 95% CI 2.56–6.87), and scores ≥7 were associated with high risk (OR 22.15, 95% CI 15.06–32.59). The influence of surgical complexity, as defined by both RVUs and surgical specialty on outcome, were not sufficiently strong to be retained in the final model. Both survivors and nonsurvivors underwent surgery of similar complexity as defined by RVUs. This suggests that the presence of major and severe CHD is

Table 9.5 Mutivariate risk stratification to predict postoperative mortality.

Variable	B (SE)	OR	95% CI	P	Risk score
Emergency procedure	0.50 (0.17)	1.66	1.19–2.31	0.003	+1
Severe CHD	0.50 (0.19)	1.65	1.15–2.39	0.007	+1
Single-ventricle physiology	0.61 (0.26)	1.83	1.10–3.06	0.020	+1
Surgery within 30 days	0.70 (0.18)	2.01	1.40–2.89	<0.001	+1
Inotropic support	0.72 (0.19)	2.05	1.40–3.01	<0.001	+1
Preoperative CPR	0.90 (0.32)	2.46	1.32–4.57	0.004	+2
Acute or chronic kidney injury	1.48 (0.40)	4.42	2.00–9.75	<0.001	+3
Mechanical ventilation	2.05 (0.18)	7.80	5.42–11.21	<0.001	+4

CHD, congenital heart disease; CPR, cardiopulmonary resuscitation; SE, standard error; OR, odds ratio; CI, confidence interval.
Source: Adapted from Faraoni et al. Anesth Analg 2016.

Figure 9.1 Systematic approach to patients with congenital heart disease presenting for noncardiac procedures.

the major determinant of mortality following noncardiac surgery regardless of surgical complexity. Incorporation of intrinsic surgical risk into this model would more precisely delineate the influence of surgical complexity on outcome in this cohort.

The risk classification of patients with CHD undergoing noncardiac procedures has recently been summarized and an algorithm defined as illustrated in Figure 9.1.

References and Further Reading

Faraoni, D., Vo, D., Nasr, V. & DiNardo, J. Development and validation of a risk stratification score for children with congenital heart disease undergoing noncardiac surgery. *Anesth Analg* **123**, 824–830 (2016).

10

Mechanical Circulatory Support

Mechanical circulatory support (MCS) can be characterized into the following categories.

- Extracorporeal membrane oxygenation (ECMO)
- Ventricular assist devices (VAD):
  - Percutaneous
  - Paracorporeal
  - Intracorporeal
- Total artificial heart (TAH)

These modalities are illustrated in Figures 10.1–10.5.

Extracorporeal Membrane Oxygenation

Extracorporeal membrane oxygenation (ECMO), also known as extracorporeal life support (ECLS), is a technology used to provide cardiopulmonary (venoarterial ECMO) or pulmonary (venovenous ECMO) support for patients with cardiac, pulmonary, and cardiopulmonary failure that is unresponsive to medical therapies.

Indications

In pediatric practice, ECMO is used to provide support in a wide variety of circumstances, including respiratory failure, circulatory failure (viral myocarditis, cardiomyopathy, post cardiac surgery [postcardiotomy support]), persistent pulmonary hypertension of the newborn, meconium aspiration syndrome, respiratory distress syndrome, group B streptococcal sepsis, asphyxia, congenital diaphragmatic hernia, and sepsis. ECMO is also used to assist cardiopulmonary resuscitation (E-CPR), and as a bridge to organ transplantation and ventricular assist device placement.

Relative Contraindications

Relative contraindications to ECMO include end-stage primary disease, severe neurologic injury, intracranial bleeding, prematurity (<34th week), uncontrolled visceral bleeding, low birth weight (<2 kg), and patient or family wishes.

Modes of ECMO Support

A typical ECMO circuit consists of a mechanical pump (centrifugal or roller), a membrane oxygenator, venous and arterial cannulas, a reservoir, heat exchanger, tubing, and pressure, flow and oxygen saturation monitors (Figure 10.1).

Two distinct modes of ECMO are available, namely venoarterial (VA) and venovenous (VV).

Venovenous (VV) ECMO
- Access is generally percutaneous via the internal jugular vein.
- Used for prolonged pulmonary support in patients with respiratory failure with preserved cardiac function.

The Pediatric Cardiac Anesthesia Handbook, Second Edition. Viviane G. Nasr and James A. DiNardo.
© 2025 John Wiley & Sons Ltd. Published 2025 by John Wiley & Sons Ltd.

Figure 10.1 ECMO circuit in venoarterial support mode. *Source:* Reproduced from Thiagarajan (2015)/with permission of Wolters Kluwer Health.

- Blood is drained from the venous circulation and returned to the venous circulation after exchange of oxygen and carbon dioxide in the membrane.

Venoarterial (VA) ECMO
- Access can be percutaneous via the internal jugular vein and the carotid artery, but generally direct surgical exposure of the vessels is required. In the postcardiotomy setting access is commonly obtained directly via the right atrium and aorta.
- Used for prolonged cardiac and pulmonary support.
- Blood is drained from the venous circulation and pumped into the arterial circulation after heat exchange and exchange of oxygen and carbon dioxide.
- Cardiac output is a combination of the native cardiac ejection and ECMO flow. Consequently, an appropriate quantity of alveolar ventilation is necessary when

venous blood transits the pulmonary circulation. When all venous drainage is captured, VA-ECMO closely resembles total CPB. When only a portion of venous return is captured, VA-ECMO resembles partial CPB.

The operational differences between VA-ECMO and VV-ECMO are summarized in Table 10.1, while functional differences in the physiologic parameters monitored are summarized in Table 10.2.

Device and Patient Complications

Device and patient complications are not uncommon occurrences with ECMO.
   Device complications include:

- embolism
- tube rupture
- oxygenator failure
- circuit thrombosis.

Table 10.1 Operational differences between VA-ECMO and VV-ECMO.

	VA-ECMO	VV-ECMO
Support type	Cardiac and pulmonary	Pulmonary
Cardiac support	Partial or complete	None
Cannulation sites	Venous and arterial	Venous

Table 10.2 Functional differences in physiologic parameters between VA-ECMO and VV-ECMO.

	VA-ECMO	VV-ECMO
Cardiac preload	Decreased	Unchanged
Cardiac afterload	Increased	Unchanged
Pulmonary blood flow	Decreased	Unchanged
Pulse pressure	May decrease	Unchanged
Coronary blood flow	Left ventricle (LV) ejection or ECMO flow	LV ejection

Patient complications include:

- thromboembolism
- bleeding
- hemolysis
- infection
- cerebral infarction and hemorrhage.

Common Terminology Used During an ECMO Run

- Adjust pump speed → changes flow rate.
- Adjust sweep (fresh gas flow) → changes $PaCO_2$.
- Adjust FiO_2 → changes PaO_2.
- Adjust temperature.

Intraoperative Considerations for Patients on ECMO

1) Particular attention during transport to and from the operating room is a must to avoid decannulation and kinking of the cannula.
2) Expect significant blood loss due to heparinization, thrombocytopenia, and coagulation factor deficits (ensure adequate vascular access and blood product availability).
3) Volatile agents have altered kinetics in patients on ECMO, and reduced alveolar ventilation may reduce volatile anesthetic delivery.
4) Hemodynamics of patients on VV-ECMO are dependent on their native heart function; it may become necessary to support the circulation with vasopressors and/or inotropes.
5) Patients on VA-ECMO are often receiving vasopressor/inotrope therapy before ECMO institution, and are likely to require vasopressor/inotrope therapy during the ECMO run.
6) During VA-ECMO ventricular ejection of blood, as indicated by a pulsatile arterial waveform, will occur whenever there is return of venous blood to the systemic ventricle **AND** when there is sufficient ventricular contractile function to open the aortic valve. Return of venous blood to the systemic ventricle in the absence of sufficient ventricular contractile function to open the aortic valve will result in ventricular distention.
7) During VV-ECMO and VA-ECMO runs, the lungs should be ventilated at low

settings to minimize barotrauma and volutrauma (RR <10, I:E ratio 2:1, FiO$_2$ <40%, PIP <25, PEEP 5–15).

8) Patients are most commonly anticoagulated with intravenous unfractionated heparin (UFH) but there is increasing use of the direct thombin inhibitors (DTIs) argatroban and bivalirudin. Multitest monitoring of UFH anticoagulation is summarized in Table 10.3 and is

Table 10.3 Summary of multitest monitoring of UFH anticoagulation during ECMO.

Laboratory tests	Frequency	Target range
ACT	Every 1 h for first six hours of ECMO, then every 2 h if stable	Range 180–220 s. If there is excessive bleeding decreases the target as per MD
PT / aPTT /INR	q 6-12 h	PT 10–13 s
		PTT 1.5–2.5 times normal (60–80 s) PT/INR normal or close to normal <1.5
Heparin assay unfractionated (anti-Xa)	q 6-12 h	0.3–0.7 IU /ml
Antithrombin (AT)	q 12 h, once level is therapeutic and stable:	50–80%
	q24 h	Start recombinant AT and follow protocol if low[a]
Fibrinogen/FDP	q 12–24 h	Fibrinogen >150 mg/dl (bleeding patient) >100 mg/dl (nonbleeding patient) FDP 10–40
Platelet count	q 6 h first 48 h, then q 12 h	50,000–100,000× 10^9/l unless VHA indicates need to give
		>100,000 × 10^9/l if bleeding.
ROTEM® /TEG®	Daily, PRN for severe bleeding or thrombosis(Compare with Heparinase sample)	Clotting time (CT) Normal: 5–10 min
		Clot formation time (CFT)
		Normal: 1–3 min
		Target: 3 × CFT of heparinase sample
		Alpha angle (LX) Normal: 53–72 degrees
		Max clot firmness/clot strength (MCF) Normal: 50–70 mm
		Target: >50 in bleeding
		Lysis Index 30 min after CT (LY30)
		Normal: 0–7%

[a] Based on manufacturer's recommendations.
ACT, activated clotting time; aPTT, activated partial thromboplastin time; FDP, fibrinogen degradation products; INR, international normalized ratio; PT, prothrombin time; ROTEM, rotational thromboelastometry; TEG, thromboelastography; VHA, viscoelastic hemostatic assay.
Source: Reproduced from Chegondi *et al.* (2022).

based on the inability of any one test to accurately define the anticoagulant effect of UFH and the lack of correlation between the various tests. Activated partial thromboplastin time (aPTT) is currently the standard test for monitoring DTIs, recognizing that at higher doses of DTIs, aPTT shows a nonlinear response to DTI dose.

When dosing medications, consideration should be given to the increased volume of distribution associated with the ECMO circuit and the possibility of drug adsorption to the ECMO tubing and oxygenator.

Ventricular Assist Devices

In 1967, DeBakey and colleagues used a left-atrial–axillary artery ventricular assist device (VAD) to provide postcardiotomy ventricular support to a 16-year-old girl. This was the earliest report of VAD use in a pediatric patient. Since then, major advances in technology have occurred, accompanied by improved outcomes. During the past decade, as device technology has matured, devices specifically designed for smaller pediatric patients have been developed for clinical use.

Indications

In pediatric practice, the size of the child, the indication for support, and the presumed duration of support are the important considerations when choosing a VAD.
    VAD use can be summarized as follows.

- *A bridge to recovery*: in this setting, devices suitable for short-term support are utilized with the intent to wean the patient off device support and remove the device after recovery of cardiopulmonary function. Myocarditis and postcardiotomy patients are suitable candidates for this type of support.
- *A bridge to decision*: in this setting, devices suitable for short-term support are utilized with the intent of determining over time whether patients with suspected severe end-organ dysfunction (particularly neurologic) are suitable candidates for recovery, longer term support, or cardiac transplantation.
- *A bridge to transplantation*: in this setting, devices suitable for long-term support are utilized with the intent of providing cardiopulmonary support until cardiac transplantation. Converting from a short-term device to a long-term device to await transplantation is known as "bridge-to-bridge."
- *Destination therapy*: in this setting, devices suitable for long-term support are utilized with the intent of providing permanent support for patients who are not deemed suitable candidates for cardiac transplantation.

Relative Contraindications

In complex situations such as concomitant respiratory failure, pulmonary hypertension and residual intracardiac shunts, VAD support may be contraindicated.

Current VAD and TAH Technologies

Current VAD and TAH technologies include pneumatic pulsatile flow and continuous non-pulsatile (axial or centrifugal) flow devices.

Pneumatic Pulsatile Flow Devices
- Berlin Heart EXCOR® VAD (Berlin Heart AG, Berlin, Germany) (Figure 10.2).
  - Paracorporeal.
  - LVAD (LA or LV apex to aorta), RVAD (RA to pulmonary artery), BiVAD.
  - Available in a variety of pump sizes (10, 15, 25, 30, 50 and 60 ml), making it widely applicable across age groups and patient sizes.
  - Short- to long-term support.
- Thoratec® PVAD (St Jude Medical, St Paul, MN).
  - Paracorporeal
  - LVAD (LA or LV apex to aorta), RVAD (RA to pulmonary artery), BiVAD.

Figure 10.2 The Berlin EXCOR, a pulsatile pnematically driven device providing mechanical support to the systemic ventricle (A), the Fontan pathway (B), and both (C) in a failing Fontan patient. This is a paracorporeal device and the dotted curved lines represent location of transit of device cannula through subcostal chest wall to the heart from the externally located device. *Source:* Reproduced from Buratto *et al.* (2017) /with permission of Taylor & Francis.

- Effective stroke volume of 65 ml and can deliver a cardiac output of 5–5.5 l min⁻¹. The device is limited to use in patients with a BSA greater than 0.7–0.8 m² and an age of seven years or older
- **Short to long-term support**.

• SynCardia® TAH (SynCardia Systems, Tucson, AZ) (Figure 10.3).
  - Intracorporeal.
  - Total artifical heart.
  - Two sizes (50 and 70 ml stroke volume); 70 ml model can deliver 9 l min⁻¹ of cardiac output. The 70 m pump is intended for patients with BSA ≥1.72 m² and 50 ml model for patients with BSA ≤1.85 m².
  - Short- to long-term support.

Pulsatile Pump Technology

A rigid case prosthetic ventricle is divided into a blood and a pneumatic chamber by a flexible, noncompliant diaphragm. Unidirectional inflow and outflow valves are located in the blood chamber. The pneumatic chamber communicates with the pneumatic drive system via the pneumatic driveline. As pressurized air is introduced into the pneumatic chamber, the diaphragm moves such that the blood chamber becomes pressurized as well. When the pressure in the blood chamber exceeds the device filling pressure, the inflow valve will close. When pressure in the blood chamber exceeds aortic or pulmonary artery pressure, the outflow valve opens and ejection commences. These processes constitute the isovolemic and ejection phases of systole in the prosthetic ventricle. Depending on the device, the driveline pressures are set approximately 80–100 mmHg higher than systemic systolic pressure for LVAD and 30–80 mmHg higher than pulmonary artey pressure for RVAD.

At the end of systole, air is vented passively from the pneumatic chamber to the atomosphere and the pressure in the blood chamber falls. This constitutes isovolemic relaxation.

Aorta

Venae
Cavae

Pulmonary
Artery

Right
Atrium

Left
Atrium

**Right
Ventricle**

**Left
Ventricle**

Figure 10.3 The SynCardia TAH, a pulsatile pnematically driven biventricular, intracorporeal device.
Source: Courtesy of SynCardia Systems, Tucson, AZ.

When the pressure in the chamber filling the prosthetic ventricle (right atrium, left atrium, or left ventricle) exceeds the pressure in the blood chamber, the inflow valve opens. The diaphragm is free to move in such a manner that virtually the entire volume of the prosthetic ventricle can fill with blood as all the air leaves the pneumatic chamber. This constitutes diastole in the prosthetic ventricle. Vacuum pressure of -20 to -40 mmHg. can be applied to the pneumatic chamber during diastole to promote filling.

The Berlin VAD always and the SynCardia TAH generally function in a fixed rate, variable stroke volume mode. In general, pump rates are kept low (60–80 bpm) with the percentage of systole set to equal one-half the device rate (percentage of systole at 60 bpm = 30%; percentage of systole at 80 bpm = 40%). These settings promote complete filling and emptying of the device, which is important because these devices function in fixed rate, variable stroke volume capacity. Increases in applied vacuum, higher driveline pressures, and reduced percent systole all increase the likelihood that blood trauma and hemolysis will occur.

The Thoratec PVAD can function in both the fixed rate, variable stroke volume mode and a fixed stroke volume, variable rate mode. This fill-to-empty mode is feasible because the movement of the pump diaphragm is monitored by a Hall sensor built into the rigid case. A small magnet mounted on the diaphragm triggers the Hall sensor when the two come in contact. This information is transmitted to the console via an electrical cable and allows the control console to know when the blood chamber is full, triggering ejection.

Axial Continuous Flow Devices
- Impella® 2.5/5.0/CP/RP (Abiomed, Andover, MA) (Figure 10.4).
  - Percutaneous (5.0 requires surgical cut-down).
  - LVAD: 2.5/5.0/CP (placed retrograde across aortic valve, impeller outflow above aortic valve, inflow in LV cavity).
    ○ Impella 2.5 can deliver 2.5 l min^{-1}.
    ○ Impella 5.0 can deliver 5.0 l min^{-1}.
    ○ Impella CP can deliver 4.3 l min^{-1}.
  - RVAD: RP (placed antegrade across tricuspid and pulmonary valves, impeller

A IABP **B** Impella **C** TandemHeart **D** ECMO

A TandemHeart with dual lumen cannula   **B** Impella RP

Figure 10.4 Available percutaneous mechanical circulatory assist devices for right and left heart support. The Impella is a continuous-flow axial device while ECMO and TandemHeart employ continuous-flow centrigual pumps. *Source:* Reproduced from Mandawat & Rao (2018)/with permission of American Heart Association, Inc.

outflow above pulmonary valve, inflow in RV cavity).

- ○ Impella RP can deliver 4.5 l min^{-1}.
- – Short-term support.
- HeartMate II^{TM} (Abbott Medical, Abbott Park, IL) (Figure 10.5).
  - – Intracorporeal.
  - – LVAD (LV apex to aorta).
  - – Flows of up to 10 l min^{-1} at pump speeds of 8000–10,000 rpm.
  - – Short to long-term support.

Axial Pump Technology

These compact pumps employ an impeller mechanism as the only moving part. At the proximal end of the pump, stationary airfoil-shaped vanes are used to straighten blood flow prior to entry into an impeller. The impeller then imparts radial velocity (kinetic energy) to the blood as it draws blood into the pump. At the distal end of the pump, a set of stationary diffuser (stator) vanes can be used to increase axial velocity by straightening flow. This improves conversion of kinetic energy to static pressure (potential energy) as blood leaves the pump. Axial pump rotating elements operate like a propeller in a pipe and can be viewed as a pusher. These pumps are small; the Impella crosses the aortic or pulmonary valve without inducing insufficiency and the HeartMate II is about the size of a D cell battery (Figure 10.5).

Figure 10.5 Detailed depiction of the working mechanism and placement of the HeartMate II axial continuous-flow pump (A) and the Heartmate 3 fully magnetically levitated centrifugal pump (B). *Source:* Reproduced from Mehra *et al.* (2017)/with permission of MASSACHUSETTS MEDICAL SOCIETY.

Pump output is determined by rpm and delta P (aortic pressure – LV pressure), also called the pressure head (H) (Figure 10.6). Axial flow pumps have steep pressure flow curves and as such, flow is inversely proportional to delta P. For a given arterial pressure during nonpulsatile flow, a higher pump differential pressure can only be generated by lowering ventricular pressure relative to aortic pressure. The increasing pressure differen-

tial generated as flow decreases results in much higher suction developed at the inlet during conditions of low LV volume or inlet cannula obstruction.This means axial pumps pull the hardest at the lowest flow, creating the potential for a self-latching condition wherein the pump continues to increase suction as flows fall, resulting in the ventricular wall being sucked in around the inlet. This results in suck-down of the ventricular wall

Figure 10.6 HQ curves (delta P versus flow) for a continuous-flow pump with a flat HQ curve demonstrating the relation between pump flow, rpm, and delta P (pump head). Illustrated here is the pump flow expected ($4\,l\,min^{-1}$) at a pump head pressure (delta P) of 75 mmHg and 2400 rpm. *Source:* Reproduced from Dalia *et al.* (2018)/with permission of Elsevier.

around the inflow cannula, leftward shift of the intraventricular septum septum, ventricular ectopy, and pump shutdown (Figure 10.7).

Centrifugal Continuous Flow Devices

- TandemHeart® (LivaNova, UK) (Figure 10.4).
  - Percutaneous.
  - Not magnetically levitated.
  - LVAD (LA via femoral vein and transatrial puncture to femoral artery).
  - 10 ml volume.
  - Flows up to $5\,l\,min^{-1}$.
  - Short-term support.
- CentriMag™ (Abbott Medical, Abbott Park, IL).
  - Paracorporeal.
  - Magnetically levitated.
  - LVAD (LA or LV to aorta).
  - RVAD (RA or RV to PA).
  - BiVAD.
  - 31 ml volume.
  - Flows up to 10 l min−1.
  - Short-term support.
- PediMag™ (Abbott Medical, Abbott Park, IL).
  - Paracorporeal.
  - Magnetically levitated.
  - LVAD (LA or LV to aorta).
  - RVAD (RA or RV to PA).

- BiVAD.
- 14 ml volume.
- Flows up to 1.5 l min−1.
- Short-term support.
- Rotaflow II (Maquet Cardiopulmonary, Rastatt, Germany).
  - Paracorporeal.
  - Not magnetically levitated.
  - LVAD (LA or LV to aorta).
  - RVAD (RA or RV to PA).
  - BiVAD.
  - 32 ml volume.
  - Flows up to 10 l min−1.
  - Short-term support.
- HeartMate 3™ (Figure 10.5).
  - Intracorporeal.
  - Magnetically levitated.
  - LVAD (LV to aorta).
  - Flows of up to 10 l min−1 at pump speeds of 5000–6000 rpm.
  - Short to long-term support.

Centrifugal Pump Technology

Centrifugal pumps use a constrained vortex to impart kinetic energy to fluid in a rotating head. The rotating head consists of a series of concentrically arranged cones or fins suspended within a rigid plastic shell (volute). Use of a fully magnetically levitated rotor

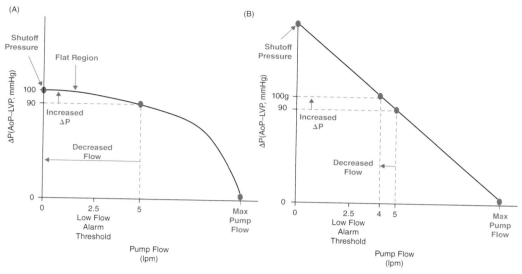

Figure 10.7 Comparison of HQ curves (delta P versus flow) for a Heartmate 3 continuous centrifugal pump (A) and a HeartMate II continuous axial pump (B). Note that the centrifugal pump has a very flat portion of its HQ curve compared to the axial pump which is consistently steep. A pump with a flat HQ curve is more sensitive to afterload (small increases in delta P lead to large reductions in pump flow) than a pump with a steep HQ curve. On the other hand, a pump with a flat HQ curve is less prone to development of a suction event and pump shutdown than a pump with a steep curve. The HeartMate 3 is unique in that it has a flatter sloped HQ curve when operating at lower flows (<4 l min^{-1}) and a steeper sloped HQ curve at higher flows (>4 l min^{-1}). *Source:* Reproduced from Belkin *et al.* (2021)/with permission of Elsevier.

creates a contact-free blood chamber due to the absence of bearings and seals, resulting in minimized blood stagnation, friction, and shear stress. Rotation of the cones or fins creates a vortex that is constrained by the rigid plastic housing. This creates lower pressure at the center of the pump than at the periphery. The pressure gradient draws blood into the center of the pump and imparts pressure to the blood as it leaves the pump at the periphery. In a centrifugal pump, its rotating elements act as a spinning disk with blades that can be viewed as a thrower.

As with axial flow pumps, centrifugal pump output is determined by rpm and inversely related to dP (aortic pressure – LV pressure). However, centrifugal flow pumps have flatter pressure–flow curves than axial pumps. A centrifugal flow pump responds only to the total differential pressure across the pump and not the absolute value of the pressures at the inlet and outlet ports. At any

given pump speed, a centrifugal pump will have the same flow at inlet and outlet pressure values respectively of 0/100, 100/200, and –50/50 mmHg, as the delta P is 100 mmHg. Because the flatter pressure–flow curve maintains a relatively fixed differential pressure even with a large drop in pump flow, no significant increase in suction pressure is generated at low-flow conditions (Figures 10.6 and 10.7).

Complications

The most common complications include bleeding, thrombosis, embolic events such as stroke, and infection.

Anesthetic Considerations for Patients Receiving VAD

End-organ dysfunction in addition to cardiac dysfunction occurs in patients supported with VAD. In particular, renal and hepatic dysfunction should be evaluated.

The preoperative evaluation includes the following factors.

- Children with a glomerular filtration rate (GFR) <60 ml min^{-1} 1.72 m^2 should be assumed to have occult renal dysfunction and are at risk for acute renal injury or failure, even if blood urea nitrogen (BUN) and creatinine levels were normal.
- A full panel of liver function tests and a full coagulation profile should be performed to rule out hepatic dysfunction.
- Levels of B-natriuretic peptide (BNP), a specific marker of elevated ventricular end-diastolic pressure, are likely to be elevated. Lethargy and anorexia in children strongly suggest the presence of a low cardiac output state.
- Particular attention should be paid during the physical examination to the assessment of arterial and venous access sites.
- A review of recent echocardiographic and cardiac catheterization data is essential.
- Pacemaker and/or implantable cardioverter defibrillators should be reprogrammed prior to surgery.
- The blood bank should be alerted to the possibility that a massive transfusion will be required. It is prudent to use leukocyte-reduced blood to minimize further antibody formation, as well as cytomegalovirus-free blood products.

Induction of Anesthesia and Pre-bypass Management

These patients have limited contractile reserve, limited preload recruitable stroke work, a limited ability to respond to acute increases or decreases in afterload, and a low cardiac output state. Thus, they require an induction that will blunt the hemodynamic response to laryngoscopy and tracheal intubation without undue myocardial depression, vasodilation, and subsequent hypotension. Detailed management of patients with severely depressed ventricular

function in covered in detail in Chapter 33 but the following basic principles apply.

- *Monitoring*: American Society of Anesthesiologists monitoring, arterial, central venous pressure catheters and transesophageal echocardiography (TEE) probe should be utilized. Preoperative inotropes should be continued.
- *Mechanical ventilation*: initiation of positive-pressure ventilation is likely to induce significant pulse pressure variation, and needs to be initiated carefully with appropriate minute ventilation provided at the lowest possible mean airway pressure. Hypoventilation and atelectasis will increase pulmonary vascular resistance.
- *Testing*: serum lactate and mixed venous oxygen saturations are monitored as indirect indicators of cardiac output. The use of the lysine analog antifibrinolytics tranexamic acid or epsilon-aminocaproic acid should be considered.

Post-VAD Placement Management

Continous-flow devices have a preload sensitivity (liters/min/mmHg) one-third to one-quarter of that seen in the native LV and an afterload sensitivity 3–4 times that seen in the native LV. Centrifugal devices are slightly less preload sensitive and slightly more afterload sensitive than axial devices. As the pump differential pressure changes between systole (smaller differential) and diastole (larger differential), pump flow is maximal during systole and lowest during diastole when LV pressure is lowest. Thus, pump flow during systole is assisted by intrinsic cardiac contraction, but flow in diastole reflects predominantly the work by the pump.

The flatter pressure–flow curves in centrifugal pumps result in larger swings in flow from ventricular systole and diastole, producing high pulsatility in pump flow in response to changing LV pressures during the cardiac cycle. Delta P is most effectively reduced by lowering aortic pressure (SVR reduction) or by increasing LV pressure (preload augmentation, LV contraction). In fact, in the presence of increased LV contractility, semipulsatile flow may occur as the result of both aortic valve opening and cyclic increases in pump output with the dP reduc-

tion that accompanies LV contraction. These differences in the performance of axial versus centrifugal continuous flow pumps are summarized in detail in Figures 10.6–10.8.

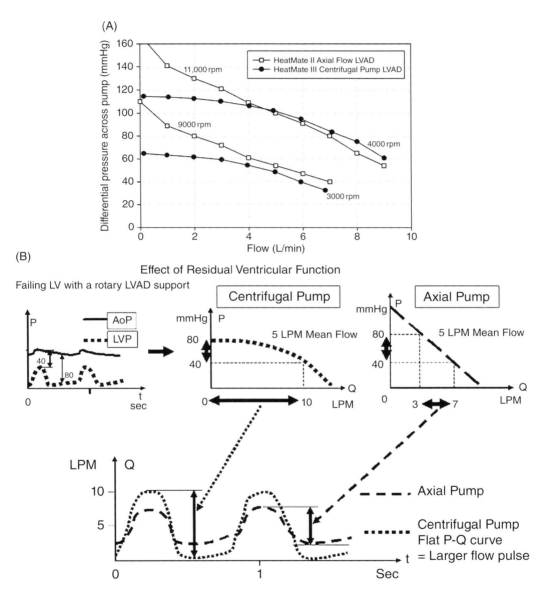

Figure 10.8 (A) Representation of the systemic arterial pressure (AoP) and left ventricular pressure (LVP) relationship is shown during continuous-flow LVAD support in a failing ventricle. Comparisons (B) of centrifugal pump and axial pump performance characteristics are shown as pressure differential across pump inlet and outlet (P here but typically called H or head) in mmHg and pump flow in liters per minute (LPM or Q). At a mean LVAD flow of 5 LPM it is quite apparent that the axial pump with the steep PQ or HQ curve exhbits a smaller variation in pump flow and less flow pulsatility due to ventricular contraction than the the centrifugal pump with a flat PQ or HQ curve, which exhibits wide flow variation and enhanced flow pulsatility.
Source: Reproduced from Pagani (2008)/with permission of Elsevier.

The pulsatility index (PI) is is a unitless measure calculated as beat-to-beat amplitude between the maximal flows and minimal flows averaged over 10–15 seconds and divided by the average flow according to the formula: 10 × [(maximum flow − minimum flow)/average flow]. From a practical perspective, pulsatility is a measure of the difference of pump flow between ventricular systole and diastole. Elevated blood pressure will increase the pressure differential across the pump and decrease flow, but the diastolic pressure gradient is affected more than the systolic gradient, and PI subsequently increases. The HeartMate 3 system utilizes the PI to recognize and avert a suction event. When the degree of pulsatility measured in the waveform falls below a preset value, the system regards this as a risk of a suction event and automatically lowers the rotor speed to a preset low speed limit and then gradually returns the rotor to its original speed.

The HeartMate 3 has an intrinsic pulsatility mechanism preprogrammed within the device, and is automatically active at a set rotor speed above 4000 rpm. The software is set to cycle every 2 seconds. Every 2 seconds, the rotor will decrease by 2000 rpm, from the set speed, for 0.15 seconds, then increase by 4000 rpm for 0.20 seconds, and finally return to the set speed. This provides for 30 pulses/ min which promotes routine washing of the pump blood surfaces, which reduces the risk of blood stasis within the pump.

Right ventricle failure results in a decreased ability to fill the LV, thus decreasing the LV preload. Because the LVAD can only sense what is occurring in the LV, the decreased LV pressure seen in RV failure will resemble the pump parameters of hypovolemia, namely, decreased preload leads to a greater pressure gradient across the pump, thus decreasing flow and increasing the PI.

Left ventricular assist device insertion results in a global impairment of RV systolic function due to loss of the LV contribution to RV function. In addition, LVAD implantation generally acutely decreases mitral regurgitation while worsening tricuspid regurgitation, both acutely and chronically. Poor apposition of the tricuspid valve leaflets after LV decompression with a LVAD occurs as the result of a leftward shift of the intraventricular septum and the increased RV volume load. There is generally dilation of the tricuspid annulus and a leftward deviation of the septal components of the tricuspid subvalvular (chordae and papillary muscles) apparatus. Normally, this is offset by an increased right ventricular preload and a reduced right ventricular afterload (due to a reduction in LA pressure and pulmonary vascular resistance [PVR]) such that right ventricular output is maintained or increased.

Treatment of right ventricular dysfunction and tricuspid regurgitation with pulmonary vasodilators (milrinone and NO) and inotropes will be necessary for patients who manifest severe right ventricular dysfunction after LVAD implantation. Severe right ventricular dysfunction will produce a low LVAD output in conjunction with a high CVP and tricuspid regurgitation. Right ventricular distension and hypokinesis seen with TEE are valuable in guiding therapy to reduce tricuspid regurgitation and improve right ventricular function. In some circumstances, a tricuspid annuloplasty may be warranted at the time of LVAD implantation. If all these maneuvers fail to support the right heart, the patient should be converted to biventricular assist or ECMO.

The following causes should be considered in decreased preload conditions.

- Hypovolemia.
- Poor positioning/obstruction of the inflow cannula.
- Impaired right ventricular function with delivery of inadequate volumes of blood across the pulmonary circulation to an LVAD.

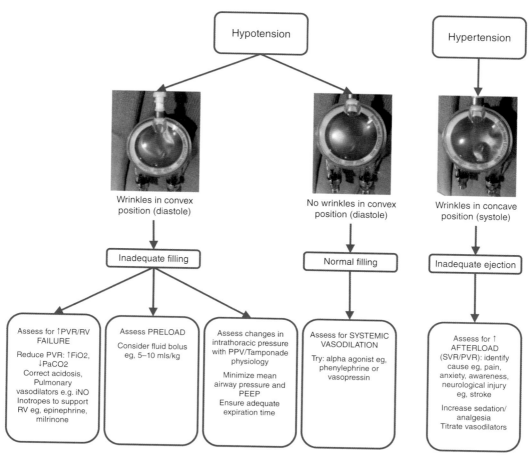

Figure 10.9 Decision algorithm for treatment of hypotension and hypertension in a patient with a pneumatic pulsatile LVAD, in this case a Berlin EXCOR, an extracorporeal device. A cellphone video played back in slow motion is the best method of seeing these changes in the device membrane. *Source:* Navaratnam et al. (2019)/ with permission of John Wiley & Sons.

It is important to realize that in patients with nonpulsatile continuous-flow devices, the arterial waveform will a nonpulsatile or minimally pulsatile representation of the mean arterial blood pressure (MAP). Given the inverse relationship between delta P and LVAD flow, it is generally desirable to keep MAP <80–90 mmHg. A detailed summary of the management of hemodynamic instability in patients following implantation of a pulsatile VAD is presented in Figure 10.9 while management of a contin- uous axial or centrifugal pump VAD is presented in Figure 10.10.

BiVAD Insertion

During BiVAD placement, the possibility of pulmonary endothelial injury, pulmonary edema, and hemorrhage exists when high flows are abruptly directed into the pulmonary vascular bed. Patients with elevated pulmonary arterial pressure due to inadequate left atrial decompression or elevated PVR are particularly at risk for this problem.

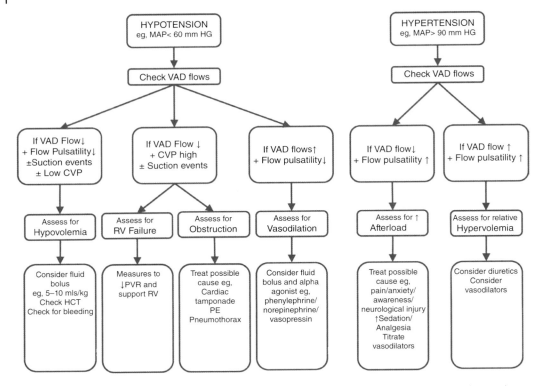

Figure 10.10 Decision algorithm for treatment of hypotension and hypertension in a patient with a axial or centrifugal continuous flow LVAD. *Source:* Reproduced from Navaratnam *et al.* (2019)/with permission of John Wiley & Sons.

References and Further Reading

Belkin, M.N., Kagan, V., Labuhn, C., Pinney, S.P. & Grinstein, J. Physiology and clinical utility of HeartMate pump parameters. *J Card Fail* **28**, 845–862 (2021).

Buratto, E., Shi, W.Y., Ye, X.T. & Konstantinov, I.E. Ventricular assist devices for the failing univentricular circulation. *Expert Rev Med Devic* **14**, 449–459 (2017).

Chegondi, M., Vijayakumar, N. & Totapally, B.R. Management of anticoagulation during extracorporeal membrane oxygenation in children. *Pediatr Rep* **14**, 320–332 (2022).

Dalia, A.A., Cronin, B., Stone, M. *et al.* Anesthetic management of patients with continuous-flow left ventricular assist devices undergoing noncardiac surgery: an update for anesthesiologists. *J Cardiothorac Vasc Anesth* **32**, 1001–1012 (2018).

Mandawat, A. & Rao, S.V. Percutaneous mechanical circulatory support devices in cardiogenic shock. *Circulation Cardiovasc Intervent* 10, e004337 (2018).

Mehra, M.R., Naka, Y., Uriel, N. *et al.* A fully magnetically levitated circulatory pump for advanced heart failure. *N Engl J Med* **376**(5), 440–450 (2017).

Navaratnam, M., Maeda, K. & Hollander, S.A. Pediatric ventricular assist devices: bridge to a new era of perioperative care. *Pediatr Anesth* **29**, 506–518 (2019).

Pagani, F.D. Continuous-flow rotary left ventricular assist devices with "3rd generation" design. *Semin Thorac Cardiovasc Surg* **20**, 255–263 (2008).

Rogers, J., Pagani, F., Tatooles, A. *et al.* Intrapericardial left ventricular assist device for advanced heart failure. *N Engl J Med* **376**, 451–460 (2017).

Thiagarajan, R.R. Extracorporeal membrane oxygenation in infants and children. In: *Cardiopulmonary Bypass and Mechanical Support: Principles and Practice*, 4th edition (eds G.P. Gravlee, R.F. Davis, J. W. Hammond, B.D. Kussman), Wolters Kluwer (2015).

11

Postoperative Cardiac Intensive Care Unit Care

Structured Hand-off from OR to CICU Team

Postoperative care commences with a structured hand-off of the patient from the OR team to the CICU team. The precise process varies from institution to institution, but the format is generally conducted as illustrated in Figures 11.1 and 11.2.

The final summary by the CICU team should include an assessment of hemodynamic goals, postoperative procedures to be performed (such as tube/line removal and chest closure), cardiopulmonary status, physiologic vulnerabilities (particularly residual lesions), and the intended duration of mechanical ventilation. Based on this assessment, the projected trajectory for each patient can be determined. Intelligent choices regarding use of sedatives, analgesics, and, if necessary, neuromuscular blocking agents (NMBA) can then be made. Since no one drug can provide analgesia, sedation, and muscle relaxation, the use of multiple agents is necessary.

Once the hand-off is complete, the CICU must carefully define the patient's anticipated postoperative trajectory and then coordinate sedation strategies, inotrope and vasodilator therapy, nutrition, hemostasis management, and ventilation strategy. For most patients, the postoperative recovery is uncomplicated. However, when the patient's clinical progress or postoperative cardiorespiratory function does not follow the expected course, myocardial function must be assessed, and the presence and significance of residual defects must be determined with echocardiography, cardiac catheterization, or both.

Sedation/Analgesia Medications

Sedation/analgesia, alone or in combination with NMBAs, is generally required for children in the CICU receiving mechanical ventilation and can be achieved with combinations of benzodiazepines, hypnotic agents such as ketamine and propofol, and the alpha-2-agonist dexmedetomidine.

An important consideration with the use of a continuous infusion of a medication in the CICU is the concept of context-sensitive half-time, which is the time required for blood or plasma concentrations of a drug to decrease by 50% after discontinuation of drug administration. During an infusion, IV drugs with multicompartmental pharmacokinetics initially distribute in the central compartment with subsequent redistribution to peripheral compartments. When these peripheral redistribution sites become saturated and the concentration of drug in them reaches equilibrium with the central compartment, the context-sensitive half-time becomes equal to the terminal elimination half-life. A practical example is fentanyl, which is highly lipophilic and initially has a short half-life due to redistribution from the central compartment to adipose tissue. Once adipose tissue becomes saturated, fentanyl loses its short-duration characteristics such

The Pediatric Cardiac Anesthesia Handbook, Second Edition. Viviane G. Nasr and James A. DiNardo.
© 2025 John Wiley & Sons Ltd. Published 2025 by John Wiley & Sons Ltd.

Operating Room to Intensive Care Unit Standardized HAND-OFF PROTOCOL

- ICU team waiting for arrival
- Room prepared
- Quiet

Hand off Team Members
- Anesthesia provider
- Surgeon/Fellow
- ICU Nurse
- ICU APP/Resident
- ICU Intensivist
- Respiratory Therapist

All team members must stay at bedside from start to end of hand off

30-45min RN-RN phone, then "on the way" call

Start: Patient enters room

1. Anesthesia provider
   ✓ Announces patient's name
   ✓ Says his/her name
   ✓ Identifies accepting RN, Intensivist, and ICU APP
   ✓ Prompts start of monitor-line setup
   ✓ Continues directing care until hand off is complete

2. Monitor-line setup
   DO NOT start report until:
   ✓ Nurse completes monitor-line setup and vitals displayed
   ✓ Fall attention of Team and all members are present

3. Surgeon gives report
   ✓ Follow checklist
   ✓ End by sharing what worries you most about this patient

4. Anesthesia provider gives report
   ✓ Follow checklist
   ✓ End by sharing what worries you the most about this patient

5. ICU provider and nurse
   ✓ Ask any questions
   ✓ Clarify remaining issues
   ✓ Announce: "Hand off is now complete"

End: Providers may leave bedside

- Receiving nurse only listens and takes notes.
- Report starts when vital signs show on ICU monitor.
- Staff anesthesiologist responsible for managing sedation and hemodynamics.
- No interruptions of handoff with questions or talking.

- Surgeon checklist
- Anesthesiologist checklist
- ICU team / RN question time.

Figure 11.1 Standardized operating room (OR)-to-intensive care unit (ICU) hand-off protocol emphasizing rigorous organization, flow of information, and uninterrupted speaking roles. *Source:* Reproduced from Chatterjee *et al.* (2019)/with permission of Elsevier.

Figure 11.2 Sample operating room (OR)-to-intensive care unit (ICU) hand-off checklists for cardiac surgery (A) and cardiac anesthesia (B). BP, blood pressure; CPB, cardiopulmonary bypass; ETT, endotracheal tube; FFP, fresh frozen plasma; HR, heart rate; IV, intravenous; LVEF, left ventricular ejection fraction; PA, pulmonary artery; PCC, prothrombin complex concentrate; PRBC, packed red blood cells; TEE, transesophageal echocardiography. *Source:* Reproduced from Chatterjee *et al.* (2019)/with permission of Elsevier.

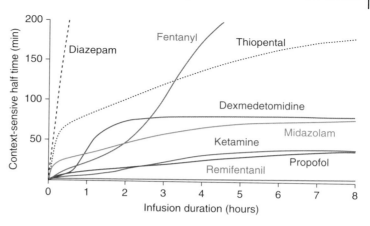

Figure 11.3 Context-sensitive half-times of commonly used CICU sedative and analgesia agents.

that after a three-hour infusion the short-acting opioid fentanyl has a longer half-time than a morphine infusion once the infusions are stopped. The context-sensitive half-times of analgesic and sedative medications commonly used in the CICU are illustrated in Figure 11.3.

Benzodiazepines

Benzodiazepines are commonly used as sedative-hypnotic agents for children in the CICU; these agents have no intrinsic analgesic activity. Midazolam is the most commonly used benzodiazepine, with a rapid onset and short duration of action, and a short context-sensitive half-life. It is generally administered via IV using either intermittent bolus doses (0.025–0.1 mg kg^{-1}) or as a continuous infusion 0.05–0.2 mg kg^{-1} h^{-1} when early extubation is not anticipated. Prolonged infusions are associated with development of tolerance and subsequent physical dependence, leading to withdrawal symptoms and delirium.

Opioids

Opioids are the mainstay of pain management in the CICU. In addition, they possess some sedative activity and are used to blunt sympathetic responses to noxious stimulation such as endotracheal tube suctioning. Morphine is the prototypical opiate and provides excellent analgesia when administered either as intermittent bolus doses (0.05–0.2 mg kg^{-1}) or as a continuous infusion (0.01–0.03 mg kg^{-1} h^{-1}) when early extubation is not anticipated. It is important to remember that a typical bolus dose of morphine achieves a peak effect in 10–20 minutes and has a duration of action of approximately 2–4 hours. Morphine has little effect on blood pressure and heart rate in normovolemic patients. However, high doses in critically ill patients can lead to decreased systemic vascular resistance (SVR), increased venous capacitance, and inhibition of baroreceptor reflexes, causing hypotension. In addition, morphine stimulates the release of histamine, which contributes to the development of hypotension.

Fentanyl is a synthetic opioid that is 70–100 times more potent than morphine. It has minimal effects on hemodynamics and is commonly administered to critically ill, hemodynamically unstable children both as a bolus doses (1–2 µg kg^{-1}) and as a continuous infusion (1-3 µg kg^{-1} min^{-1}). Tolerance to fentanyl develops more rapidly and the risk of dependence and withdrawal phenomena is greater than with morphine.

Sufentanil is 5–10 times more potent than fentanyl and 1000 times more potent than morphine. It has excellent context-sensitive half-time kinetics but is rarely used as a continuous infusion in the CICU due to extremely rapid development of tolerance. Remifentanil is a very short-acting, pure μ-receptor agonist that is equipotent to fentanyl. Its rapid onset and offset times and lack of significant hemodynamic effects make it particularly useful as a continuous infusion (0.4–1 μg kg^{-1} min^{-1}) for procedural analgesia and anesthesia, and less useful for prolonged sedation in the CICU, and its context-sensitive half-time remains constant at four minutes regardless of infusion duration.

Propofol

Propofol is an IV-administered sedative-hypnotic agent. It has no intrinsic analgesic properties. Propofol has a fast onset time with an effect seen within 40 seconds of injection. It has a large volume of distribution and an increased clearance in children when compared with adults. It takes 1–3 minutes for blood–brain equilibration to occur and therefore dose adjustments are not recommended sooner than 3–5 minutes, allowing time for a clinical effect. The context-sensitive half-time for an infusion duration of up to eight hours is less than 40 minutes, allowing rapid emergence from its effects. Unfortunately, the very narrow therapeutic index of this drug leaves little margin for error with sedation, rapidly progressing to unconsciousness and apnea. Despite this and other risks that accompany the use of propofol in critically ill cardiac patients, including bradycardia, decreased SVR, hypotension, and reduced clearance, it is commonly used in early tracheal extubation protocols.

The current package insert for propofol contains the following language: "Propofol injectable emulsion is not indicated for use in PICU sedation since the safety of this regimen has not been established." Nonetheless, propofol is used at low doses (<4 mg kg^{-1} h^{-1} or 67 μg kg^{-1} min^{-1}) alone or in combination with other drugs, generally in older patients, to provide short sedation. Enthusiasm for the use of propofol in critically ill children must be tempered by the concern for the development of the propofol infusion syndrome, the risk factors for which appear to be an infusion rate of 4 mg kg^{-1} h^{-1} or 67 μg kg^{-1} min^{-1} for longer than 48 hours, young age, critical illness, concomitant catecholamine infusions, and concomitant steroid supplementation. Many institutions do not encourage or allow propofol infusions for sedation of children for more than 24–48 hours.

Dexmedetomidine

Dexmedetomidine is a highly selective central nervous system alpha-2-adrenergic receptor agonist with a large volume of distribution (necessitating a loading dose), an initial short half-life allowing titration during continuous infusion, and a prolonged context-sensitive half-time (four hours after an eight-hour infusion). It produces sedation and benzodiazepine-sparing effects as well as weak analgesia/opioid-sparing effects by increasing GABA inhibition in the central nervous system and spinal cord. The central nervous system effects of therapeutic plasma levels of dexmedetomidine resemble those of nonrapid eye movement stage 2 (light) sleep. Dexmedetomidine has minimal effect on respiratory function.

Therapeutic plasma levels of dexmedetomidine obtained during continuous infusion (0.5–1.5 μg kg^{-1} h^{-1}) allow lower amounts of opioid and benzodiazepine infusions to be utilized. As such, dexmedetomidine may help avoid the development of opioid and benzodiazepine dependence, ameliorate withdrawal symptoms, and prevent postoperative delirium. Sedation in children with dexmedetomidine alone is not practical in the intensive care setting given that large doses of dexmedetomidine (2–3 μg kg^{-1} h^{-1}), with their associated hemodynamic effects, are necessary. Withdrawal following prolonged dexmedetomidine infusions is problematic, with the most common manifestations being transient hypertension, agitation, and tachyarrhythmias. Slow weaning with transition to a nonparenteral alpha-2-adrenergic receptor agonist such as a clonidine transdermal patch is usually necessary.

There is some evidence that the prevalence of perioperative junctional ectopic tachycardia and supraventricular tachycardia is lower in patients receiving dexmedetomidine and that dexmedetomidine administration may be useful in terminating arrhythmias.

Ketamine

Ketamine is structurally related to phencyclidine and blocks the N-methyl-D-aspartate receptor. It acts on the cortex and limbic system, leading to a dissociative anesthetic state with strong analgesic, sedative, and antegrade amnestic effects during which there is maintenance of the airway reflexes. While multiple routes of administration are available, IV and intramuscular administrations are preferred for procedural sedation and analgesia. Ketamine has a short context-sensitive half-time (40 min after discontinuation of an eight-hour infusion), making it an ideal agent for a continuous infusion. Ketamine infusions ($0.5-1.5$ mg kg^{-1} h^{-1}) can be utilized in the CICU to provide analgesia, sedative, and a dissociative state, as well as to provide opioid and benzodiazepines "holidays" in patients requiring long-term sedation.

Management of Sedation/ Analgesia

Management of sedation, analgesia, and NMB agents, and prevention of the development of delirium and iatrogenic withdrawal syndrome (IWS) are major challenges in critically ill pediatric patients, particularly those who require prolonged CICU stays. In patients six years old and older who can communicate, pain assessment via self-report can be performed using the Visual Analog Scale, the Numeric Rating Scale, the Oucher Scale, or the Wong-Baker Faces pain scale. The Faces, Legs, Activity, Cry, and Consolability (FLACC) or COMFORT-B scales can be used in assessing pain in noncommunicative pediatric patients. The COMFORT-B Scale or the State Behavioral Scale (Figure 11.4) can be used to assess the level of sedation in mechanically ventilated

pediatric patients. The Cornell Assessment of Pediatric Delirium (CAPD) for children $0-18$ years and the Pediatric Confusion Assessment Method for the ICU (pCAM-ICU) for children older than five years are the most widely used assessment tools for delirium. The Sophia Observation Scale and the Withdrawal Assessment Tool-1 are both pediatric withdrawal symptom grading scales. An example of a coordinated approach utilizing these various scales and the complex interplay between the various components is illustrated in Figure 11.5.

Detection and Treatment of Low Cardiac Output Syndrome

Low cardiac output syndrome (LCOS) is defined as clinical signs or symptoms (tachycardia, oliguria, poor perfusion, or cardiac arrest) with or without a widened arterial-mixed venous oxygen saturation difference or metabolic acidosis, and with or without elevated blood lactate or rapid increase in blood lactate. Strictly defined LCOS is a cardiac index (CI) ≤ 2 l min^{-2} m^2. Once LCOS is identified, the following factors must be considered.

- Residual anatomic defects such as a large VSD or severe RV or LV outflow tract obstruction.
- Postcardiotomy dysfunction such as RV dysfunction following a right ventriculotomy.
- Compromised coronary artery from anatomic causes.
- Supraventricular or ventricular dysrhythmias or loss of atrioventricular conduction.
- Low preload due to ongoing bleeding.
- Systemic vasoconstriction and high SVR.
- Metabolic derangements such as hypocalcemia and hypomagnesemia.
- Pulmonary hypertension.
- Low hematocrit and compromise of systemic oxygen delivery (Chapter 7).

Nevertheless, a cardiac output decline of approximately 30% should be anticipated

State Behavioral Scale (SBS)

Score as patient's response to voice then gentle touch then noxious stimuli (planned endotracheal suctioning or <5 seconds of nail bed pressure)

Score	Description	Definition
−3	Unresponsive	No spontaneous respiratory effort No cough or coughs only with suctioning No response to noxious stimuli Unable to pay attention to care provider Does not distress with any procedure (including noxious) Does not move
−2	Responsive to noxious stimuli	Spontaneous yet supported breathing Coughs with suctioning/repositioning Responds to noxious stimuli Unable to pay attention to care provider Will distress with a noxious procedure Does not move/occasional movement of extremities or shifting of position
−1	Responsive to gentle touch or voice	Spontaneous but ineffective nonsupported breaths Coughs with suctioning/repositioning Responds to touch/voice Able to pay attention but drifts off after stimulation Distresses with procedures Able to calm with comforting touch or voice when stimulus removed Occasional movement of extremities or shifting of position
0	Awake and able to calm	Spontaneous and effective breathing Coughs when repositioned/Occasional spontaneous cough Responds to voice/No external stimulus is required to elicit response Spontaneously pays attention to care provider Distresses with procedures Able to calm with comforting touch or voice when stimulus removed Occasional movement of extremities or shifting of position/increased movement (restless, squirming)
+1	Restless and difficult to calm	Spontaneous effective breathing/Having difficulty breathing with ventilator Occasional spontaneous cough Responds to voice/No external stimulus is required to elicit response Drifts off/Spontaneously pays attention to care provider Intermittently unsafe Does not consistently calm despite 5 minute attempt/unable to console Increased movement (restless, squirming)
+2	Agitated	May have difficulty breathing with ventilator Coughing spontaneously No external stimulus required to elicit response Spontaneously pays attention to care provider Unsafe (biting ETT, pulling at lines, cannot be left alone) Unable to console Increased movement (restless, squirming or thrashing side-to-side, kicking legs)

Figure 11.4 The State Behavioral Scale (SBS).

within 9–12 hours after surgery, even if the surgical repair is adequate. Vasoactive infusions are often needed to mitigate the decreased cardiac output in these patients. Dopamine and epinephrine are commonly used for inotropy, while milrinone may be added to reduce ventricular afterload. Ideally, afterload reduction, or the reduction in systolic intraventricular wall tension, is initiated to improve ventriculoarterial coupling. That is, afterload reduction strategies are intended to achieve better matching of ventricular contractility to the impedance characteristics of the arterial circulation such that stroke volume (SV), CI and systemic oxygen delivery (DO_2) can be optimized. Ideally, myocardial O_2 demands should be minimized, while preload, heart rate and rhythm, and myocardial contractility (if possible) should be optimized to derive the most benefit from a hemodynamic support strategy emphasizing systemic afterload reduction.

To better understand the use of inodilator therapy, a thorough grasp of ventriculoarterial coupling is required. The most illustrative way to approach this analysis is with the use of ventricular pressure–volume loops (Figure 11.6). The slope of the straight line generated by connecting the ventricular end-systolic pressure–volume points defines time-varying ventricular elastance, which represents the contractile state and stiffness of the ventricle. Effective arterial elastance (Ea) derived from ventricular pressure–volume loops is a measure of afterload. Ea lumps the nonpulsatile and pulsatile components of arterial load into a single number but does not provide information on their relative contributions.

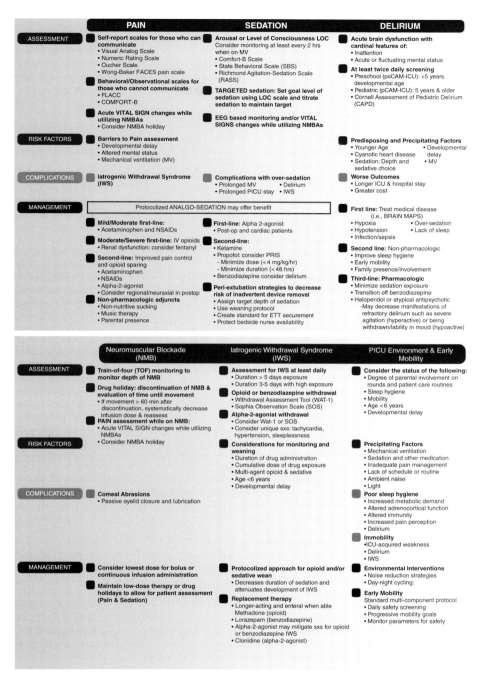

Figure 11.5 Summary of the key pain, agitation, neuromuscular blockade, and delirium scales used in critically ill pediatric patients with consideration of the PICU Environment and Early Mobility (PANDEM) recommendations. Summarized is the interplay between sedative and analgesic choice on unintended but related outcomes. BRAIN MAPS, Bring oxygen, Remove/Reduce deliriogenic drugs, patient Atmosphere, Immobilization, New organ dysfunction, Metabolic disturbances, Awake, Pain, Sedation; CAPD, Cornell Assessment of Pediatric Delirium; COMFORT-B, COMFORT-Behavior; EEG, electroencephalogram; ETT, endotracheal tube; FLACC, Faces, Legs, Activity, Cry, and Consolability; IWS, iatrogenic withdrawal syndrome; MV, mechanical ventilation; NMBA, neuromuscular blocking agent; NSAID, nonsteroidal antiinflammatory drug; pCAM-ICU, pediatric Confusion Assessment Method for the ICU; PRIS, propofol-related infusion syndrome; psCAM-ICU, preschool Confusion Assessment Method for the ICU; RASS, Richmond Agitation-Sedation Scale; SBS, State Behavioral Scale; SOS, Sophia Observation Scale; TOF, train-of-four; WAT-I, Withdrawal Assessment Tool-1. *Source:* Reproduced from Smith et al. (2022)/with permission of the Society of Critical Care Medicine.

Figure 11.6 A family of four left ventricular pressure–volume loops was generated by increasing preload (ventricular end-diastolic volume) in a ventricle with fixed contractility and fixed afterload. Joining the ventricular end-systolic pressure and volume points from the four loops defines the slope's fixed contractility. Fixed afterload is the slope of the line defined by joining ventricular end-diastolic volume to ventricular end-systolic pressure for each loop. The slope for fixed afterload is the same for each loop. This can be seen in loop 2 and loop 4. Despite fixed afterload and fixed contractility, augmentation of preload results in an elevation of ventricular end-systolic pressure. The intersection point of fixed contractility and fixed afterload uniquely defines ventricular end-systolic pressure for each loop. Ventricular end-systolic pressure will remain constant with an augmentation of preload only if fixed afterload simultaneously decreases (shallower slope). A subtle increase in SV can be seen as preload is progressively increased. Ea, afterload; Ees, end-systolic elastance (contractility); LV, left ventricle; Pes, ventricular end-systolic pressure; SV, stroke volume; Ved, ventricular end-diastolic volume.

The effects of vasodilator therapy on SV and blood pressure in a particular patient will be dependent on the existing ventriculoarterial coupling. This concept is illustrated in Figure 11.7 by observing the effects of utilizing milrinone or sodium nitroprusside as a vasodilator in two patients with very different ventriculoarterial coupling characteristics: one with depressed ventricular contractility, such as a heart failure patient or a patient with postcardiotomy LCOS, and the other with hyperdynamic ventricular function, such as a patient with left ventricular concentric hypertrophy following relief of LVOT obstruction (coarctation repair, subaortic membrane resection, aortic valve surgery for AS). Sodium nitroprusside reduces afterload by reducing peripheral resistance and increasing large vessel compliance, which reduces pulse-wave velocity and wave reflection. When ventricular function is reduced, vasodilator therapy that reduces Ea results in substantial improvements in SV and cardiac output with little or no change in blood pressure and a substantial

reduction in left atrial pressure. This left atrial pressure reduction then produces a significant reduction in pulmonary artery pressure regardless of the pulmonary vascular resistance. When the left ventricle is hyperdynamic and stiff, as occurs in concentric hypertrophy, vasodilator therapy that reduces Ea results in profound hypotension with no substantial improvement in SV or cardiac output. Such hypotension is exacerbated in cases of hypovolemia (such as bleeding postoperative patients) and is especially disadvantageous to these patients because it compromises subendocardial perfusion, particularly in cases of reflex tachycardia.

There are numerous approaches to treatment of LCOS but regardless of the initial choice of agents, there must be a consistent reassessment of CI and DO_2. For example, combining low-dose epinephrine or dopamine with an IV afterload-reducing agent such as milrinone is frequently beneficial to support patients with significant ventricular dysfunction accompanied by elevated

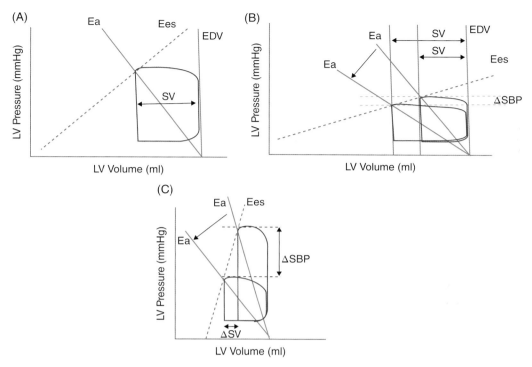

Figure 11.7 (A) A left ventricular pressure–volume loop from a normal patient with an ejection fraction of 50% and a normal fixed afterload/fixed contractility ratio of 1. (B) A left ventricular pressure–volume loop with depressed contractility; fixed contractility is shifted down and rightward. A reduction in fixed afterload, as indicated by the arrow, results in a significant increase in stroke volume with essentially no changes in LVESP and blood pressure. (C) A left ventricular pressure–volume loop from a patient with a hyperdynamic, stiff left ventricle; fixed contractility is shifted up and leftward. A decrease in afterload, as indicated by the arrow, results in significant decreases in LVESP and blood pressure with essentially no change in stroke volume. Ea, afterload; Ees, end-systolic elastance (contractility); LV, left ventricle; LVESP, left ventricular end-systolic pressure; SV, stroke volume.

afterload. If a patient does not respond adequately to dopamine (up to 7.5 μg kg^{-1} min^{-1}) and has persistent signs of a low CO state, including poor extremity perfusion, hypotension (>30% decrease in mean arterial blood pressure for age), tachycardia, elevated atrial filling pressure, oliguria, and lactic acidemia, treatment with epinephrine should be considered. An epinephrine infusion can be added to dopamine at a starting dose of 0.05–0.1 μg kg^{-1} min^{-1} and subsequently titrated to achieve the target systemic blood pressure. At high doses, epinephrine can produce significant renal and peripheral vasoconstriction as well as tachycardia. It may be necessary to normalize SVR in this situation with a vasodilator. The advantage of milrinone (0.5–1.0 μg kg^{-1} min^{-1}) over nitroprusside or nicardipine (both 0.5–2.0 μg kg^{-1} min^{-1}) is its weak inotropic effects and steady-state plasma levels (hours) compared to nitroprusside or nicardipine (minutes). Patients who persistently require high doses of epinephrine should be evaluated for the initiation of mechanical circulatory support.

Norepinephrine (0.25–1.0 μg kg^{-1} min^{-1}), titrated to normalize a persistently low SVR, can be considered in patients with severe hypotension (warm distributive shock), inadequate coronary artery perfusion, or inadequate pulmonary blood flow with a systemic-to-pulmonary artery shunt.

Additionally, in patients with persistent LCOS, efforts should be made to optimize the balance between oxygen delivery and demand. Metabolic demand should be minimized by maintaining adequate analgesia, sedation, and NMBA to avoid movement and reduce muscle tone and oxygen debt. While hyperthermia from any cause must be treated and mild hypothermia may be preferable in some instances, care must be taken to avoid inducing peripheral vasoconstriction, which will increase myocardial oxygen demand.

Mechanical Ventilation

The requirement for postoperative mechanical ventilation is determined by the extent of altered lung mechanics, ventilation/perfusion abnormalities and intrapulmonary shunt present. When initiated, the effects of positive-pressure ventilation (PPV) on intrathoracic pressure and subsequently on cardiac function and ventricular interaction must be considered. These changes as compared to spontaneous ventilation are summarized in Figure 11.8 and are as follows.

- PPV increases pleural pressure and produces changes opposite to those seen during spontaneous breathing.
- During the inspiratory phase of PPV, RV preload is reduced and RV afterload is increased.
- During the inspiratory phase of PPV, LV preload increases as positive pressure enhances blood flow from the pulmonary veins.
- During the inspiratory phase of PPV, LV afterload is reduced due to a decrease in the transmural pressure of the LV relative to the extrathoracic aorta.

As a result, LV stroke volume and MAP increase at the end of the inspiratory phase of PPV. At the end of the expiratory period, both LV stroke volume and MAP decrease consequent to a reduction in LV preload. This delayed reduction in LV preload is due to the 2–3-second transpulmonary blood transit time for the decreased venous return and RV preload during late inspiration/early expiration to manifest as a reduction of LV preload during end-expiration.

Patients with normal RV compliance and without residual volume load or pressure load on the ventricle after surgery usually show little change in RV function from the alteration in preload and afterload with PPV. However, these effects can be magnified in patients with restrictive RV physiology after congenital heart surgery. Neonates with diastolic dysfunction following a right ventriculotomy such as necessary to repair TOF, pulmonary atresia, or truncus arteriosus, or those with concentric RV hypertrophy due to RVOT obstruction are especially sensitive to increased RV afterload from PPV. In this setting, an increase in RV afterload can lead to RV distention, septal shift, and reduced LV compliance and filling.

The effects of PPV on LV function are most evident in patients with LV dysfunction with elevated preload and afterload. Here, the reduction in preload and afterload can result in an increase in the cardiac output and a reduction in myocardial oxygen demand. In addition, patients with LV dysfunction may have impaired pulmonary mechanics secondary to increased lung water, decreased lung compliance, and increased airway resistance. Neonates and infants fatigue early because of limited respiratory reserve. Furthermore, a significant proportion of total body oxygen consumption is directed at the increased work of breathing in neonates and infants with LV dysfunction, contributing to poor feeding and failure to thrive. PPV has an additional benefit in these patients by reducing the work of breathing and oxygen demand. In general, with their limited physiologic reserve, neonates and infants should not be weaned from mechanical ventilation until hemodynamic stability is accompanied by resolution of intrapulmonary shunt and altered respiratory mechanics.

Most patients wean from PPV without difficulty but some patients with borderline cardiac function and a significant residual lesion burden may require prolonged mechanical ventilation and a slower weaning process. Most

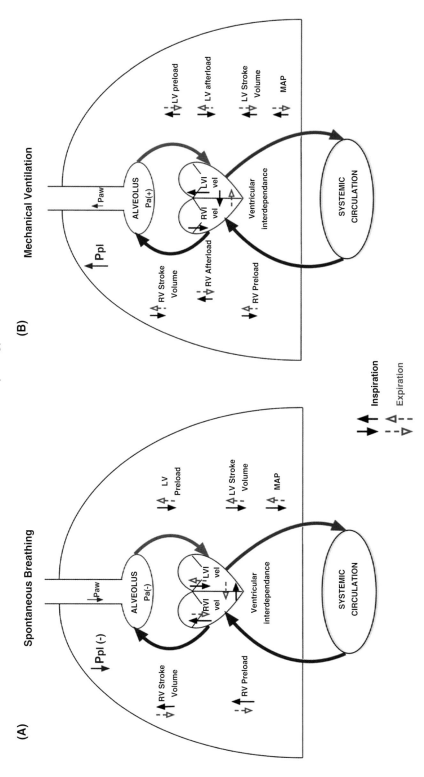

Figure 11.8 Heart lung interactions and hemodynamic changes during (A) spontaneous breathing; (B) mechanical ventilation. ↑, increase; ↑, decrease; →, leftward shift; ←, rightward shift; green solid arrows, inspiratory event; orange dashed arrows, expiratory event. RV, right ventricle; LV, left ventricle; RVI, right ventricle inflow; LVI, left ventricle inflow; Vel, velocity; Syst BP, systolic pressure. *Source:* Reproduced from Madhivathanan et al. (2020)/with permission of Elsevier.

patients can be weaned using either a volume- or pressure-limited mode by simply decreasing the intermittent mandatory ventilation rate. The mechanical ventilator rate is gradually decreased while observing physical examination, hemodynamics, respiratory pattern, and arterial blood gas measurements. In patients with a limited hemodynamic and respiratory reserve or in those who exhibit significant dyssynchrony with the ventilator, the addition of pressure- or flow-triggered pressure support (PSV) of 8–15 cmH$_2$O above positive end-expiratory pressure (PEEP) is often beneficial in reducing the work of breathing. One major advantage of PSV is that it facilitates weaning of sedation and analgesic medications.

Enhanced Recovery after Surgery and Early Tracheal Extubation

Common enhanced recovery after surgery (ERAS) components include minimization of preoperative fasting, multimodal opioid-sparing analgesic agents such as acetaminophen and ketorolac, regional anesthesia techniques, postoperative nausea and vomiting prevention, temperature control, hemostasis, fluid management, nutrition, early surgical chest tube removal, and early mobilization. Early tracheal extubation, either immediately in the operating room or within two hours after arrival in the intensive care unit, or alternatively within 4–8 hours after arrival in the intensive care unit, is an integral component of ERAS programs. Patients undergoing selected nonbypass cardiac surgery and thoracic procedures are usually suitable for early extubation. These surgeries include patent ductus arteriosus closure and vascular ring ligation in infants and older children. In addition, infants and older children undergoing repair of coarctation of the aorta may benefit from early extubation to avoid hypertension and tachycardia that often accompanies a slow wean from mechanical ventilation in the CICU after surgery.

The risk for rebound hypertension and the need to protect high-pressure surgical suture lines often dictates early blood pressure control with vasodilating and beta-blocking drugs. However, mild-to-moderate hypothermia is commonly induced during surgery to optimize spinal cord protection while the aorta is cross-clamped, and tracheal extubation should be delayed until patients are normothermic.

Children undergoing relatively short bypass procedures using mild-to-moderate hypothermia, such as ASD repair, small VSD closure, and right ventricle-to-pulmonary artery conduit replacement, are often suitable for weaning and extubation in the operating room or early after CICU admission. These patients generally have a stable preoperative clinical status, demonstrate few complications related to CPB, and have an uncomplicated postoperative course.

Infants undergoing complete repair of a VSD, balanced common atrioventricular canal defect, or tetralogy of Fallot are often suitable for extubation in the first 6–12 hours after surgery. Such patients should typically have been in stable clinical condition preoperatively and have adequate postoperative cardiac output, gas exchange, and hemostasis before considering early extubation. Nevertheless, if there was a large volume load on the ventricle before surgery with significant congestive heart failure or labile pulmonary vascular resistance secondary to increased pulmonary blood flow, management should be guided by postoperative hemodynamic and respiratory function.

Infants and older children undergoing some types of LV outflow tract repair, including subaortic stenosis repair with the Konno operation or subaortic membrane resection, and aortic valvuloplasty or replacement, usually have either preserved or hyperdynamic ventricular systolic function. Hypertension and tachycardia are frequently a management concern in these patients in the immediate postoperative period, particularly during emergence from anesthesia. Not only will hypertension and tachycardia increase the risk for disruption of suture lines, but the increased myocardial work can contribute to ischemia and increase the likelihood of ventricular tachyarrhythmias. If ventricular function is stable, hemostasis has been secured, and there are no concerns for ventricular tachyarrhythmias, it is often preferable for these patients to be extubated within 6–12 hours after surgery rather than undergoing a more prolonged weaning process. The combination of esmolol (100–300 µg kg^{-1} min^{-1}) and sodium nitroprusside or nicardipine (0.5–1.0 µg kg^{-1} min^{-1}) can be used to control blood pressure and reduce reflex contractility increases in patients with preexisting increased LV mass following procedures to relieve LVOTO. This combination prevents the development of tachycardia and diastolic hypotension that potentially compromises subendocardial perfusion in patients with LVH.

Early tracheal extubation can be of benefit to a subset of patients following a cavopulmonary connection surgery such as a BDG or a Fontan procedure. Spontaneous ventilation is certainly of benefit to these patients compared to PPV due to a lower mean intrathoracic pressure and improved delivery of preload to the systemic ventricle, particularly in Fontan patients. However, more important is the recognition that to prevent ventilator–patient dyssynchrony during PPV, moderate to deep sedation +/− NMBA is often utilized. This regimen significantly increases unstressed venous volume and, without very aggressive intravascular volume replacement and use of venocontrictor agents, results in a decrease in gradient to deliver preload to the systemic ventricle across the pulmonary vascular bed. After an uncomplicated BDG or Fontan procedure, it is usually possible to extubate the trachea within 6–12 hours after surgery.

Extended CICU Care

In certain circumstances, delayed extubation and the need for an extended CICU stay are both predictable and necessary. Neonates undergoing two-ventricle repairs are usually initially managed with deep sedation +/− NMBA in the immediate postoperative period until hemodynamic and respiratory stability has been attained. However, there are clear differences depending on diagnosis and procedure. For example, many neonates are sufficiently stable to start to wean from mechanical ventilation and be extubated by the first or second postoperative day after procedures such as an uncomplicated arterial switch operation for d-transposition.

On the other hand, neonates who have undergone a right ventriculotomy, such as after neonatal repair of TOF or truncus arteriosus, commonly demonstrate restrictive RV diastolic function in the immediate postoperative period. A low cardiac output state with increased right-sided filling pressure may be evident, and continuing sedation and mechanical ventilation may be necessary for the first 48–72 hours until diastolic function improves.

Neonates and infants who require surgical limitation of pulmonary blood flow with a pulmonary artery band or augmentation of pulmonary blood flow with a systemic-to-pulmonary artery shunt generally require meticulous management of ventilation and augmentation of cardiac output in the immediate postoperative period. They are not candidates for early extubation. PPV and deep sedation for at least the first 24 hours post operation are usually required to attain cardiorespiratory stability.

Neonates undergoing a Norwood or Sano procedure for hypoplastic left heart syndrome or other forms of single ventricle anatomy with aortic arch obstruction require a carefully coordinated management strategy in the immediate postoperative period to address the potential for cardiopulmonary instability and ongoing blood loss. Sedation and NMBA should be continued after surgery to mitigate the stress response and any imbalance between oxygen supply and demand should be managed until a stable circulation and gas exchange have been achieved. Inotropic and vasoactive support is usually required, often combined with afterload reduction to reduce myocardial work and improve systemic perfusion. Volume replacement to maintain preload is essential, and monitoring mixed venous O_2 saturation as an indicator of cardiac output is beneficial. There is likely to be institutional variation in the individual components of a postoperative management strategy of a patient following Stage 1 palliation. However, it is important that all components be goal directed and coordinated with the other components as illustrated in Figure 11.9.

Oliguria, both pre-renal and renal in origin, in the first 24 hours after cardiac surgery and CPB is common particularly in neonates and infants. Intravascular volume depletion results from capillary leak, interstitial fluid accumulation, and a significant increase in total body water after surgery due to an ongoing inflammatory response. In addition, a fall in cardiac output and increased antidiuretic hormone secretion contribute to delayed water clearance. RV dysfunction and/or tricuspid valve dysfunction associated with an elevated CVP will result in elevated renal venous pressure, further compromising renal perfusion, particularly in the case of diminished arterial blood pressure. Significant body wall edema in a neonate or infant with a closed sternum can result in high intrathoracic pressure due to poor chest wall compliance, resulting in hemodynamic and respiratory compromise.

Figure 11.9 An example of a coordinated, goal-directed postoperative management strategy for a neonate following Stage 1 palliation. *Source:* Reproduced from Mills et al. (2016)/with permission of the American Heart Association, Inc.

Consequently, the cardiac output should be enhanced with volume replacement and vasoactive drug infusions as necessary before diuretics or can be effective. Dopamine at low doses ($0.3–5$ μg kg^{-1} min^{-1}) stimulates DA$_1$ and DA$_2$ receptors, inducing natriuresis and diuresis and enhancing renal blood flow by renal vasodilation. At higher doses, dopamine increases renal blood flow through an increase in cardiac output. Fenoldopam mesylate, a selective dopamine (DA$_1$) receptor agonist, is a smooth muscle relaxant with enhanced activity in the renal and splanchnic beds and is used in some institutions to enhance renal perfusion. Because fenoldopam has a hemodynamic profile similar to sodium nitroprusside, the advantages of selective renal vasodilation may be offset by systemic hypotension.

Diuretics are a mainstay of fluid management and agents of different classes are commonly used in combination. The loop diuretics furosemide and bumetanide must be excreted into the renal tubular system before producing diuresis; therefore, low cardiac output reduces their efficacy. These agents are commonly used in conjunction with hydrochlorothiazide, which acts on the distal convoluted tubules and inhibits the sodium chloride cotransporter system, leading to diuresis and loss of potassium in the urine. Spironolactone is a potassium-sparing diuretic that competitively inhibits mineralocorticoid receptors in the distal convoluted tubule to promote sodium and water excretion and potassium retention.

In some institutions, neonates and infants undergoing complex surgical repairs who are deemed at risk for fluid retention have a peritoneal dialysis catheter placed in the operating room to manage fluid balance and improve renal blood flow by reducing intraabdominal pressure from ascites. The catheter can be used solely for drainage, in which case large-volume losses may require replacement with albumin or fresh frozen plasma to treat hypovolemia and hypoproteinemia. Should oliguria occur in conjunction with acute kidney injury (AKI), the catheter can be used to perform low-volume dialysis.

References and Further Reading

Chatterjee, S., Shake, J., Arora, R. *et al.* Handoffs from the operating room to the intensive care unit after cardiothoracic surgery: from the Society of Thoracic Surgeons Workforce on Critical Care. *Ann Thorac Surg* **107**, 619–630 (2019).

Madhivathanan, P.R., Corredor, C. & Smith, A. Perioperative implications of pericardial effusions and cardiac tamponade. *BJA Educ* **20**, 226–234 (2020).

Mills, K., Kaza, A., Walsh, B. et al. Phosphodiesterase inhibitor-based vasodilation improves oxygen delivery and clinical outcomes following Stage 1 palliation. *J Am Heart Assoc* **5**, e003554 (2016).

Nasr, V.G. & DiNardo, J.A. Sedation and analgesia in pediatric cardiac critical care. *Pediatr Crit Care Med* **17**, S225–S231 (2016).

Smith, H.A.B., Besunder, J., Betters, K. *et al.* Society of Critical Care Medicine Clinical Practice Guidelines on Prevention and Management of Pain, Agitation, Neuromuscular Blockade, and Delirium in Critically Ill Pediatric Patients With Consideration of the ICU Environment and Early Mobility. *Pediatr Crit Care Med* **23**, e74–e110 (2022).

Part II

Specific Lesions

12

Patent Ductus Arteriosus

Introduction

Dr Robert Gross's first successful ligation of a patent ductus arteriosus (PDA) on 8th August 1938, at the Children's Hospital in Boston, marked the beginning of pediatric cardiac surgery. Currently, PDAs represent about 10% of congenital heart defects, and in preterm infants the overall incidence is 20–30%.

Anatomy

A PDA connects the main pulmonary trunk near the origin of the left pulmonary artery with the proximal descending aorta just distal to the origin of the left subclavian artery (Figure 12.1).

Physiology

A PDA is a simple shunt. When the PDA is large, there is little or no pressure gradient across the duct and shunting becomes dependent on the ratio of pulmonary vascular resistance (PVR) to systemic vascular resistance (SVR). Initially, the high PVR present after birth tends to limit the shunt magnitude of even the largest PDAs until the PVR begins to decrease. As the PVR decreases, a left-to-right (L-R) shunt with increased pulmonary blood flow develops. In order for systemic blood flow to be maintained, the left ventricular output must increase and a volume load must be imposed on the left ventricle. The increased pulmonary blood flow increases the pulmonary venous return and left atrial pressure. These factors may, in turn, increase the PVR and the work of breathing, and ultimately lead to the development of pulmonary artery hypertension. Diastolic run-off of blood from the proximal aorta into the pulmonary artery can result in a holodiastolic flow reversal in the descending aorta that compromises both proximal and distal organ perfusion, and may be associated with necrotizing enterocolitis, renal failure, and intraventricular hemorrhage (IVH). The reduction in aortic diastolic blood pressure also compromises coronary perfusion pressure.

Surgical Therapy

The surgical approach to PDA closure is via a left thoracotomy or video-assisted thoracoscopic surgery (VATS). Cardiopulmonary bypass (CPB) is not used. The ductus is either ligated or ligated and transected. The left pulmonary artery, left mainstem bronchus, or descending aorta are at risk of being inadvertently ligated if the PDA is misidentified. Injury to the recurrent laryngeal nerve is also a recognized complication.

The Pediatric Cardiac Anesthesia Handbook, Second Edition. Viviane G. Nasr and James A. DiNardo.
© 2025 John Wiley & Sons Ltd. Published 2025 by John Wiley & Sons Ltd.

Figure 12.1 Patent ductus arteriosus (PDA).

Catheterization Laboratory Intervention

Closure of a PDA in the cardiac catheterization laboratories was introduced by Portsmann in 1967, using a conical Ivalon* plug, and in 1979 Rashkind and Cuaso used an umbrella-type device. In 1992, Cambier and Moore introduced the use of coils for the occlusion of small PDAs. In 2003, the Amplatzer™ became the first device to be approved by the Food and Drug Administration for PDA closure. The transcatheter closure of PDA can be performed safely and effectively in premature infants as small as 700 g or smaller using the Amplatzer Piccolo Occluder. The symmetrical configuration allows the device to be delivered either antegrade via the femoral vein or retrograde via the femoral artery. In children ≤2 kg, this obviates the need for femoral artery access and the potential for significant vascular compromise.

Because patient immobility greatly facilitates the deployment of PDA occlusion devices, a general anesthesia is commonly utilized in children incapable of cooperation.

Embolization of the device downstream into the pulmonary artery or aorta requires catheter-based or surgical retrieval.

Anesthetic Management

The anesthetic management goals are summarized in Table 12.1. There are a few additional considerations. Surgical retraction of the left lung may necessitate high-inspired oxygen concentrations to prevent hypoxemia. Blood pressure should be monitored in both an upper and lower extremity; the right arm is preferable to the left arm because the surgeon may have to place a clamp on the aorta if control of the aortic end of the PDA is lost during dissection or ligation. In patients with a large left-to-right shunt, there will be an increase in aortic diastolic blood pressure following ligation, due to the cessation of run-off of blood into the pulmonary circulation. An upper- and lower-extremity blood pressure should be compared following ligation to assure that a coarctation has not been created.

Induction and Maintenance

Most patients presenting for PDA ligation are premature infants with respiratory distress syndrome. Age and the likelihood that congestive heart failure exists make these patients poor candidates for inhalational anesthesia. A technique using fentanyl in combination with a benzodiazepine or low inspired concentration of inhalation agent is well tolerated.

Table 12.1 Anesthetic management goals for a patent ductus arteriosus.

---

1) Maintain HR, contractility, and preload to maintain cardiac output.
2) Avoid decreases in PVR:SVR to maintain systemic blood flow.
3) Avoid increases in PVR:SVR. An increase in PVR increases the right-to-left shunting.
4) Bubble precautions.

For older children with an isolated PDA and no pulmonary venoocclusive disease, early extubation or extubation in the operating room after ligation is possible. In this age group, thoracotomy can be avoided using VATS. An inhalational induction with sevoflurane, followed by placement of an IV and administration of rocuronium and fentanyl $10–15$ µg kg^{-1} is commonly performed. Alternatively, a remifentanil infusion ($0.5–1.0$ µg kg^{-1} min^{-1}) can be utilized. Anesthesia is supplemented with isoflurane ($0.5–1.0\%$) or sevoflurane ($1.0–2.0\%$). Regional anesthesia (paravertebral block, intercostal block) can be used to treat postoperative pain.

Postligation Cardiac Syndrome

Postligation cardiac syndrome, defined as hypotension requiring inotropic support and failure of oxygenation and ventilation, may occur $6–12$ hours following ligation. An increase in LV afterload leads to left ventricular systolic contractility/afterload mismatch, reduced stroke volume and cardiac output, and LV diastolic dysfunction.

The result is hypotension, elevated LA pressure, interstitial pulmonary edema, and reduced lung compliance.

Noncardiac Surgery

Patients with a repaired PDA can present with laryngeal nerve injury. They may also present with pulmonary hypertension and ventricular dysfunction if the repair was delayed.

References and Further Reading

Giesinger, R.E., Bischoff, A.R. & McNamara, P.J. Anticipatory perioperative management for patent ductus arteriosus surgery: understanding postligation cardiac syndrome. *Congenit Heart Dis* **14**, 311–316 (2019).

Sathanandam, S.K., Gutfinger, D., O'Brien L. *et al*. Amplatzer Piccolo Occluder clinical trial for percutaneous closure of the patent ductus arteriosus in patients ≥700 grams. *Catheter Cardiovasc Interv* **96**, 1266–1276 (2020).

13

Aortopulmonary Window

Introduction

Aortopulmonary window (AP) is a rare disorder making up <0.1% of congenital heart lesions. It results from a failure of fusion of the two opposing conotruncal ridges that are responsible for separating the truncus arteriosus into the aorta and pulmonary artery.

Anatomy

Aortopulmonary window is associated with other cardiac abnormalities in one-third to one-half of cases, but may occur as an isolated lesion. The most common associated lesions are arch abnormalities, specifically interrupted aortic arch, and coarctation of the aorta. Other associated cardiac anomalies include abnormal origin of the coronary arteries, ventricular septal defects, tetralogy of Fallot, and transposition of the great arteries. Noncardiac-associated anomalies include VATER, CHARGE, and 22q11.2 deletion syndrome.

AP windows are classified into four types (Figure 13.1).

- Type I: proximal defect; occurs between the ascending aorta and main pulmonary artery, above the sinus of Valsalva.
- Type II: distal defect; the distal ascending aorta opens into the origin of the right pulmonary artery.
- Type III: total defect; the largest defect involving most of the ascending aorta with complete absence of the aortopulmonary septum.
- Type IV: intermediate defect; this defect has adequate superior and inferior rims and is the most suitable for possible device closure.

Physiology

As pulmonary vascular resistance (PVR) decreases after birth, these patients present in the neonatal period with a large nonrestrictive left-to-right (L-R) physiologic shunt with high pulmonary blood flow and congestive heart failure. Tachypnea and diaphoresis are common. A systolic murmur can be heard along the left sternal border; however, unlike patients with a patent ductus arteriosus (PDA), a diastolic component to the murmur is rare. Diagnosis is routinely made with echocardiography.

Surgical Management

The presence of an AP is an indication for early surgical repair to prevent the development of pulmonary artery hypertension (PAH). A median sternotomy is performed and the procedure is carried out using cardiopulmonary bypass (CPB). The area of the AP window is exposed and a patch is used to close the defect and separate both circulations.

Early mortality following the repair of simple AP approaches zero, and long-term outcomes are excellent. Follow-up is

The Pediatric Cardiac Anesthesia Handbook, Second Edition. Viviane G. Nasr and James A. DiNardo.
© 2025 John Wiley & Sons Ltd. Published 2025 by John Wiley & Sons Ltd.

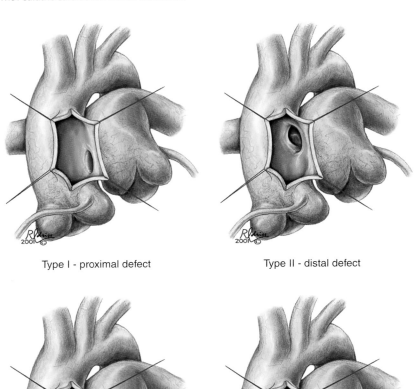

Type I - proximal defect

Type II - distal defect

Type III - total defect

Intermediate defect

Figure 13.1 Classification of aortopulmonary window by the Society of Thoracic Surgeons Congenital Heart Surgery Database Committee. *Source:* Reproduced from Backer and Mavroudis(2002)/with permission of Oxford University Press.

indicated to detect residual aortopulmonary septal defects and the development of branch pulmonary artery stenosis.

Catheterization Laboratory Intervention

Device closure of the AP window may be possible for very small defects not associated with anomalous coronary artery origin.

Anesthetic Management

The anesthetic management is similar to the management of the large L-R physiologic shunt lesion truncus arteriosus. Monitoring includes intraarterial and central venous catheters. High-dose opioids and muscle relaxant with low-dose inhalation is an adequate technique for the induction and maintenance of anesthesia. Maintenance of a balanced PVR:systemic vascular resistance

(SVR) ratio to avoid excessive pulmonary blood flow and systemic hypoperfusion is a must.

Noncardiac Surgery

Patients with AP window may have residual pulmonary stenosis and/or pulmonary vascular disease that need to be evaluated prior to noncardiac surgery.

References and Further Reading

Backer, C.L. & Mavroudis, C. Surgical management of aortopulmonary window: a 40-year experience. *Eur J Cardiothorac Surg* **21**, 773–779 (2002).

Barnes, M.E., Mitchell, M.E. & Tweddell, J.S. Aortopulmonary window. *Semin Thorac Cardiovasc Surg Pediatr Card Surg Annu* **14**, 67–74 (2011).

14

Coarctation of the Aorta

Introduction

Coarctation of the aorta is present in 5–10% of patients with congenital heart disease (CHD). It is more commonly found in males and is the most common lesion in patients with Turner syndrome. Almost half of all cases have associated cardiac and noncardiac anomalies.

Anatomy

Coarctation of the aorta is a focal narrowing of the aorta. The anatomic pathology is remarkably consistent, with a discrete posterior shelf or invagination in the aortic wall just opposite the insertion of the ductus arteriosus (juxtaductal) and distal to the left subclavian artery. In some instances this shelf may be circumferential. Longer segment coarctation and coarctation of the abdominal aorta are also seen (Figure 14.1).

It has been postulated that coarctation develops as the result of fetal blood flow patterns which reduce antegrade aortic blood flow, with a proportionate increase in pulmonary artery and ductus arteriosus blood flow. Coarctation can be associated with aortic valve stenosis (most commonly bicuspid aortic valve), with hypoplasia of other left-heart structures such as the mitral valve and left ventricle, and with hypoplasia of the aortic arch. Hypoplasia of the aortic isthmus (the region of the aortic arch from the left subclavian to the ductus arteriosus) is the isolated aortic arch lesion most commonly associated with coarctation. Ventricular septal defects (VSDs), particularly posterior malalignment VSDs that cause left ventricular outflow tract (LVOT) obstruction and divert flow from the ascending aorta into the pulmonary artery, are also associated with coarctation. In contrast, coarctation is virtually never found in association with obstructive right-heart lesions.

Physiology

Despite remarkably consistent anatomic pathology, the pathophysiology of coarctation is varied and depends on the severity of the coarctation and the location of associated lesions. These variations in pathophysiology have led to the use of confusing terms such as "infantile" and "adult" coarctation or pre- and postductal coarctation, which are of little practical significance. Coarctation of the aorta produces left ventricular pressure overload and a reduction in lower body perfusion (Figure 14.2).

The physiologic consequences of a coarctation will depend on several factors.

- The severity of the coarctation.
- The extent of antegrade aortic blood flow afforded by a patent or partially patent ductus arteriosus (PDA).
- The extent of collateralization to the distal aorta.
- The type and severity of associated heart lesions.

The Pediatric Cardiac Anesthesia Handbook, Second Edition. Viviane G. Nasr and James A. DiNardo.
© 2025 John Wiley & Sons Ltd. Published 2025 by John Wiley & Sons Ltd.

(A)   (B)

Figure 14.1 Echocardiography of coarcation in a neonate (A) and a 12 year old (B). Panel A shows imaging of neonatal coarctation from the suprasternal notch view. Coarctation ridge (COA) located ~5 mm below the origin of left subclavian artery. Descendent thoracic aorta (DAO) below obstruction is dilated. AOA, aortic arch. Panel B shows the discrete shelf partly occluding the aortic isthmus (COA) and marked poststenotic dilation of thoracic aorta. AOA, aortic arch; DAO, descendent aorta; PA, pulmonary trunk.

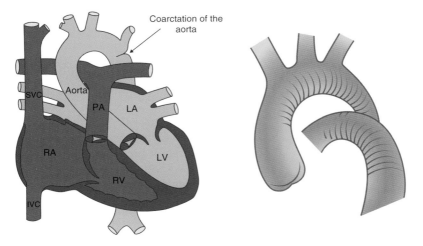

Figure 14.2 Typical appearance of coarctation of the aorta.

The ductus arteriosus plays a critical role in pathophysiology. Closure of the ductus arteriosus after birth initially occurs at the pulmonary end, with constriction of the aortic orifice normally delayed for several weeks or months. Closure of the aortic end of the ductus arteriosus may abruptly impede blood flow around the aortic shelf lesion and increase the severity of the lesion (Figure 14.3). Ductal closure may also be

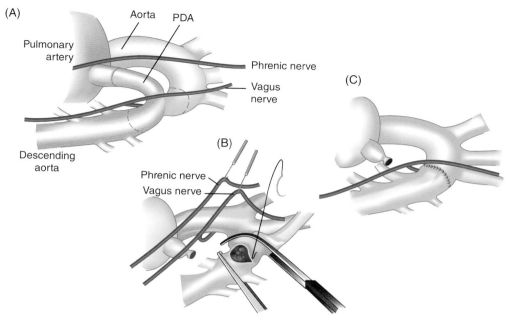

(A) Pulmonary artery — Aorta — PDA — Phrenic nerve — Vagus nerve — Descending aorta

(B) Phrenic nerve — Vagus nerve

(C)

Figure 14.3 Anatomy of a coarctation of the aorta involving a small patent ductus arteriosus (PDA). The repair shown is resection of the coarcted segment, ligation of the PDA, and primary end-to-end reanastomosis of the aorta. *Source:* Reproduced from DiNardo and Zvara (2008)/with permission from John Wiley & Sons.

associated with constriction of the aorta at the level of the ductus arteriosus, presumably due to the presence of ductal tissue in this area. When coarctation is severe, distal aortic perfusion will, in part, be supplied with blood from the pulmonary artery via a PDA (Figure 14.4). This will result in differential cyanosis with a higher arterial saturation proximal to the coarctation compared to distal to the coarctation. When the development of aortic obstruction is gradual, collateral flow to the distal aorta will be established via the intercostal, internal thoracic, subclavian, and scapular arteries.

Presentation will be in infancy for all patients except those capable of tolerating ductal closure without overt hemodynamic compromise. In general, presentation beyond infancy is limited to patients with an isolated coarctation of mild to moderate severity, or those with rapid compensatory collateral formation. In these patients there is a secondary phase of fibrosis that occurs during the first 2–3 months of life. As the child grows, the ligamentum arteriosum develops a thick fibrous shelf within the lumen of the aorta.

In the presence of severe coarctation, and particularly in association with left-heart and aortic arch hypoplasia, patency of the ductus arteriosus is necessary to provide blood flow to the aorta distal to the coarctation (right-to-left physiologic shunt). In this ductal-dependent physiology, right ventricular pressures are systemic.

Ductal closure in patients with a severe coarctation will result in a near loss of distal perfusion. Left ventricular dilation from the acute afterload increase, left atrial hypertension, and pulmonary edema may ensue. The reduction in left ventricular output may be so severe that proximal hypertension will not be present. The infant may present in a profound low-cardiac output state or following cardiopulmonary arrest. In the case of a less severe coarctation, ductal closure will result in a diminution of distal perfusion and evidence of left atrial hypertension.

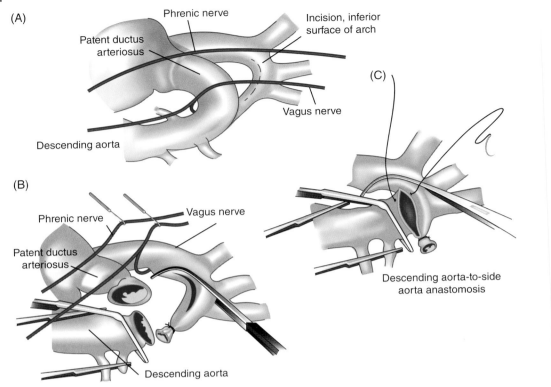

Figure 14.4 Anatomy of the coarctation of the aorta involving a large patent ductus arteriosus and hypoplasia of the aortic isthmus. The repair is a resection of ductal tissue and mobilization of the descending aorta and aortic arch to perform a primary reanastomosis. During this procedure, clamp placement may compromise left carotid artery flow. Cerebral blood will be dependent on right carotid flow and an intact circle of Willis. *Source:* Reproduced from DiNardo and Zvara (2008)/with permission from John Wiley & Sons.

If an anatomic intracardiac shunt lesion, such as an atrial septal defect (ASD) or VSD, is also present, the increased impedance to aortic ejection induced by the coarctation will enhance physiologic left-to-right (L-R) shunting. Reductions in pulmonary vascular resistance (PVR) will increase pulmonary blood flow, thereby diverting flow from the distal aorta. Left atrial hypertension will be exacerbated by the increase in pulmonary blood flow.

In all these instances, the institution of prostaglandin (PGE) E_1 (0.01–0.05 µg kg^{-1} min^{-1}) to reestablish ductal and aortic patency can be life saving. Mechanical ventilatory support, inotropic support, and diuretic therapy are usually necessary to stabilize the sickest infants following the administration of PGE$_1$. These patients often present with a profound metabolic acidosis and suffer transient renal and hepatic dysfunction following initial resuscitation.

Patients presenting in childhood with coarctation will not be ductus dependent and will have well-developed collaterals. In addition, they will have developed the concentric left ventricular hypertrophy that accompanies chronic left ventricular pressure overload lesions. These patients will have proximal aortic hypertension.

Surgical Therapy

Three basic types of repair are used for correction of coarctation of the aorta: (i) reverse subclavian patch angioplasty; (ii) synthetic patch angioplasty; and (iii) end-to-end anastomosis of the aorta after resection of the coarctation segment (Figures 14.3 and 14.4). These procedures are performed via a left thoracotomy. It is necessary to cross-clamp the aorta to perform these procedures. For older children, partial cardiopulmonary bypass (CPB) or a shunt from proximal to distal aorta may be used if the adequacy of the collateral circulation is in question.

Presentation as an infant generally leads to medical stabilization followed by surgical intervention. Complete excision of the area of coarctation and surrounding ductal tissue with end-to-end anastomosis is indicated. In the case of coarctation associated with a hypoplastic aortic isthmus, complete excision in conjunction with an extended end-to-end or end-to-side anastomosis is recommended. The descending aorta is anastomosed to the underside of the aortic arch in an end-to-end or end-to-side fashion.

Dacron* patch aortoplasty following resection of the posterior coarctation ridge is associated with the late development of hypertension and aneurysm formation, compared to end-to-end anastomosis. Reverse subclavian patch angioplasty is rarely utilized, as the rate of recoarctation is high. In adult patients, placement of an interposition graft is usually necessary as there is insufficient mobility of the aorta to allow resection and the creation of an end-to-end anastomosis.

The incidence of paraplegia secondary to spinal cord ischemia is quite low (0.14– 0.4%). Several factors are associated with an increased risk of developing paraplegia, including hyperthermia, prolonged aortic cross-clamp time, elevated cerebral spinal fluid (CSF) pressures, low proximal and distal aortic blood pressures, and poorly developed collaterals to the descending aorta.

Catheterization Laboratory Intervention

Balloon intervention to the coarctation was initially described during the early 1980s. Endovascular stent placement is an alternative therapy for treatment of coarctation in older children and adults, with results superior to balloon dilation alone. This technique allows for subsequent percutaneous stent dilations over time as needed. Uncommon but devastating complications include neurologic injury, uncontrolled aortic tear/ rupture, aortic aneurysms and dissections.

Anesthetic Management

The goals of anesthetic management are as follows.

- To maintain heart rate, contractility, and preload to maintain cardiac output. The high afterload faced by the left ventricle makes it particularly vulnerable to reductions in contractility.
- For neonates and infants with coarctation, continuation of PGE_1 (0.01– 0.05 µg kg^{-1} min^{-1}) to maintain ductal patency may be necessary to prevent cardiovascular collapse.
- If there is an associated ASD or VSD, reduction in the PVR:SVR ratio should be avoided. Such reductions will increase pulmonary blood flow and will necessitate an increase in cardiac output to maintain systemic blood flow.
- Avoid increases in SVR. An increased SVR will worsen left ventricular pressure overload, which may cause large reductions in left ventricular output.
- Cross-clamping of the aorta may produce impressive proximal hypertension or left ventricular dysfunction. This is less likely in the presence of well-developed collaterals.

The arterial line should be in the right arm. The left arm is an unreliable blood pressure source during clamping because the proximal clamp may occlude or compromise the origin of the left subclavian artery. This is particularly true if the left subclavian patch technique is utilized. The surgeon may also request that a femoral arterial catheter be placed to assess the adequacy of the repair by way of comparison of proximal and distal blood pressures. In circumstances where the adequacy of distal collateralization is in question, measurement of femoral arterial pressure after test occlusion of the descending aortic may be helpful. At a minimum, a pulse oximeter probe and a noninvasive blood pressure (NIBP) cuff should be applied to a lower extremity. A pulse oximeter probe should also be placed on the right hand. During aortic cross-clamping, this site will yield the only reliable plethysmographic waveform and oxygen saturation data. The use of cerebral near-infra-red spectroscopy (NIRS) may be helpful in assessing the adequacy of cerebral blood flow, and flank NIRS may be used to indirectly assess somatic blood flow.

Permissive hypothermia, with rectal and nasopharyngeal temperatures allowed to drift down to 34–35 °C, is used by many centers to afford some degree of spinal cord protection during aortic cross-clamping. Careful attention to patient temperature is necessary to avoid excessive hypothermia during the cross-clamp period. Sufficient rewarming of the patient after cross-clamp removal to allow extubation in the operating room can be a challenge.

Induction and Maintenance

Neonates and infants presenting for coarctation repair generally are PGE_1 dependent, with compromised distal perfusion and pulmonary congestion. A technique using high-dose fentanyl in combination with a benzodiazepine or low inspired concentration of an inhalation agent is well tolerated by these patients. In older children with only proximal systemic hypertension, intravenous or inhalational techniques are well tolerated.

Regardless of the technique chosen, it should be appreciated that proximal blood pressure response to stimulation will be exaggerated.

Management after Cross-clamp Removal

Cross-clamping of the thoracic aorta has been shown to produce increases in both proximal aortic blood pressure and CSF pressure, and decreases in distal aortic blood pressure. The use of sodium nitroprusside to normalize proximal aortic blood pressure results in further increases in CSF pressure and further decreases in distal aortic blood pressure. This combination of increased CSF pressure and reduced aortic blood pressure reduces spinal cord blood perfusion pressure and may place the spinal cord at greater risk for ischemia. Therefore, vasodilators should be used cautiously to control extreme proximal hypertension and left ventricular dysfunction.

Transesophageal echocardiography (TEE) is useful during cross-clamping, particularly for infants with coexisting cardiac lesions. Left ventricular function and the extent of intracardiac shunting can be monitored. In some instances of severe coarctation in infants – particularly those with proximal tubular hypoplasia – vasodilator therapy may be insufficient to prevent left ventricular dilation, and inotropic support may be necessary. Ventilatory control of the PVR will be complicated by the fact that the left lung must be retracted for exposure. It is important to know which arch vessels are clamped during the surgical procedure. At least one of the carotid arteries must be patent for cerebral perfusion (Figures 14.3 and 14.4).

Removal of the cross-clamp will result in reactive hyperemia in distal tissues, with subsequent vasodilation and transient hypotension. Release of lactic acid will cause the $PaCO_2$ to rise, but volume expansion and an increase in minute ventilation just before clamp removal diminish these effects. The cross-clamp times for these repairs are relatively short (<15 min), which reduces the hemodynamic consequences of clamp removal. Many of these patients will have hyperdynamic left ventricular function and will be hypertensive post CPB. Pure vasodilators such as sodium nitroprusside and nicardipine widen the pulse pressure by decreasing diastolic blood pressure, and induce a reflex tachycardia. This combination of hemodynamic changes increases sheer forces on the aorta and jeopardizes subendocardial perfusion. Judicious doses of sodium nitroprusside ($0.25–1.0 \mu g\, kg^{-1}\, min^{-1}$) or nicardipine ($0.25–1.0 \mu g\, kg^{-1}\, min^-$) in combination with esmolol ($100–300 \mu g\, kg^{-1}\, min^-$) is a more appropriate choice.

Postoperatively, rebound hypertension may occur and persist for up to one week. Initially this is likely to be due to an altered baroreceptor response that results in very high circulating levels of catecholamines. Later, there may be involvement of the renin–angiotensin–aldosterone system. Beta-blockers and vasodilators, particularly angiotensin converting enzyme (ACE) inhibitors, are used to control this hypertension.

Older children without coexisting diseases are candidates for early extubation using the technique described for PDA ligation.

Noncardiac Surgery

Patients with repaired coarctation may present for noncardiac surgery with residual or recoarctation, persistent hypertension and myocardial hypertrophy, or associated berry aneurysms.

References and Further Reading

DiNardo, J.A. & Zvara, D.A. *Anesthesia for Cardiac Surgery*, 3rd edn. Blackwell, Massachusetts (2008).

Lipton, G., Nagler, J. & Geva, T. Coarctation of the aorta. *J Pediatr* **152**, 737 (2008).

15

Atrial Septal Defect

Introduction

Atrial septal defects (ASDs) are the second most common congenital heart disease in children, with an incidence of 0.07–0.2%, and have a female-to-male ratio of about 2:1. Approximately 15% of ASDs close spontaneously by the age of four years, whereas others decrease in size and are of no major clinical significance. However, about 1% of infants with moderate to large isolated ASDs experience symptoms which usually do not occur until late childhood, or older.

Anatomy

An ASD is a communication between the left and right atrium due to a defect in the intraatrial septum (IAS). The IAS consists of a central membranous portion and a thicker inferior and superior fatty limbus. The central membranous portion is formed by tissue of the septum primum ultimately forming the fossa ovalis. This membrane lies posterior to the superior aspect of the fatty limbus.

Atrial septal defects, like ventricular septal defects (VSDs), are classified by their location. There are four morphological types of ASD: (i) ostium secundum defects; (ii) ostium primum defects; (iii) inferior and superior sinus venosus defects; and (iv) coronary sinus (CS) defects (Figure 15.1). Although they are classified as ASDs, sinus venosus and CS defects are not truly defects in the IAS.

Ostium Secundum ASD

These defects comprise 80% of ASDs. While a patent foramen ovale (PFO) results from incomplete fusion of an intact fossa ovalis membrane with the superior aspect of the fatty limbus, an ostium secundum ASD is the result of actual deficiencies in the membrane (septum primum) of the fossa ovalis.

Ostium Primum ASD

Isolated ostium primum ASDs, also known as partial atrioventricular (AV) canal defects, develop when a partial fusion of the endocardial cushions separates the two AV valves and closes the ventricular septal communication, but fails to close the ostium primum (Figure 15.2). This defect occurs inferiorly at the level of the AV valves outside the fossa ovalis. The isolated ostium primum defect extends from the inferior IAS fatty limbus to the crest of the interventricular septum (IVS).

A characteristic finding of this lesion is insertion of the septal portions of both AV valves on the IVS at the same level. Normally, insertion of the tricuspid valve to the IVS is inferior to the insertion of the mitral valve, producing the ventriculoatrial septum (VAS) that separates the right atrium from the left ventricle. Isolated ostium primum defects are commonly associated with a cleft anterior mitral valve leaflet and mitral regurgitation (MR) resulting from a partial fusion of the leftward portions of the anterosuperior and inferoposterior bridging leaflets that

The Pediatric Cardiac Anesthesia Handbook, Second Edition. Viviane G. Nasr and James A. DiNardo.
© 2025 John Wiley & Sons Ltd. Published 2025 by John Wiley & Sons Ltd.

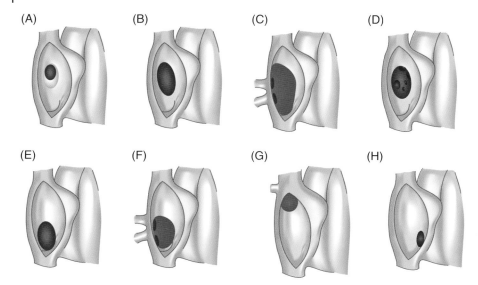

Figure 15.1 Various types of ASD seen from the right atrium. (A) Patent foramen ovale; (B) complete septal rim; (C) missing septal rim; (D) multiple fenestrations of the fossa ovalis; (E) large fossa ovalis extending to the orifice of the inferior vena cava; (F) posterior ASD; (G) sinus venosus defect; (H) coronary sinus ASD. *Source:* Reproduced from Stark and Tsang (2006)/with permission of John Wiley & Sons.

Figure 15.2 An ostium primum atrial septal defect (ASD) in a midesophageal four-chamber view. RA, right atrium; LA, left atrium; RV, right ventricle; LV, left ventricle.

normally fuse to form the anterior mitral valve leaflet. See Chapter 17 for more details regarding these partial atrioventricular canal defects.

Sinus Venosus Defects

These defects are located either superiorly at the junction of the right atrium and the superior vena cava (SVC), or inferiorly at the junction of the right atrium and the inferior vena cava (IVC) (Figure 15.3). Both defects are located posterior to the fossa ovalis. Superior defects comprise the majority, and inferior defects are rare. Strictly speaking, these are not defects in the true atrial septum, but are believed to result from a deficiency in the common wall that normally separates the right pulmonary veins/left atrium junction from the right atrium/SVC or right atrium/ IVC junction, rather than a defect in the IAS or a change in the position of the pulmonary veins *per se*. Unroofing of the posteriorly located pulmonary vein(s) produces drainage of the left atrium into the SVC and right atrium, creating a left-to-right (L-R) shunt. The interatrial communication is the orifice of the pulmonary veins rather than a defect in the atrial septum.

Sinus venosus defects can also be associated with partially anomalous pulmonary venous return (PAPVR). The distinction between an anomalous connection (drainage of a pulmonary vein into a structure other than the left atrium) and anomalous drainage (drainage of normally positioned pulmonary

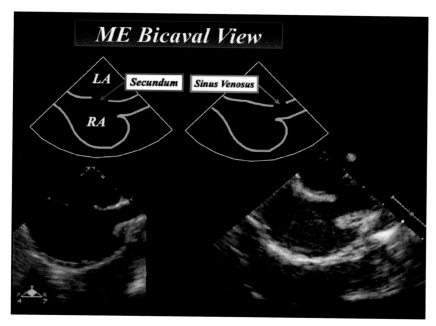

Figure 15.3 Comparison of an ostium secundum atrial septal defect (ASD) and superior sinus venosus ASD seen in a bicaval view. LA, left atrium; RA, right atrium; ME, midesophageal. *Source:* Reproduced from Burch et al. (2012)/with permission of Wolters Kluwer Health, Inc.

veins across the defect into the SVC/right atrium junction or IVC/right atrium junction) must be made.

The most common type of anomalous pulmonary connection is the RUPV draining directly into the lateral wall of the SVC above the SVC/right atrium junction at the level of the right pulmonary artery. In the case of the inferior defect, Scimitar syndrome (an anomalous connection of the right pulmonary veins to the IVC/right atrium junction, aortopulmonary collaterals to the right lower lobe, and hypoplasia of the right lung) can be seen.

Coronary Sinus Defect

Unroofing of the CS (posterior) allows direct communication with the left atrium (anterior). At its entry into the right atrium, the CS orifice becomes the connection between the left atrium and right atrium. CS defects are commonly associated with a persistent left superior vena cava (LSVC) draining to a large dilated CS.

Physiology

An ASD is a simple shunt. A small, restrictive defect will allow minimal shunt flow. A large defect (at least 1 mm in diameter) is unrestrictive. Flow across the defect occurs predominantly in diastole, and thus is largely determined by the relative compliances of the right ventricle and left ventricle, which in turn are influenced by PVR and SVR. Because the high PVR present after birth declines such that PVR is 1/10 to 1/20 that of SVR, the right ventricle is able to pump a large volume of blood across the pulmonary vascular bed into the pulmonary veins and left atrium, elevating the left atrial pressure. This physiologic L-R shunting results in a recirculation of oxygenated venous blood into the pulmonary artery and back into the left atrium. The L-R diminishes the effective forward left ventricular outflow and results in a volume overload of the right atrium, right ventricle, and left atrium. Right ventricular volume overload (RVVO) is typically reported on echocardiograms in patients with ASD.

A large defect will greatly increase pulmonary blood flow; however, unlike a VSD, systemic pressures are not transmitted to the pulmonary vasculature. In fact, the pulmonary artery pressure may remain normal for many years due to the distensibility of the pulmonary arteries. In contrast to a patient with VSD, the onset of pulmonary vascular disease and elevated pulmonary vascular resistance may not occur until the third or fourth decade of life for a patient with ASD.

Surgical Therapy

Some small ostium secundum ASDs can be primarily closed, whereas larger defects are patched, usually with pericardium. Primum ASDs generally require patch closure and suture closure of the anterior leaflet mitral cleft. Sinus venosus defects without anomalous venous connections can be closed primarily with a patch.

Alternative procedures must be performed when the pulmonary vein(s) anomalously enter the SVC. When the anomalous vein(s) enter the SVC near the SCV/right atrium junction, the SVC is transected above the origin of the anomalous vein(s). The proximal end of the SVC is oversewn, and the SVC orifice is directed across the defect into the left atrium with a pericardial patch. The distal end of the SVC is then anastomosed end to end to the roof of the right atrial appendage, recreating SVC to right atrium continuity. This is known as the Warden procedure. When the anomalous vein(s) enter the SVC remote from the SCV/right atrium junction, it may be necessary to create a baffle within the SVC to direct pulmonary venous blood across the defect into the left atrium. In this case, the anterior wall of the SVC is enlarged with a patch to allow unrestricted SVC return to the right atrium. This is known as the two-patch technique.

Surgical correction of CS defects depends on the presence or absence of LSVC. In the absence of LSVC the orifice of the CS is oversewn, allowing coronary sinus blood to drain to the left atrium (a very small physiologic right-to-left shunt). When the LSVC is present and drains to the CS with a connecting vein between the two cavae, the LSVC is ligated below the connecting vein and the CS is oversewn.

Catheterization Laboratory Intervention

An alternative is nonoperative device closure of secundum ASDs in the cardiac catheterization laboratory. It is generally performed with transesophageal echocardiographic guidance (Figure 15.4). Case-specific risks include: (i) air embolization during device deployment or manipulation; (ii) device embolization which on occasion may necessitate surgical intervention for retrieval; and (iii) transient electrocardiogram changes and rarely high-grade AV block.

Anesthetic Management

The anesthetic management goals include: (i) maintain the heart rate, contractility, and preload to maintain cardiac output and systemic perfusion; (ii) avoid increases in the PVR:SVR ratio as this may induce a right-to-

Figure 15.4 Device closure in the catheterization laboratory with transesophageal echocardiography guidance.

left shunt with potential for reduced arterial oxygen saturation; and (iii) avoid a decrease in the PVR:SVR ratio as this will cause a L-R shunt, an increase in pulmonary blood flow, and potential for reduced systemic perfusion and oxygen delivery.

Induction and Maintenance

Most children with ASDs have excellent cardiac reserve and will tolerate an inhalation induction without problems. Good airway management is necessary to allow manipulation of the PVR and prevent any reversal of L-R shunting. The presence of an enlarged atrium may predispose to atrial dysrhythmias, though these are usually well tolerated.

For children with an isolated ASD and low PVR, early extubation in the intensive care unit or extubation in the operating room after repair is possible. If a mini-sternotomy is performed, defibrillator pads should be placed. An inhalational induction with sevoflurane, followed by placement of an IV and administration of rocuronium 0.6–1.2 mg kg^{-1} and fentanyl 10–15 µg kg^{-1} can be used. If an IV line is in place, propofol, etomidate or ketamine, in conjunction with rocuronium and fentanyl, can be used for induction. In either case, anesthesia is maintained with isoflurane (0.5–1.0%) or sevoflurane (1.0–2.0%) supplementation. Caudal morphine (70 µg kg^{-1} in 5–10 ml of preservative-free saline), although not performed routinely, can be administered after induction. A vaporizer on the cardiopulmonary bypass (CPB) circuit, along with supplemental opioids and muscle relaxants, can be used for maintenance during CPB.

Post-CPB Management

The post-CPB management goals are to: (i) maintain an age-appropriate heart rate to maintain cardiac output; (ii) reduce the PVR, especially in cases where an elevated PVR exists (e.g., milrinone); and (iii) provide inotropic support to the right ventricle if needed (e.g., dopamine).

Separation from CPB is generally not problematic. In primum defects, there is the possibility of heart block, as the patch must be sutured to the crest of the IVS. In addition, the possibility of residual mitral regurgitation exists. If partial anomalous venous drainage is unrecognized during sinus venous defect closure, a residual L-R shunt may exist after repair. Intraoperative transesophageal echocardiography can be used to detect this defect. In the rare patient with an elevated PVR, the pulmonary vasculature is likely to be hyper-reactive in the post-CPB period. Therefore, it is necessary to use ventilatory measures to reduce post-CPB PVR. These manipulations will prevent right ventricular dysfunction secondary to increased afterload.

In most cases, there is no need for prolonged ventilation and early extubation is feasible with adequate titration of anesthetics and paralysis intraoperatively.

Noncardiac Surgery

Children and adult patients following ASD repair can present for noncardiac surgery. The history should include the timing of the repair, the type of repair (device or surgical), and any associated arrhythmias or other cardiac defects. Endocarditis prophylaxis is recommended for patients during the first six months after device or patch closure. Persistent right ventricular dilation or pulmonary hypertension should be considered in patients who present for repair at a later age.

References and Further Reading

Burch, T.M., Mizuguchi, K.A. & DiNardo, J.A. Echocardiographic assessment of atrial septal defects. *Anesth Analg* **115**, 772–775 (2012).

Gaynor, J.W. Management of sinus venosus defects. *Semin Thorac Cardiovasc Surg Pediatr Card Surg Annu* **9**, 35–39 (2006).

Stark, M. & Tsang, V.T. *Surgery for Congenital Heart Defects*, 3rd edn. Wiley & Sons Ltd, Oxford (2006).

16

Ventricular Septal Defect

Introduction

Ventricular septal defect (VSD) is the most common congenital heart disease, with an incidence that varies between 1.5–3 per 1000 term infants and 4.5–7 per 1000 preterm infants. VSDs have a high rate of spontaneous closure (30–40%). The most common associated chromosomal syndromes include trisomy 13, 18, and 21.

Anatomy

A VSD is an opening in the ventricular septum that permits communication between the right and left ventricles. It may exist in one or more locations in the ventricular septum, and is classified by its location in the septum (Figures 16.1 and 16.2).

Subpulmonary or Supracristal Defects

These are located in the infundibular septum just below the pulmonary valve. The lesions may be associated with aortic insufficiency due to a lack of support for the right coronary cusp of the aortic valve and prolapse of this leaflet.

Membranous or Perimembranous Defects

These defects comprise approximately 80% of all VSDs, and are located in the subaortic region of the membranous septum. Such defects are located near or under the septal leaflet of the tricuspid valve, and communicate with the left ventricle just below the aortic valve. These defects are commonly partially closed by a collection of tricuspid valve and membranous septal tissue, which gives an aneurysmal appearance to the septum.

Conoventricular Defects

These defects involve the same area as perimembranous defects, but extend anteriorly and superiorly into the septum.

Inlet or Canal-type Defects

These defects involve the posterior septum near the atrioventricular (AV) valves.

Muscular Defects

These defects are located in the lower trabecular septum, and may appear deceptively small on inspection from the right ventricular aspect of the septum due to heavy trabeculation. They may be apical, mid-muscular, anterior, or posterior.

Physiology

A VSD is an example of a simple shunt. The size of the defect is the critical determinant of the magnitude of shunting. If the defect is small (restrictive shunt), flow through the defect will be limited and there will be a large pressure gradient across the defect. However,

The Pediatric Cardiac Anesthesia Handbook, Second Edition. Viviane G. Nasr and James A. DiNardo.
© 2025 John Wiley & Sons Ltd. Published 2025 by John Wiley & Sons Ltd.

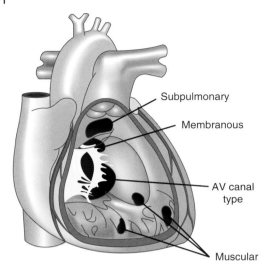

Figure 16.1 Different locations of ventricular septal defects. *Source:* Reproduced from DiNardo and Zvara (2008)/with permission of John Wiley & Sons.

Figure 16.2 Apical four-chamber view with anterior angulation demonstrates a large VSD with posterior malalignment of conal septum. The aortic valve is aligned entirely over the left ventricle without the normal slight over-ride above the ventricular septum and is hypoplastic.

as the orifice becomes larger (approximating the size of the aortic valve orifice) and the pressure gradient across the orifice decreases, the magnitude and direction of shunting become more dependent on the relative resistances of the systemic and pulmonary vascular beds.

Because the ratio of pulmonary vascular resistance (PVR) to systemic vascular resistance (SVR) is normally 1:10 to 1:20, VSDs generally result in the production of a left-to-right (L-R) shunt. In some instances, however, the PVR:SVR ratio may be higher, resulting in near-normal pulmonary blood flow or, in extreme cases, the production of a right-to-left (R-L) shunt.

The infant with a large VSD may have near-normal pulmonary blood flow as a result of high PVR present at birth. By the second week of life, the PVR begins to fall to near-normal levels and pulmonary blood flow increases dramatically. Continued decreases in PVR after birth may be delayed by the elevated left atrial pressure that accompanies increased pulmonary blood flow.

All patients with large, nonrestrictive VSDs have elevated, often systemic or near-systemic, pulmonary artery pressures. As a consequence, large VSDs predispose to the development of pulmonary artery hypertension (PAH) during the first few years of life due to exposure of the pulmonary vasculature to high flows and systemic blood pressures. The increases in PVR that accompany PAH will ultimately produce bidirectional and R-L shunts. Patients with advanced PAH and markedly increased PVR (Eisenmenger complex) generally are not candidates for VSD closure, because closure will result in an enormous increase in right ventricle afterload and right ventricle afterload mismatch. In older patients with large VSDs and elevated pulmonary artery pressures, cardiac catheterization to measure PVR is necessary to distinguish high pulmonary blood flow into a pulmonary bed with normal or slightly elevated PVR (candidate for VSD closure) from pulmonary blood flow into a pulmonary bed with significantly elevated PVR (potentially not a candidate for closure). For this reason, large VSDs (Q_p:Q_s >2:1) are corrected early in childhood.

An increase in left atrial volume and pressure parallels the increase in pulmonary blood flow seen with a large VSD. The resultant pulmonary venous congestion increases the work of breathing, decreases pulmonary compliance, and increases airway resistance. All of these factors predispose to recurrent pulmonary infections. Left ventricular end-diastolic volumes are increased in parallel with the increase in pulmonary blood flow. Although the majority of L-R shunting across VSDs occurs during ventricular systole, significant diastolic and isovolumic shunting occurs in the presence of large VSDs to result in an increased right ventricular end-diastolic volume.

In VSDs with a large L-R shunt, systemic blood flow is maintained at the expense of a large volume load on both the right and left ventricles. This limits the capacity of the patient to meet increased cardiac output demands, and may result in pulmonary and systemic venous congestion at rest. The timing of surgery often is dictated by failure of medical therapy to control this congestion.

Surgical Therapy

Ventricular septal defects generally are closed with a patch via a variety of approaches, depending on their location. Most defects in the perimembranous and conoventricular septum are approachable through the right atrium and tricuspid valve. A small right ventriculotomy may be necessary to visualize the most superior aspect of a conoventricular defect. Subpulmonary or supracristal defects are usually approached via an incision in the right ventricle and proximal pulmonary artery. To avoid postoperative compromise of a small ventricle, with its poor compliance and limited capacity for tension development, a ventriculotomy to approach and correct VSDs should be avoided whenever possible. Less commonly, assessment and closure of some muscular defects will require a left ventriculotomy. Because a left ventriculotomy may seriously compromise myocardial function in the infant, palliation with pulmonary artery banding may be preferable to a left ventriculotomy for small infants.

Nonoperative device closure of muscular VSDs remote from atrioventricular or semilunar valves is possible in the cardiac catheterization laboratory.

Catheterization Laboratory Intervention

Under guidance of fluoroscopy and echocardiography while avoiding sternotomy and cardiopulmonary bypass (CPB), VSDs may be closed in the catheterization laboratory based on the location and size of the lesion. This approach can be associated with adverse events such as arrhythmia, device embolism, and vascular complications. More recently, a hybrid perventricular device closure of VSDs (muscular and premembranous) has been described which combines the advantages of both surgical and percutaneous approaches.

Anesthetic Management

Induction and Maintenance

As discussed previously, control of ventilation is the most reliable way to manipulate PVR. For infants and children without congestive heart failure (CHF), an inhalational induction is well tolerated. For neonates and patients with CHF, an intravenous induction with fentanyl or sufentanil will provide better hemodynamic stability. In particular, for patients with reactive pulmonary vasculature, high opioid doses will be useful in blunting increases in PVR associated with surgical stimulation. In the absence of intravenous access, intramuscular ketamine or gentle inhalation induction may be used, followed by placement of an intravenous catheter.

The anesthetic management goals are to: (i) maintain heart rate, contractility, and preload to maintain cardiac output; (ii) avoid decreases in the PVR:SVR ratio to maintain systemic blood flow; and (iii) avoid large increases in the PVR:SVR ratio.

In instances in which a R-L shunt exists, ventilatory measures to decrease the PVR should be used. In addition, SVR must be maintained or increased. These measures will reduce the magnitude of the R-L shunt.

Post-CPB Management

Closure of the VSD will prevent further exposure of the pulmonary vasculature to high flows and pressures. This usually will result in some immediate decrease in pulmonary artery pressures. For patients with small defects and those with large VSDs in whom PAH has not yet developed, near-normal pulmonary artery pressures may result. In these patients, inotropic support post CPB is rarely necessary. In fact, reduction in the large volume load on the left ventricle usually results in post-CPB hypertension. Direct vasodilators such as sodium nitroprusside (0.5–1.0 µg kg^{-1} min^{-1}) or nicardipine (0.5–1.0 µg kg^{-1} min^{-1}) in conjunction with esmolol (100–300 µg kg^{-1} min^{-1}) may be necessary.

Pulmonary artery pressures and PVR will remain elevated in patients with underlying PAH. In addition, the pulmonary vasculature of these patients will remain hyper-responsive to vasoconstricting stimuli due to medial hypertrophy that accompanies PAH. Therapy to reduce PVR in the post-CPB period may be necessary for these patients to avoid right ventricle afterload mismatch.

Separation from CPB may be complicated by a variety of surgical problems. Inadequate closure of the VSD or the presence of an unrecognized VSD may prevent separation from CPB. Assessment of the presence and location of such defects in the operating room can be accomplished using transesophageal echocardiography. In addition, tricuspid valve damage due to a difficult transatrial approach may produce tricuspid regurgitation. Distortion of the aortic annulus or direct damage to the right coronary valve cusp may result in leaflet prolapse and aortic insufficiency. Patch closure of the VSD may create subaortic or subpulmonic obstruction. Because the atrioventricular node and the bundle of His are often near the area where the surgeon is working, transient heart block may occur. Temporary epicardial A-V sequential pacing may be necessary to terminate CPB.

Noncardiac Surgery

Patients with repaired VSD can present for noncardiac surgery with residual ventricular dysfunction and PAH. They may also suffer from dysrhythmias and conduction defects (e.g., right bundle branch block, ventricular arrhythmias, and heart block).

References and Further Reading

DiNardo, J.A. & Zvara, D.A. *Anesthesia for Cardiac Surgery*, 3rd edn. Blackwell, Massachusetts (2008).

Penny, D.J. & Vick, G.W. Ventricular septal defect. *Lancet* **377**, 1103–1112 (2011).

Richter, E.W., Sniecinski, R.M. & Sumler, M.L. Echocardiographic assessment of ventricular septal defects. *A&A Practice* **14**, 31–34 (2019).

17

Atrioventricular Canal Defects

Introduction

Atrioventricular canal defects (AVCs) or endocardial cushion defects constitute 4–5% of congenital heart diseases (CHDs).

Anatomy

Embryologically, there are four endocardial cushions that contribute to the development of the lower ostium primum portion of the atrial septum and the upper, posterior inlet portion of the interventricular septum (IVS) where the atrioventricular valves (AVs) insert. The cushions also contribute to the tissue that forms the septal leaflets of the mitral and tricuspid valves. Therefore, cushion defects, or AVC defects, include abnormalities in all of these structures. The components of these lesions are summarized in Figures 17.1 and 17.2.

Partial AVC

There is an ostium primum atrial septal defect (ASD) in association with a cleft mitral valve. There are two separate AV (mitral and tricuspid) annuli. No inlet ventricular septal defect (VSD) is present.

Transitional AVC

There is an ostium primum ASD, common AV valve orifice, common anterosuperior and posteroinferior bridging leaflets with dense chordal attachments to the crest of the IVS creating functionally separate mitral and tricuspid valve orifices; the mitral valve is cleft. There is a very small or absent inlet VSD.

Intermediate AVC

There is an ostium primum ASD and a moderate to large inlet VSD but a tongue of tissue divides the common AV valve into distinct right and left orifices; the mitral valve is cleft.

Complete AVC (CAVC)

There is an ostium primum ASD, common AV valve orifice, common anterosuperior and posteroinferior bridging leaflets with varying chordal attachments to the crest of the IVS. There is a moderate to large inlet VSD (Figure 17.3).

The types of chordal attachments present in a CAVC are summarized as follows (Figure 17.4).

- *Rastelli A*: the anterosuperior bridging leaflet is effectively divided into left (mitral) and right (tricuspid) anterosuperior leaflets by chordal attachments to the crest of the IVS. There is also usually an attachment of the posteroinferior leaflets to the crest of the IVS. The majority (70%) of CAVCs are of this type.
- *Rastelli B*: there are chordal attachments from the right side of the IVS (right ventricular septal papillary muscle) to the left side of the anterosuperior bridging leaflet.

The Pediatric Cardiac Anesthesia Handbook, Second Edition. Viviane G. Nasr and James A. DiNardo.
© 2025 John Wiley & Sons Ltd. Published 2025 by John Wiley & Sons Ltd.

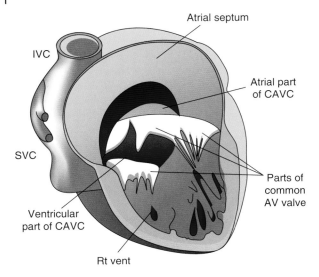

Atrial septum

IVC

Atrial part of CAVC

SVC

Parts of common AV valve

Ventricular part of CAVC

Rt vent

Figure 17.1 Components of a complete atrioventricular canal defect. AV, atrioventricular; CAVC, complete atrioventricular canal; IVC, inferior vena cava; RT vent, right ventricle; SVC, superior vena cava. *Source:* Reproduced from DiNardo and Zvara (2008)/with permission from John Wiley & Sons.

AVSD Summary

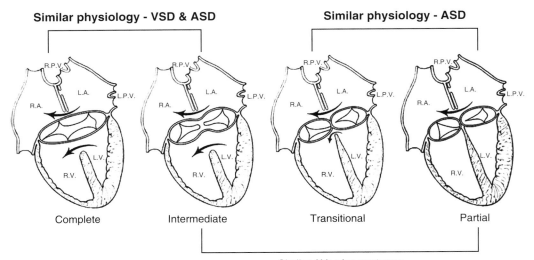

Similar physiology - VSD & ASD

Similar physiology - ASD

Complete   Intermediate   Transitional   Partial

Similar AV valve anatomy:
A tongue of tissue divides the common AV valve into a right and left component by connecting the anterior and posterior "bridging" leaflets centrally

Figure 17.2 Anatomic characterization of atrioventricular canal (AVC) defects and associated physiology are illustrated. CAVC defects have one annulus with a large ASD and VSD component. Intermediate defects have a large ASD and VSD component but a tongue of tissue divides the single valve annulus into two distinct valve orifices. Transitional defects are associated with a small or absent inlet VSD and two distinct valve orifices. In partial defects there is an ostium primum ASD in association with a cleft mitral valve. There are two separate AV (mitral and tricuspid) annuli. No inlet ventricular septal defect (VSD) is present. AV, atrioventricular; LA, left atrium; LPV, left pulmonary vein; LV, left ventricle; RA, right atrium; RPV, right pulmonary vein; RV, right ventricle. *Source:* Reproduced from Robert E. Shaddy et al. (2021)/with permission of Wolters Kluwer Health – Lippincott Williams & Wilkins.

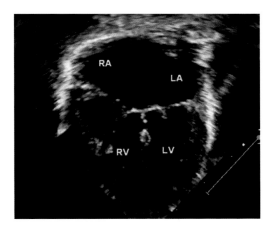

Figure 17.3 Apical four-chamber view demonstrating a large atrial and large ventricular communication in a patient with complete CAVC. The common AV valve is closed but can be identified as a single common valve. More superior or inferior location of the valve alters the size of the atrial and ventricular communications. LA, left atrium; LV, left ventricle; RA, right atrium; RV, right ventricle. *Source:* Reproduced from Cohen (2016)/with permission of John Wiley & Sons.

There are no choral attachments to the crest of the IVS.

- *Rastelli C*: there are no chordal attachments of the anterosuperior bridging leaflet to any portion of the IVS; there is usually an attachment to a right ventricular free wall papillary muscle. This creates what appears to be a free-floating common AV valve. This type is seen most commonly in conjunction with other lesions such as tetralogy of Fallot (TOF).

Unbalanced AVC

In this lesion there is relative hypoplasia of either the right ventricle (left dominant) or left ventricle (right dominant) and the corresponding outflow tract.

Physiology

These defects can result in communication between all four heart chambers, as well as in abnormalities of the mitral and tricuspid valves. The physiology associated with the various types of CAVC defects is summarized in Figure 17.2. While complete and intermediate defects have physiology similar to a large ASD and VSD, transitional and partial canal defects have physiology similar to a large ASD. Because the orifice between the chambers tends to be large, these lesions produce dependent simple shunts. When a large VSD component is present, there is:

- the production of a large left-to-right physiologic shunt
- increased pulmonary blood flow
- the transmission of systemic pressures to the right ventricle and pulmonary arteries
- volume overloading of the right and left ventricles.

With large VSD components, intermediate and CAVC defects predispose to the early development of precapillary pulmonary hypertension or true pulmonary arterial hypertension (PAH). This may increase

Figure 17.4 Types of complete atrioventricular canal. (A) Rastelli type A; (B) Rastelli type B; (C) Rastelli type C. LIL and RIL, left and right inferior (posterior) leaflets; LLL and RLL, left and right lateral leaflets; LSL and RSL, left and right superior (anterior) leaflets; SL, superior anterior bridging leaflet. *Source:* Reproduced from DiNardo and Zvara (2008)/with permission from John Wiley & Sons.

the pulmonary vascular resistance (PVR):systemic vascular resistance (SVR) ratio such that a bidirectional or right-to-left (R-L) shunt develops. This is a particular concern for patients with trisomy 21, who are prone to the early development of PAH. These defects are generally repaired at about three months of age when there is sufficient maturation of AV valve tissue to facilitate a good surgical repair and before the development of pulmonary vascular changes and PAH. In some CAVC defects, the presence of severe mitral insufficiency results in regurgitation of left ventricular blood directly into the right atrium (left ventricle to right atrium shunt). This increases the left-to-right (L-R) shunt. In addition, mitral regurgitation increases the volume work of the left ventricle.

In children presenting for repair at a later age, in those without symptoms of congestive heart failure (CHF) and in those with episodes of cyanosis, the possibility that PVR is elevated may be investigated with a preoperative cardiac catheterization to directly determine PVR.

Surgical Therapy

The repair of these defects involves:

- septation of the common AV valve tissue into two separate competent, nonstenotic tricuspid and mitral valves
- closure of the ostium primum ASD
- closure of the inlet VSD.

This can usually be accomplished using a one-patch technique wherein a single patch is used to close both the VSD and ASD, and the reconstructed AV valves are resuspended by sutures to the patch. When the VSD is large and extends to other areas of the septum (as in TOF), two patches (atrial and ventricular) may be necessary. When the inlet VSD component is small, the AV valve tissue can be sutured down to the crest of the ventricular septum, essentially closing the VSD. A patch is then sutured to the crest of the ventricular septum and is used to close the ASD. This is often referred to as the Australian technique.

Anesthetic Management

Induction and Maintenance

Anesthetic management is similar to that for large VSDs (Table 17.1). However, the child with CAVC also may have severe mitral regurgitation and a highly reactive pulmonary vasculature. Because control of ventilation is the most reliable way to manipulate PVR, a prompt and reliable control of the airway at induction is important. The goal should be to use a reduced FiO_2 and to maintain $PaCO_2$ at 35–40 mmHg. Despite aggressive medical management with diuretics and ACE inhibitors, many of these patients present for surgery with pulmonary vascular congestion and poor lung compliance. This may make mask ventilation without insufflation of the stomach with air difficult. Inhalational induction should be reserved for infants and children with small defects, no mitral regurgitation, and no PAH. Cardiac reserve often is limited or exhausted in patients with large shunts and high pulmonary blood flow. Moreover, the additional volume load

Table 17.1 Anesthetic management goals for surgical repair of CAVC.

Intraoperatively	Post CPB
Maintain heart rate, contractility and preload to maintain cardiac output	Maintain age-appropriate heart rate and sinus rhythm
Avoid decreases in PVR:SVR ratio	Reduce PVR, especially in cases of PAH. Consider nitric oxide
Avoid large increases in PVR:SVR ratio to avoid an increase in R-L shunt	Inotropic support (e.g., dopamine 5–10 µg kg^{-1} min^{-1}, epinephrine 0.05–0.1 5 µg kg^{-1} min^{-1} +/- milrinone 0.5 µg kg^{-1} min^{-1})

imposed on the left ventricle by mitral regurgitation will further limit cardiac reserve.

An intravenous induction and maintenance with fentanyl will provide better hemodynamic stability. In particular, for patients with a reactive pulmonary vasculature, high doses of fentanyl will be useful in blunting increases in PVR associated with surgical stimulation. High doses of fentanyl will also blunt stimulation-induced increases in the SVR, which will increase the mitral regurgitant fraction.

Post-CPB Management

Closure of the defects will prevent further exposure of the pulmonary vasculature to high blood flows and pressures. This usually will result in some immediate decrease in pulmonary artery pressures. In patients with small defects and patients with large defects in whom PAH has not yet developed, near-normal pulmonary artery pressures may result. However, the pulmonary artery pressures and PVR will remain elevated in patients with underlying PAH. In addition, the pulmonary vasculature of these patients (especially trisomy 21 patients) will remain hyper-responsive to vasoconstricting stimuli due to medial hypertrophy that accompanies PAH. Therapy to reduce PVR in the post-CPB period may be necessary for these patients to avoid right ventricular afterload mismatch.

Separation from CPB may be complicated by a variety of surgical problems. Inadequate closure of the defects or persistent mitral regurgitation may prevent separation from CPB. An assessment of the presence and location of such defects in the OR can be accomplished using transesophageal echocardiography (TEE). The presence of large V-waves on the pressure trace obtained from a left atrial catheter may be helpful in assessing the degree of mitral regurgitation, whereas TEE will provide definitive information. Because the AV node is near the area of patch placement, heart block may occur. Temporary epicardial A-V sequential pacing may be necessary to terminate CPB.

In patients with unbalanced canal defects, restrictive diastolic function and reduced ventricular chamber size and stroke volume may be limiting factors in maintaining cardiac output. In these patients the appropriate heart rate is a balance between the competing priorities of reduced diastolic filling time and the requirement for an increased heart rate in the setting of reduced stroke volume.

Noncardiac Surgery

Patients with repaired CAVC may present with residual mitral valve disease, pulmonary hypertension and right ventricle dysfunction and arrhythmias (heart block, sinus node dysfunction).

References and Further Reading

Cohen, M.S. Common Atrioventricular Canal Defects. In: Lai, W., Mertens, L., and Cohen, M.S. (eds) *Echocardiography in Pediatric and Congenital Heart Disease* (pp. 259–278). John Wiley & Sons (2016).

DiNardo, J.A. & Zvara, D.A. *Anesthesia for Cardiac Surgery*, 3rd edn. Blackwell, Massachusetts (2008).

Mendeloff, E.N. Correction of partial atrioventricular canal defects. *Oper Techn Thorac Cardiovasc Surg* **7**, 29–37 (2002).

Moss, A.J. & Allen, H.D. *Moss and Adams' Heart Disease in Infants, Children, and Adolescents: Including the Fetus And Young Adult*, 7th edn. Wolters Kluwer Health/ Lippincott Williams & Wilkins (2008).

18

Double Outlet Right Ventricle

Introduction

Double outlet right ventricle (DORV), a clinically significant congenital heart defect, occurs in 1–3% of individuals with congenital heart defects. It is associated with trisomy 13 and 18 but only rarely with chromosome 22q11 deletions.

Anatomy

In the Congenital Heart Surgery Nomenclature and Database Project, the consensus definition of DORV is "…DORV is a type of ventriculoarterial connection in which both great vessels arise either entirely or predominantly from the right ventricle." It results from a failure of counterclockwise rotation of the distal conus and a leftward shift of the conoventricular septum. It is almost always associated with a ventricular septal defect (VSD). In DORV it is generally not the position of the VSD that is variable; rather, it is the rotation of the great arteries driven by the conal development that is variable.

Given the morphologic and physiologic diversity of DORV, determining the following anatomic features is important in the evaluation of DORV.

- Ventricular septal defect size and its relationship to the semilunar valves (Figure 18.1). The VSD is generally cradled within the limbs of the septomarginal trabeculation or septal band with the relationship to the great arteries described as subaortic (50%), subpulmonary (30%), or doubly committed (10%). Atrioventricular (AV) canal-type VSDs are more remote from the great arteries with the relationship described as uncommitted (10%).
- Conal morphology (Figure 18.2). In the normal heart the infundibulum or conus is a right ventricular structure, a fibromuscular tube that separates the tricuspid valve (AV valve) from the pulmonary valve (semilunar valve). In DORV there may be bilateral conus, subaortic conus with absent subpulmonary conus, subpulmonary conus with absent subaortic conus, or bilaterally absent conus. The size and location of conus are determinants of the distance from the VSD to each semilunar valve, and of the distance between the AV valve and the semilunar valve. This is important because the width of an intracardiac baffle connecting the left ventricle to the aorta via a VSD is limited to the distance between the tricuspid valve (TV) and the pulmonary valve. In order for the baffle not to be the source of subaortic stenosis, the distance between the tricuspid valve and the pulmonary valve must be adequate.
- Relationship of the great arteries to each other (Figure 18.3). The great artery trunks commonly have a side-by-side orientation but may occasionally have a normal, spiraled orientation.

The Pediatric Cardiac Anesthesia Handbook, Second Edition. Viviane G. Nasr and James A. DiNardo.
© 2025 John Wiley & Sons Ltd. Published 2025 by John Wiley & Sons Ltd.

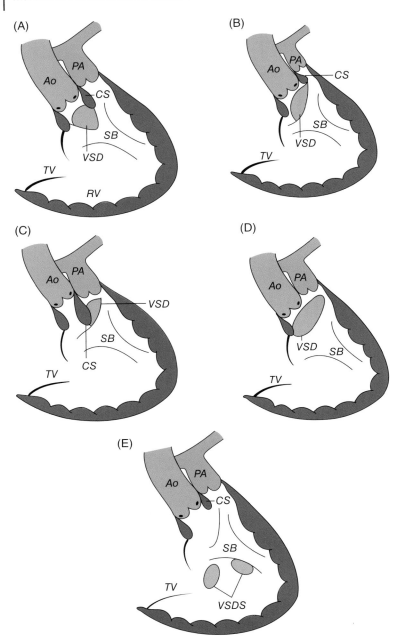

Figure 18.1 Different variants of double outlet right ventricle (DORV). (A) DORV with a subaortic ventricular septal defect (VSD) where the conal septum is attached to the anterosuperior limb of the septal band. (B) DORV with a subaortic VSD and pulmonary stenosis secondary to significant anterior attachment of the conal septum to the anterosuperior limb of the septal band. (C) DORV with a subpulmonary VSD where the conal septum is attached to the right ventriculoinfundibular fold. (D) DORV with a doubly committed VSD and absent conal septum. (E) DORV with a remote VSD. Ao, aorta; CS, conal septum; PA, pulmonary artery; RV, right ventricle; SB, septal band; TV, tricuspid valve; VSD, ventricular septal defect. *Source:* Adapted from Lopez and Geva (2016).

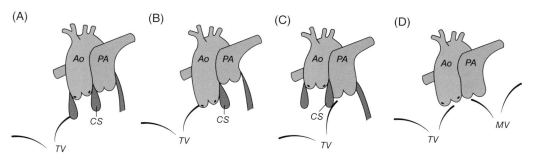

Figure 18.2 Four categories of conal morphology. (A) Bilateral conus; (B) absent subaortic conus; (C) absent subpulmonary conus; (D) bilaterally absent conus. Ao, aorta; CS, conal septum; MV, mitral valve; PA, pulmonary artery; TV, tricuspid valve. *Source:* Adapted from Lopez and Geva (2016).

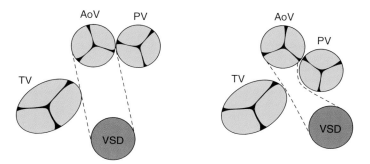

Figure 18.3 How the distance from the tricuspid valve (TV) to the pulmonary valve (PV) can affect the potential baffle pathway from the left ventricle (LV) to the aorta. AoV, aortic valve; VSD, ventricular septal defect. *Source:* Adapted from Lopez and Geva (2016).

- Associated cardiac lesions, including outflow tract obstruction, AV valve anomalies, and ventricular hypoplasia.
- Coronary artery anatomy.

Physiology

The pathophysiology of DORV is determined by the magnitude and direction of intracardiac physiologic shunting which in turn is determined by the interplay of:

- VSD size
- VSD relationship to the great arteries
- the presence of right ventricular outflow tract (RVOT) or left ventricular outflow tract (LVOT) obstruction
- pulmonary vascular resistance
- associated cardiovascular anomalies.

The common pathophysiologic variants are summarized below.

- *VSD physiology*: DORV with a large subaortic VSD and no pulmonary stenosis.
- *Tetralogy of Fallot (TOF) physiology*: DORV with a subaortic or doubly committed VSD and pulmonary stenosis.
- *Transposition of the great arteries (TGA) physiology*: DORV with a subpulmonary VSD. This physiology is seen in the Taussig–Bing anomaly where there is a subpulmonary VSD, side-by-side great vessels, and bilateral conus.
- *Noncommitted VSD physiology*: remotely located VSD commonly associated with AV canal defects and/or heterotaxy syndrome, where the distance from the VSD to the aortic valve or pulmonary valve is greater than the aortic diameter. These

patients have a physiology similar to that of patients with complete AV canal defects.

- *Single-ventricle physiology*: DORV with mitral atresia or significant ventricular hypoplasia, often in association with an unbalanced AV canal defect and/or heterotaxy syndrome.

Surgical Therapy

Surgical options for DORV include the following broad approaches, as dictated by the complex relationship between the ventricles, VSD, and great arteries (Figure 18.4).

- Intracardiac baffle from the left ventricle to the aortic valve via the VSD, with or without resection of the conal septum while ensuring unobstructed intracardiac flow from the right ventricle to the pulmonary artery.

- Intracardiac baffle from the left ventricle to the aortic valve, with or without resection of the conal septum as well as a RVOT reconstruction with options such as transannular patch augmentation, placement of a homograft or conduit from the right ventricle to the pulmonary artery (Rastelli procedure), or direct anastomosis of the pulmonary trunk to the right ventricle free wall (réparation á l'étage ventriculaire known as the REV or Lecompte procedure).

- Intracardiac baffle from the left ventricle to the pulmonary valve in conjunction with an arterial switch operation, aortic translocation and RVOT reconstruction

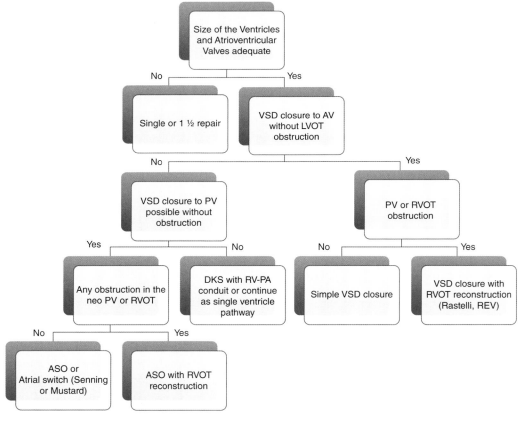

Figure 18.4 Surgical management for patient with double outlet right ventricle (DORV). See text for details of repairs.

(Nikaidoh), double root translocation, or truncal block translocation (Yamagishi).

- Intracardiac baffle to both aortic and pulmonary valves in conjunction with a Damus–Kaye–Stansel (DKS) anastomosis and a right ventricle to pulmonary artery conduit (Yasui procedure) can be used to create a biventricular circulation when an unobstructed pathway from the VSD to either the pulmonary or aortic outflow tract alone cannot be created.
- Single-ventricle palliation.
- Most patients with a DORV undergo surgical intervention within the first year of life. Transthoracic echocardiography provides the information necessary for surgical planning in all but the most complex anatomy, in which case cardiac magnetic resonance imaging or cardiac catheterization may be necessary. Surgical management of DORV with noncommitted VSD physiology is very challenging, since long intracardiac baffles with multiple potential points of obstruction are often necessary.

Anesthetic Management

Induction and Maintenance

Anesthetic management is based on the physiologic variant of DORV (TOF, TGA, single ventricle) present. The anesthetic management of each lesion is described in detail in Chapters 24, 27, and 28, respectively.

Post-CPB Management

Post-CPB management is described in Chapters 24, 27, and 28. Given the complexity of many of the biventricular repairs, transesophageal echocardiography, epicardial echocardiography, and determination of $Q_p{:}Q_s$ by blood gas oximetry may be necessary to rule out residual lesions, particularly residual VSD and LVOT obstruction, and baffle obstruction.

References and Further Reading

Ebadi, A., Spicer, D.E., Backer, C.L., Fricker, F.J. & Anderson, R.H. Double-outlet right ventricle revisited. *J Thorac Cardiovasc Surg* **154**, 598–604 (2017).

Lopez, L. & Geva, T. Double outlet ventricle. In: Lai, W.W., Mertens, L.L., Cohen, M.S. & Geva, T. (eds) *Echocardiography in Pediatric and Congenital Heart Disease: From Fetus to Adult*, 2nd edn. John Wiley & Sons, Chichester (2016).

Yamagishi, M. Half-turned truncal switch operation for transposition of the great arteries with left ventricular outflow obstruction. *Oper Tech Thorac Cardiovasc Surg* **26**, 588–604 (2022).

19

Truncus Arteriosus

Introduction

Truncus arteriosus (TA) occurs in approximately 1–4% of patients with congenital heart defects.

Anatomy

Truncus arteriosus is characterized by a single great vessel arising from the base of the heart and giving rise to the pulmonary, coronary, and systemic arteries. There is a single semilunar valve, which is usually abnormal, and invariably a large (nonrestrictive) ventricular septal defect (VSD) is present. The truncus usually straddles this large VSD. The VSD is of the conoventricular type, similar to that seen in tetralogy of Fallot (TOF). The truncal valve is tricuspid in 60–70% of patients, but multiple cusps can be seen and the valve itself may be regurgitant (50%) or stenotic (30%). Extracardiac anomalies are seen in approximately 30% of patients. TA is classified based on the origin of the pulmonary arteries; typically, there are two classifications (Figure 19.1). Collett and Edwards (1949) classified TA into four major types based on the sources of pulmonary blood supply.

- *Type I*: a short main pulmonary artery segment gives rise to both branch pulmonary arteries (Figure 19.2).
- *Type II*: both branch pulmonary arteries arise from the common arterial trunk adjacent to one another, with a rim of truncal tissue between them (Figure 19.3).
- *Type III*: the branch pulmonary arteries arise from either side of the truncus and are somewhat remote from one another.
- *Type IV (previously termed pseudotruncus)*: the pulmonary circulation is supplied by collateral vessels from the descending aorta. This anomaly is considered a form of TOF with pulmonary atresia rather than TA.

The classification of Van Praagh and Van Praagh, as devised in 1965, is as follows.

- *Type A1*: the branch pulmonary arteries arise from a short main pulmonary artery.
- *Type A2*: the branch pulmonary arteries arise directly from the arterial trunk through separate orifices.
- *Type A3*: only one branch pulmonary artery arises from the ascending segment of the arterial trunk. Collateral vessels usually supply the contralateral lung.
- *Type A4*: truncus arteriosus with aortic arch hypoplasia, coarctation or interruption of the aortic arch (IAA), usually a type B interruption distal to the left common carotid artery. In this anatomic variant there is usually a well-formed main pulmonary artery and a small ascending aorta. The associated cardiac lesions include right-sided aortic arch (33%), interrupted aortic arch (19% of type A4), left superior vena cava (SVC) (12%), and partial anomalous pulmonary venous return (PAPVR) (1%).

The Pediatric Cardiac Anesthesia Handbook, Second Edition. Viviane G. Nasr and James A. DiNardo.
© 2025 John Wiley & Sons Ltd. Published 2025 by John Wiley & Sons Ltd.

Collett and Edwards

Van Praagh

Figure 19.1 Classification of truncus arteriosus. Upper panel: Collett and Edwards' system. Lower panel: Van Praagh and Van Praagh's system. *Source:* Reproduced from Slesnick and Sachdeva, (2021)/with permission of John Wiley & Sons.

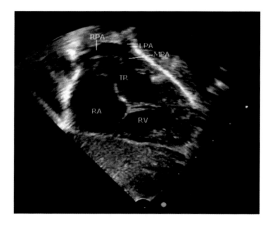

Figure 19.2 Subcostal coronal view showing the truncal root and the origin of the main pulmonary artery segment from the left lateral aspect of the truncus, with subsequent bifurcation into right and left pulmonary arteries. LPA, left pulmonary artery; MPA, main pulmonary artery segment; RA, right atrium; right pulmonary artery; RV, right ventricle; TR, truncal root. *Source:* Reproduced from Slesnick and Sachdeva, (2021)/with permission of John Wiley & Sons.

Figure 19.3 Parasternal short-axis view demonstrating separate origins of the pulmonary artery branches from the posterior aspect of the truncal root (truncus arteriosus type II). LPA, left pulmonary artery; RPA, right pulmonary artery; TR, truncal root. *Source:* Reproduced from Slesnick and Sachdeva, (2021)/with permission of John Wiley & Sons.

Physiology

Truncus arteriosus is a simple shunt with a common chamber and single-ventricle physiology. The large (nonrestrictive) VSD allows equalization of pressures in the right and left ventricles. As a result, there is bidirectional shunting and complete mixing of systemic and pulmonary venous blood in a functionally common ventricular chamber. This blood is then ejected into the truncal root, which gives rise to the pulmonary, systemic, and coronary circulations. Q_p:Q_s is determined by the ratio of pulmonary vascular resistance (PVR) to systemic vascular resistance (SVR).

In TA, as in all single-ventricle physiology lesions, the pulmonary and systemic circulations are supplied in parallel from a single vessel, and increases in flow to one circulatory system are likely to produce reductions in flow to the other. Under normal circumstances, as the PVR decreases following birth, the balance of PVR and SVR is such that pulmonary blood flow is high and the patient with TA has symptoms of congestive heart failure (CHF) with mild cyanosis. After the cardiac reserve has been exhausted, further decreases in PVR will increase pulmonary blood flow at the expense of systemic and coronary perfusion. This will produce a progressive metabolic acidosis.

If PVR is increased relative to SVR, systemic blood flow will increase at the expense of pulmonary blood flow and severe hypoxemia will result. This second scenario is particularly likely in older patients in whom pulmonary arterial hypertension (PAH) has developed in response to high pulmonary blood flow and the transmission of systemic arterial pressures to the pulmonary vasculature.

Finally, if truncal valve insufficiency is present, this will impose an additional volume load on the ventricles.

Surgical Therapy

Because of the risk of early development of PAH from high pulmonary blood flow and pressure, prompt surgical intervention is recommended. A definitive repair of TA requires patch closure of the VSD, detachment of the pulmonary arteries from the truncus, and establishment of right ventricular-to-pulmonary artery continuity with a valved homograft. The right ventricular-to-pulmonary artery conduit requires placement of the proximal end of the conduit over a ventriculotomy in the right ventricle free wall. The truncal valves must be assessed at the time of surgery.

In some instances, valve replacement or valve repair is necessary to address valvular insufficiency or stenosis. Considering the problems with valve replacement in a growing child, valvuloplasty is preferred over valve replacement. The valved right ventricular-to-pulmonary artery conduit will eventually require replacement as the child grows. End-to-side anastomosis is generally used to repair TA in association with type B IAA.

Catheterization Laboratory Intervention

Most patients with a TA undergo surgical intervention based entirely on information obtained from transthoracic echocardiography.

Anesthetic Management

Goals

Management principles are based on those described in Chapter 28.

- Maintain heart rate, contractility, and preload to maintain cardiac output. A reduction in cardiac output will compromise systemic perfusion, despite a relatively high pulmonary blood flow. A decrease in cardiac output will also reduce systemic venous saturation. As with all mixing lesions, a reduction in systemic venous saturation will reduce arterial oxygen saturation.

- For patients without PAH, avoid decreases in the PVR:SVR ratio. The increase in pulmonary blood flow that accompanies a reduced PVR:SVR ratio is likely to occur at the expense of systemic and coronary blood flow. Ventilate with a reduced FiO_2 (<30%) and maintain PCO_2 at 35–40 mmHg.
- For patients with severe CHF, inotropic support of the ventricles in combination with normocarbia or slight hypercarbia to reduce pulmonary blood flow may be necessary.
- For patients with PAH and reduced pulmonary blood flow, ventilatory interventions to reduce the PVR will be necessary. A high PVR will increase systemic and coronary blood flow at the expense of pulmonary blood flow, resulting in hypoxemia.

Induction and Maintenance

The neonate with TA often will be intubated and ventilated, requiring inotropic support to manage CHF due to high pulmonary blood flow. Cardiac reserve is very limited due to ventricular volume overload. Subendocardial perfusion will be compromised by the low aortic diastolic blood pressure that results from diastolic flow into the lower-resistance pulmonary vascular bed. Consequently, ventricular fibrillation can be seen during routine maneuvers, such as opening the pericardium in the precardio-pulmonary bypass (CPB) period. Ventilatory control of PVR will help reduce pulmonary blood flow and prevent systemic and coronary hypoperfusion.

Patients with TA are unlikely to tolerate the myocardial depression associated with inhalational anesthetics. Fentanyl in high doses, combined with a muscle relaxant, will provide hemodynamic stability without myocardial depression.

Post-CPB Management

Post-CPB management may be complicated by ventricular failure. Left ventricular volume overload may occur secondary to truncal valve insufficiency. Right ventricular systolic dysfunction may result from a right ventricular afterload mismatch due to the high pulmonary vascular resistance in patients with PAH, the right ventriculotomy required for conduit placement, and poor protection of the right ventricle during CPB.

Goals

- Maintain heart rate (preferably sinus rhythm) at an age-appropriate rate. Cardiac output is likely to be more heart rate dependent during the post-CPB period.
- Reduce PVR when necessary through ventilatory interventions.
- Inotropic support of the left and right ventricles may be necessary for the reasons addressed previously. Dopamine (5–10 µg kg^{-1} min^{-1}) or epinephrine (0.05–0.1 µg kg^{-1} min^{-}1) intravenously is useful in this instance as it provides potent inotropic support without increasing PVR.

References and Further Reading

Collett, R.W. & Edwards, J.E. Persistent truncus arteriosus; a classification according to anatomic types. *Surg Clin North Am* **29**, 1245–1270 (1949).

Naimo, P.S. & Konstantinov, I.E. Surgery for truncus arteriosus: contemporary practice. *Ann Thorac Surg* **111**, 1442–1450 (2020).

Slesnick, T.C., Sachdeva, R., Kreeger, J.R. & Border, W.L. Truncus arteriosus and aortopulmonary window. In: Lai, W.W., Mertens, L.L., Cohen, M.S. & Geva, T. (eds) *Echocardiography in Pediatric and Congenital Heart Disease: From Fetus to Adult*, 2nd edn. John Wiley & Sons, Chichester (2016).

Van Praagh, R. & Van Praagh, S. The anatomy of common aorticopulmonary trunk (truncus arteriosus communis) and its embryologic implications. A study of 57 necropsy cases. *Am J Cardiol* **16**, 406–425 (1965).

20

Total Anomalous Pulmonary Venous Return

Introduction

The incidence of total anomalous pulmonary venous return (TAPVR) ranges from 0.6 to 1.2 per 10,000 live births. Among patients born with congenital heart disease (CHD), the incidence of TAPVR ranges between 0.7% and 1.5%. It is the fifth most common cause of cyanotic CHD.

Total anomalous pulmonary venous return arises from a failure of the left atrium to connect the pulmonary venous plexus, which results in the retention of connections to the primitive cardinal and umbilicovitelline drainage systems. The anatomic variants of TAPVR are dependent upon which connections are retained. The cardinal venous system provides connections to the innominate vein, right atrium, superior vena cava, or azygous vein, and the umbilicovitelline system to the portal or hepatic vein, or inferior vena cava (IVC).

Anatomy

Total anomalous pulmonary venous return is characterized by drainage of all the pulmonary veins into the systemic venous system rather than directly into the left atrium. In this lesion, there is usually a single common pulmonary venous confluence with no direct connection to the left atrium. The pulmonary vein confluence then drains into the systemic venous circulation via one of the following four types of drainage patterns (Figure 20.1).

- *Supracardiac (type 1)*: in 46% of patients, drainage of the pulmonary vein confluence is into a supracardiac structure. Most commonly, drainage is to the superior vena cava (SVC) via a vertical vein that connects the pulmonary vein confluence with the innominate vein, which then empties into the SVC.
- *Intracardiac (type 2)*: in 24% of patients, drainage of the pulmonary vein confluence is directly into the right atrium via the coronary sinus.
- *Infracardiac (type 3)*: in 22% of patients, drainage is into an infracardiac structure such as the IVC, portal vein, or hepatic vein. A vertical pulmonary vein passes through the esophageal hiatus of the diaphragm to connect the pulmonary vein confluence to one of these infracardiac vessels.
- *Mixed (type 4)*: in 8% of patients, pulmonary venous drainage is some combination of types 1, 2, and 3.

In general, the greater the distance the vertical connecting vein travels, the greater the likelihood that this pathway will be stenotic or compressed and that there will be pulmonary venous obstruction. For this reason, infracardiac drainage is most commonly associated with pulmonary venous obstruction. Some patients with supracardiac TAPVR have compression of the vertical vein between the left mainstem bronchus and left

The Pediatric Cardiac Anesthesia Handbook, Second Edition. Viviane G. Nasr and James A. DiNardo.
© 2025 John Wiley & Sons Ltd. Published 2025 by John Wiley & Sons Ltd.

Figure 20.1 Total anomalous pulmonary venous connection. (A) Supracardiac; (B) cardiac; (C) infracardiac; (D) mixed connections. *Source:* Reproduced from Brown (2016)/with permission of John Wiley & Sons.

pulmonary artery. As the pulmonary artery pressure rises due to the obstruction of pulmonary venous return, the connecting vein may become further compressed between the left mainstem bronchus and left pulmonary artery, leading to near-complete compression of the connecting vein. This has been described as a "hemodynamic vice."

Physiology

The delivery of all pulmonary venous blood to the right atrium results in a large physiologic left-to-right (L-R) shunt. There is complete mixing of systemic and pulmonary venous blood in the right atrium. There must be an anatomic right-to-left (R-L) shunt and delivery of effective systemic blood flow if there is to be filling of the left heart and survival outside the uterus. Normally, an atrial septal defect (ASD) or patent foramen ovale (PFO) exists as the communication with the left heart. The magnitude and direction of shunting across the ASD or PFO are determined by the principles of simple shunting. Normally, a nonrestrictive or mildly restrictive atrial level communication exists in these patients. The delivery of blood across the atrial septum can be impeded by the poor compliance of the left atrium and left ventricle, as these structures tend to be small due to reduced blood flow to the left side of the heart *in utero*. As a result, in the absence of any obstruction, neonates will have a $Q_P:Q_S$ close to 1:1. As the pulmonary vascular resistance (PVR) falls following birth, there will be a preferential delivery of the mixed systemic and pulmonary venous blood to the pulmonary circuit. The pulmonary artery pressures will be near systemic because, although the PVR is near-normal, the $Q_P:Q_S$ will be high (>2–3:1).

Compression or stenoses along the vertical vein pathway will produce an obstructed TAPVR, leading to pulmonary venous hypertension, an elevated PVR, and systemic or suprasystemic right ventricular and pulmonary artery (PA) pressures. Some of these patients may also develop pulmonary arterial hypertension (PAH) *in utero*. In addition, pulmonary edema may occur, further elevating the PVR, much as it does with mitral stenosis. These patients have a small heart and congested lung fields on chest radiography.

The cardiac output can be severely compromised in these patients. Systemic or suprasystemic right ventricular pressures will result in a leftward septal shift that "pancakes" the left ventricle, thereby further reducing the compliance of the small left ventricle. This will impede the delivery of blood across the atrial septum to the left ventricle. There is likely to be a right ventricle afterload mismatch with right ventricular distension and tricuspid regurgitation. The systemic cardiac output will be largely dependent on a physiologic R-L shunt across the ductus arteriosus supplied by a failing right ventricle.

These patients will be hypoxemic because all the determinants of SaO_2 with complete mixing will be reduced.

- Pulmonary edema will induce intrapulmonary shunt and V/Q mismatch, leading to low $SpvO_2$.
- $Q_P:Q_S$ will be reduced by the presence of a high PVR.
- Low cardiac output will reduce SvO_2.

Efforts to increase pulmonary blood flow in these patients will only worsen the pulmonary edema, and inhaled pulmonary vasodilators (e.g., NO) are clearly contraindicated.

In patients with severe pulmonary venous obstruction leading to suprasystemic right ventricular and PA pressures, ductal patency with R-L shunting is necessary to maintain cardiac output because the left ventricle is pancaked due to leftward shift of the intraventricular septum and underfilled. In patients with less severe obstruction and subsystemic right ventricular and PA pressures, ductal flow will be bidirectional or L-R. In these patients ductal patency may exacerbate pulmonary edema. Patients with obstructed TAPVR present at birth with hypoxemia and poor systemic perfusion. In many cases there is an ongoing metabolic acidosis and evidence of end-organ (hepatic and renal) dysfunction. Obstructed TAPVR is a surgical emergency, one of the few remaining in the era of prostaglandin E_1 (PGE_1) therapy.

Surgical Therapy

Definitive repair involves anastomosis of the pulmonary venous confluence to the posterior wall of the left atrium, ligation of the vertical vein, and closure of the ASD. "Sutureless" techniques, which use the pericardial reflection behind the LA distal from the pulmonary vein orifices as the site for suture lines, have evolved to mitigate the risk of developing pulmonary vein stenosis.

Anesthetic Management

Goals

- Maintain heart rate, contractility, and preload to maintain cardiac output. Decreases in cardiac output will reduce systemic venous saturation. In a complete mixing lesion, this will reduce arterial saturation.
- For patients with TAPVR and pulmonary venous obstruction, emergency surgery is necessary. Efforts to increase pulmonary blood flow through ventilatory interventions

and pulmonary vasodilators will worsen pulmonary edema.

- For patients with increased pulmonary blood flow, decreases in the PVR:SVR ratio should be avoided. The increase in pulmonary blood flow that accompanies a reduced PVR:SVR ratio necessitates an increase in cardiac output to maintain systemic blood flow.
- For patients with increased pulmonary blood flow and right ventricular volume overload, ventilatory interventions should be used to increase the PVR, reduce pulmonary blood flow, and decrease the volume load on the right ventricle.

Induction and Maintenance

Neonates with pulmonary venous obstruction generally arrive in the operating room intubated, ventilated, and on inotropic support. These patients are best anesthetized with a high-dose opioid technique using fentanyl or sufentanil. Older patients without obstruction and compensated right ventricular volume overload may be candidates for an inhalational induction. Patients with TAPVR, particularly those with venous obstruction, have a highly reactive pulmonary vasculature. High doses of fentanyl and sufentanil will be useful for blunting increases in PVR associated with surgical stimulation.

Post-CPB Management

Goals

- Maintain heart rate (preferably sinus rhythm) at an age-appropriate rate. Cardiac output is likely to be more heart rate dependent during the post-CPB period.
- In the presence of postoperative pulmonary venous obstruction, efforts to increase pulmonary blood flow may worsen pulmonary edema. Surgical revision may be necessary.

- For patients with PAH and reactive pulmonary vasculature:
  - blunting of stress-induced increases in PVR with opioids is warranted
  - ventilatory interventions to reduce PVR and use of selective pulmonary vasodilators such as NO are warranted.
- Inotropic support of the right ventricle may be necessary, even in the face of aggressive therapy to reduce PVR. Dopamine (5–10 µg kg^{-1} min^{-1}) is useful because it provides potent inotropic support without increasing the PVR. In the absence of systemic hypotension, milrinone (0.5–1.0 µg kg^{-1} min^{-1}) can be considered.

Right ventricular and PA hypertension is the most common problem encountered following CPB. This may be the result of one or more of the following.

- Residual pulmonary venous obstruction may exist due to the technical difficulty of constructing a nonrestrictive surgical anastomosis.
- In the presence of a nonrestrictive surgical anastomosis, an appropriate cardiac output may produce left atrial hypertension due to the presence of a small, noncompliant left atrium and left ventricle, or left ventricular dysfunction.
- Reactive pulmonary vasoconstriction (precapillary) may cause labile increases in PVR.
- Preexisting PAH.

The use of transesophageal echocardiography (TEE) and surgically placed PA and left atrial lines is helpful in sorting out these etiologies (Figure 20.2). The PA line can be advanced and "wedged" to determine the pulmonary artery occlusion pressure. TEE is valuable in assessing the patency of the pulmonary venous to left atrial anastomosis, and in assessing ventricular function. In some institutions, epicardiac echocardiography is preferred in neonates and infants given concern that the TEE probe in the esophagus may result in compression of the left atrium and pulmonary venous confluence, to the detriment of hemodynamics.

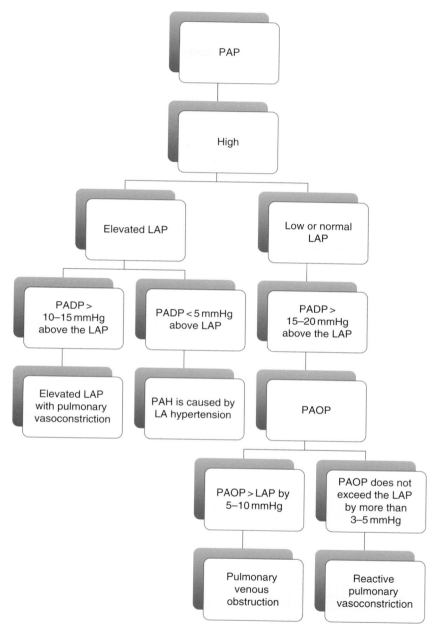

Figure 20.2 Etiologies of pulmonary hypertension. LAP, left atrial pressure; PADP, pulmonary artery diastolic pressure; PAH, pulmonary artery hypertension; PAOP, pulmonary artery occlusion pressure; PAP, pulmonary arterial pressure.

Long-term Outcomes

Following a successful surgical repair, medical or catheterization interventions are normally not needed. A subset of children with repaired TAPVR develop restenosis of the pulmonary vein anastomosis site and may require reoperation in the form of a "sutureless repair," wherein the atrial wall is sutured to the pericardium in a suture line remote from the divided edge of the pulmonary veins. Some children develop a form of progressive pulmonary vein stenosis proximal to the anastomosis site that can only be remedied with catheter-based balloon dilation and stenting.

References and Further Reading

Brown, D. Pulmonary venous anomalies. In: Lai, W.W., Mertens, L.L., Cohen, M.S. & Geva, T. (eds) *Echocardiography in Pediatric and Congenital Heart Disease: From Fetus to Adult*, 2nd edn. John Wiley & Sons, Chichester (2016).

Feins, E.N., Callahan, R. & Baird, C.W. Pulmonary vein stenosis – evolving surgical management of a challenging disease. *Children* **8**, 631 (2021).

Shi, G., Zhu, Z., Chen, J. *et al.* Total anomalous pulmonary venous connection. *Circulation* **135**, 48–58 (2017).

21

Left Ventricular Outflow Tract Obstruction

Introduction

Several categories of congenital left ventricular outflow tract (LVOT) obstruction exist, including valvular aortic stenosis, subaortic stenosis, and supravalvar stenosis (Figures 21.1 and 21.2).

Anatomy

Valvular aortic stenosis is most commonly caused by a bicuspid (bicommissural) aortic valve. Most of these patients will remain asymptomatic until the fourth or fifth decade of life. In infants presenting with valvular aortic stenosis, the left ventricle and aortic annulus may be small. These patients may represent a milder form of hypoplastic left heart syndrome.

Subaortic stenosis occurs secondary to a discrete membranous ring located 1–2 cm below the aortic valve or a fibromuscular overgrowth of the LVOT that produces a tunnel-like stenosis. It may also occur late following ventricular septal defect (VSD) closure due to the fibrous nature of the patch material in the subaortic region.

Supravalvular aortic stenosis (SVAS) is caused by an elastin gene microdeletion in the q11.23 region of chromosome 7, and is most commonly associated with Williams–Beurin syndrome, although it can occur in both sporadic and familial forms in the absence of the other manifestations of Williams–Beurin syndrome. SVAS is due to a characteristic hourglass narrowing of the aorta at the sinotubular junction; in a smaller percentage of cases (approximately 30%) there is a diffuse tubular narrowing of the ascending aorta which often extends to the arch and the origin of the brachiocephalic vessels. There may also be localized stenoses in the renal and mesenteric arteries.

The aortic valve may also be pathologically involved in SVAS, creating an additional source of LVOT obstruction. A tissue ridge at the sinotubular junction is the usual location of aortic wall constriction, and, importantly, it is also the peripheral attachment point of the aortic valve commissures. The sinotubular junction normally expands during systole, allowing the free edge of the leaflets to assume a position parallel to flow during ejection. The narrowed, nondistensible sinotubular junction renders the aortic valve leaflets redundant relative to the size of the aorta and inhibits alignment of the leaflets with blood flow. This mechanism is felt to be responsible for the development of the thickened aortic valve leaflets which have been reported in association with SVAS.

The mechanical impairment of coronary blood flow is a frequent and often unappreciated

The Pediatric Cardiac Anesthesia Handbook, Second Edition. Viviane G. Nasr and James A. DiNardo.
© 2025 John Wiley & Sons Ltd. Published 2025 by John Wiley & Sons Ltd.

(A)   (B)

Figure 21.1 These two echocardiographic images illustrate a supravalvar and subvalvar aortic stenosis. (A) Parasternal long-axis view of a supravalvar aortic stenosis. The line represents the dimension of the narrowest region of the aorta at the level of the sinotubular junction. (B) Discrete area of stenosis below the aortic valve. LA, left atrium; LV, left ventricle; STJ, sinotubular junction. Ao, aorta; AoV, aortic valve; SM, subaortic membrane. *Source:* Reproduced from Simpson and Miller (2021)/with permission from John Wiley & Sons.

Figure 21.2 Long-axis view of the left ventricle demonstrating aortic valve stenosis with an eccentric jet across the aortic valve. Use of color flow Doppler permits optimization of the angle of insonation to obtain the most accurate values of pressure drop across the valve. The dashed line represents the distance between the hinge points of the aortic valve, which is employed for balloon sizing for aortic valvuloplasty. Ao, aorta; LA, left atrium; LV, left ventricle. *Source:* Reproduced from Simpson and Miller (2021)/with permission from John Wiley & Sons.

feature of Williams–Beurin and nonsyndromic SVAS. Adhesion of the right or left aortic leaflet edge to the narrowed sinotubular junction can restrict coronary blood flow into the sinus of Valsalva. The thickened aortic wall may narrow the coronary artery orifice itself. Coronary artery dilation and tortuosity due to exposure of the coronary arteries to high prestenotic pressures, and coronary artery structural changes consistent with elastin arteriopathy, may further compromise coronary flow. Finally, the SVAS impairs coronary diastolic flow, as the pressure in the prestenotic region is lower than in the poststenotic region during diastole.

Although peripheral pulmonary artery stenoses are characteristically associated with SVAS, it is not uncommon for there to be central pulmonary artery (pulmonary artery proximal to the hilum) stenoses as well. In approximately 40% of SVAS patients, severe pulmonary stenosis and right ventricular pressure overload exist in conjunction with SVAS and LV pressure overload and hypertrophy. These patients may have right ventricular systolic pressures as high 200 mgHg and right ventricular to descending aortic pressure ratios as high as 2.0.

QTc prolongation has been noted in 13% of Williams–Berurin syndrome patients and the QTc interval is seen to increase with age, heart rate, and severity of severe obstructive lesions.

Physiology

Infants with aortic stenosis tend to have a small left ventricle and varying degrees of endocardial fibroelastosis secondary to prolonged subendocardial ischemia. When aortic stenosis is severe and there is reduced antegrade aortic blood flow in the neonatal period, systemic blood flow and survival may be dependent on right-to-left (R-L) shunting across a patent ductus arteriosus (PDA). This will result in perfusion of the aorta distal to the ductus largely with systemic venous blood, producing differential cyanosis (higher arterial oxygenation saturation in the upper extremities than in the lower extremities). In the absence of antegrade aortic blood flow, the coronary arteries will be perfused retrograde down the aortic arch with desaturated ductal blood. This, combined with the high left ventricular end-diastolic pressure (LVEDP) that accompanies aortic stenosis, will exacerbate myocardial ischemia.

Williams–Beurin and nonsyndromic SVAS

The normal presence of elastin is responsible for the distensibility of the aorta during systole and its subsequent recoil during diastole. This allows storage of hydrodynamic energy during systole and its release during diastole, a phenomenon known as the Windkessel effect. Loss of the Windkessel effect, as occurs normally with aging, produces a wide pulse pressure with elevated systolic and reduced diastolic aortic pressures. In addition, loss of aortic distensibility results in a reduction in the diastolic component of phasic coronary blood flow. Although the loss of aortic distensibility alone is sufficient to elevate left ventricular (LV) afterload, the major impedance to LV ejection in SVAS is the development of the obstructive aortic lesions.

Right ventricular and LV hypertrophy induced by outflow tract obstruction is a risk factor for development of subendocardial ischemia. Myocardial oxygen consumption is increased by the mass of the myocardium, the prolonged ejection phase and a high-pressure isovolumic contraction phase. Myocardial oxygen delivery is compromised by a reduced diastolic interval (prolonged ejection phase), absence of systolic coronary perfusion particularly in the right ventricle due to elevated right ventricular systolic pressure, elevated LV end-diastolic pressure due to reduced LV compliance, low aortic diastolic pressure due to loss of the Windkessel effect, and compression of subendocardial vessels. The presence of obstructed coronary blood flow via any of the mechanisms previously described further increases this risk.

Surgical Therapy

Isolated aortic valve stenosis is approached by transecting or opening the ascending aorta. A decision can then be made about repairing or replacing the aortic valve.

Subaortic lesions are approached across the aortic valve. Resection of discrete subvalvular or supravalvular membranes is relatively straightforward, but the treatment of fibromuscular tunnel-like stenosis is difficult. Resection of the fibromuscular tissue is limited by the potential damage to surrounding structures such as the conduction system, mitral valve, and septum.

In some instances of LVOT hypoplasia, the repair of subaortic and aortic stenosis may require widening of the LVOT with a patch and performing an aortic valve replacement. A Konno procedure is performed to enlarge the aortic annulus and subaortic area. This procedure involves enlarging the aortic annulus in the region of the interventricular septum with graft material (essentially creating and closing a VSD). This procedure allows the placement of an appropriately sized aortic valve (mechanical or bioprosthetic) or the performance of a Ross procedure. The Ross procedure involves harvesting a patient's normal-sized pulmonary valve to be used as an aortic valve; the right ventricular outflow tract (RVOT) is then reconstructed with a valved conduit. Increasingly, aortic valve reconstruction such as the Ozaki procedure which utilizes autologous pericardium to reconstruct the valve is being performed

Supravalvular aortic stenosis is best repaired by symmetrical reconstruction of the aortic root using two or three patches to widen the aortic sinuses. In instances where diffuse tubular hypoplasia of the aorta and arch exists, symmetrical reconstruction of the ascending aorta with extension of the patch to the underside of the aortic arch is necessary. In some circumstances, surgical relief of coronary ostial stenosis may be necessary.

Postrepair transesophageal echocardiography (TEE) can be used to detect residual gradients and rule out damage to the mitral valve and ventricular septum. In particular, the presence of a small VSD should be ruled out.

Catheterization Laboratory Intervention

Aortic valve balloon dilation in the catheterization laboratory can be performed. Ideally, the procedure is intended to substantially reduce the peak and mean aortic valve gradients without producing hemodynamically significant aortic regurgitation.

Anesthetic Management

Tachycardia in patients with LVOT obstruction is detrimental because, although there is adequate time in systole to allow ejection across the stenotic area, the diastolic time and subendocardial perfusion are drastically reduced. Bradycardia in these patients is also detrimental because the valve pressure gradient increases as the square of the flow across the stenotic area. Maintaining CO at a reduced heart rate requires increased flow across the valve as stroke volume (SV) (cardiac output = heart rate × SV) at the expense of an increase in the transvalvular gradient.

Goals

- Sinus rhythm is essential. Atrial contraction may contribute up to 40% of LV filling.
- Maintain heart rate at baseline.
- Maintain a LAP high enough to ensure adequate LVEDV; more full rather than less full.
- Maintain afterload. Decreases in diastolic blood pressure reduce coronary perfusion.
- Maintain contractility.
- An additional concern in Williams–Beurin and nonsyndromic SVAS patients is avoidance of factors which increase PVR when bilateral outflow tract obstruction is present.

Attempts to risk stratify patients with Williams–Beurin and nonsyndromic SVAS have largely focused on noncardiac surgical

Table 21.1 Risk factors for major adverse cardiac events in children with Williams–Beurin syndrome receiving anesthesia.

Low risk	Moderate risk	High risk
Age >20 years	Hypertension	Age <3 years
No cardiac involvement greater than mild supravalvar or branch pulmonary artery stenosis	Moderate supravalvar or branch pulmonary artery stenosis	History of adverse cardiovascular event
Normal ECG	Mild bilateral outflow tract obstruction	Preprocedural arrhythmia
No renal artery involvement	Renal artery stenosis	Bilateral outflow tract obstruction of ≥ moderate severity
	Renal dysfunction	SVAS gradient of ≥40 mmHg and the presence of left ventricular hypertrophy
	QTc on ECG >450 ms but <500 ms	Coronary artery involvement
	Airway abnormalities, lung disease, or severe gastroesophageal reflux	Diffuse stenosis of the thoracic aorta
		≥Moderate left of right ventricular hypertrophy Symptoms or ECG signs of ischemia
		QTc on ECG ≥500 ms

ECG, electrocardiogram; QTc, corrected QT interval; SVAS, supravalvular aortic stenosis.

Source: Reproduced from Collins et al. (2017)/with permission of John Wiley & Sons.

procedures and none of the risk stratification schemes have been validated. A example of such a scheme is shown in Table 21.1. Given the premise that every one of these patients should be managed as though they are at high risk for myocardial ischemia, it is unclear how risk stratification would alter management.

Induction and Maintenance

There is no one anesthetic technique superior to another. Induction agents must be chosen based on their ability to achieve the anesthetic goals outlined above. Etomidate or ketamine in combination with opioids are appropriate. Both short-acting (remifentanil) and longer acting (fentanyl and sufentanil) opioids can be utilized. Propofol may cause a severe reduction in blood pressure and should be used with great caution in patients with LVOT obstruction. A high-dose opioid

induction is indicated in some critically ill patients. Generally, a balanced technique of opioids and inhalational agents for maintenance of anesthesia is appropriate.

Fentanyl (10–25 μg kg^{-1}) can be used as the primary anesthetic for maintenance before cardiopulmonary bypass (CPB). These agents have no effect on myocardial contractility and cause a reduction in peripheral vascular resistance only through a diminution in central sympathetic tone. For patients who are poorly beta-blocked and for those not taking beta-blockers, fentanyl in combination with muscle relaxant is a good choice.

Tachycardia requires aggressive treatment to avoid subendocardial ischemia and hemodynamic compromise. The first strategy should be to terminate any noxious stimuli and increase the depth of anesthesia if appropriate. Esmolol is an excellent agent to acutely reduce heart rate in a patient with LVOT obstruction. Esmolol is a beta-1-selective agent with an elimination half-life of 9 minutes. This short half-life renders esmolol quite useful for patients with poor ventricular function or bronchospastic disease because, if it is not tolerated, therapy is terminated quickly. Furthermore, unlike longer-acting beta-blockers, esmolol can be used aggressively during the pre-CPB period without fear that it will compromise termination of CPB.

If hypotension due to reduced peripheral vascular resistance occurs during induction, small doses of phenylephrine and volume infusion to increase preload to preinduction levels usually will correct the problem. TEE is very useful at this point. If TEE reveals a dilated, hypokinetic left ventricle or if the patient fails to respond with a prompt increase in aortic blood pressure, an inotropic agent may be indicated. Dopamine $5-10$ µg kg^{-1} min^{-1} is a reasonable choice.

If surgical stimulation (skin incision, sternotomy, sternal spreading, or aortic manipulation) produces hypertension, additional doses of fentanyl ($5-15$ µg kg^{-1}) and/or inhalational agents may be necessary.

Post-CPB Management

After LVOT obstruction repair, the obstruction to forward flow is eliminated. As regards AS, with allograft replacement, the valve gradients are usually normal, and with mechanical valves there is a small peak gradient of $10-20$ mmHg. Many of these patients will have hyperdynamic left ventricular function and will be hypertensive post CPB. Pure vasodilators such as sodium nitroprusside and nicardipine widen the pulse pressure by decreasing diastolic blood pressure, and induce a reflex tachycardia. This combination of hemodynamic changes increases sheer forces on the aorta and jeopardizes subendocardial perfusion. Judicious doses of sodium nitroprusside ($0.25-1.0$ µg kg^{-1} min^{-1}) or nicardipine ($0.25-1.0$ µg kg^{-1} min^{-1}) in combination with esmolol ($100-300$ µg kg^{-1} min^{-1}) is a more appropriate choice.

As with any procedure requiring cardioplegia, the left ventricular systolic function may be compromised by inadequate myocardial protection during CPB. It may therefore be necessary to rely on inotropic agents for augmentation of systolic function, despite the dramatic reduction in afterload. Epinephrine $0.01-0.1$ µg kg^{-1} min^{-1} or dopamine $3-5$ µg kg^{-1} min^{-1} are reasonable choices, providing inotropic support with little concomitant vasoconstriction and afterload increase.

Because the surgical procedure requires an aortotomy with subsequent repair, it is helpful to avoid hypertension, which places undue stress on the aortic suture line. The atrioventricular node lies proximal to the aortic valve annulus and may be transiently or permanently damaged after valve replacement. Ventricular pacing may be necessary.

References and Further Reading

Burch, T.M., McGowan Jr, F., Kussman, B.D., Powell, A.J. & DiNardo, J.A. Congenital supravalvular aortic stenosis and sudden death associated with anesthesia: what's the mystery? *Anesth Analg* **107**, 1848–1854 (2008).

Collins, R.T.C., Collins, M.G., Schmitz, M.L. & Hamrick, J.T. Peri-procedural risk stratification and management of patients with Williams syndrome. *Congenit Heart Dis* **12**, 133–142 (2017).

Ozaki, S., Kawase, I., Yamashita, H. *et al.* A total of 404 cases of aortic valve reconstruction with glutaraldehyde-treated autologous pericardium. *J Thorac Cardiovasc Surg* **147**, 301–306 (2014).

Simpson, J. & Miller, O. Anomalies of the left ventricular outflow tract and aortic valve. In: Lai, W.W., Mertens, L.L., Cohen, M.S. & Geva, T. (eds) *Echocardiography in Pediatric and Congenital Heart Disease: From Fetus to Adult*, 3rd edn. John Wiley & Sons, Chichester (2021).

22

Mitral Valve

Mitral Valve Stenosis

Introduction

Isolated congenital mitral valve disease is a rare entity. Most commonly, mitral valve stenosis is associated with mitral valve hypoplasia or occurs as part of Shone syndrome.

Anatomy

The mitral valve acquired its name in the sixteenth century because of its resemblance to a bishop's miter. In a normal heart, the mitral valve separates the left ventricle from the left atrium, pulmonary circulation, and entire right side of the heart, and has an anterior leaflet and a posterior leaflet. The anterior leaflet is the larger of the two, accounting for two-thirds of the surface area of the valve. The anterior leaflet base-to-coaptation distance is longer than the posterior leaflet base-to-coaptation distance. The posterior leaflet wraps around the anterior leaflet, accounting for only one-third of the valve's surface area and two-thirds of the annular circumference.

The mitral annulus is a fibrous ring surrounding the mitral valve. The anterior leaflet portion of the annulus is part of the heart's fibrous skeleton. This skeleton also has a common attachment to the left coronary and noncoronary cusps of the aortic valve. The coaptation points of the anterior and posterior leaflets at the annulus are called the anterolateral and posteromedial commissures. The leaflets themselves are attached to the anterolateral and posteromedial papillary muscles via the chordae tendineae. During ventricular systole, contraction of the papillary muscles prevents mitral leaflet prolapse.

The Carpentier classification divides the three scallops of the posterior leaflet into P1, P2, and P3. The anterior leaflet is similarly divided into the three segments A1, A2, and A3, which oppose the corresponding scallops of the posterior valve. The coaptation of A1/P1 at the annulus forms the anterolateral commissure, while the coaptation of A3/P3 at the annulus forms the posteromedial commissure (Figure 22.1).

Several congenital causes of obstruction to left ventricular filling exist.

- *Valvular mitral stenosis*: isolated congenital mitral stenosis is very rare and usually is caused by short, fused chordae tendineae.
- *Parachute mitral valve*: in this lesion, two mitral valve leaflets are attached to shortened chordae that insert on the same papillary muscle.
- *Supravalvular mitral stenosis*: in this lesion, an obstructive ring of thickened endocardium is found above the mitral valve, downstream from the atrial appendage.
- *Cor triatriatum*: in this lesion, an obstructive membrane is located upstream of the atrial appendage.

The severity of mitral stenosis based on the *mean* Doppler gradient is: mild (less than

The Pediatric Cardiac Anesthesia Handbook, Second Edition. Viviane G. Nasr and James A. DiNardo.
© 2025 John Wiley & Sons Ltd. Published 2025 by John Wiley & Sons Ltd.

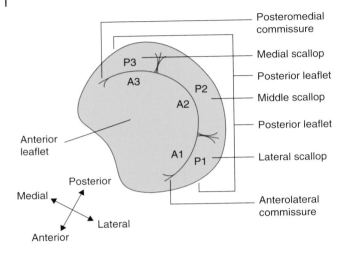

Figure 22.1 Anatomy of the mitral valve leaflets. A1, lateral segment; A2, middle segment; A3, medial segment; P1, lateral scallop; P2, middle scallop; P3, medial scallop.

4–5 mmHg), moderate (6–12 mmHg) or severe (more than 13 mmHg). It is important to note that a structurally normal mitral valve can be functionally stenotic because of underdevelopment. The z-score in such a case is less than 2.5–3.0.

Physiology

All the above-mentioned lesions have the same physiologic consequences as valvular mitral stenosis, namely obstruction to left ventricular diastolic filling and pulmonary venous congestion (Figure 22.2). A notable finding is elevated pulmonary artery pressure (PAP) and right ventricular pressure. This will be associated with a failure to thrive.

Surgical Therapy

Resection of a supravalvular ring or of the membrane in cor triatriatum normally suffices. Repair of the mitral valve is a superior alternative to mitral valve replacement in infants and children. If a valve replacement is performed, a low-profile valve must be used to prevent LVOT obstruction. Mechanical valves require long-term anticoagulation, which may be problematic for growing,

active children. Bioprosthetic valves do not require anticoagulation but tend to degenerate rapidly in children and implantation has been associated with shorter time to reoperation.

Recently, the off-label surgical implantation of the Melody^{TM} valve (Medtronic, Minneapolis, MN) and Sapien S3 valve (Edwards LifeSciences, Irvine, CA) has gained popularity, especially in small patients. These valves can be serially dilated with catheter-based techniques to match somatic growth. Unfortunately, implantation can be associated with LVOT obstruction and these valves deteriorate in function similar to other bioprosthetic valves.

Catheterization Laboratory Intervention

Mitral valve dilation for congenital mitral stenosis is commonly used as a palliative procedure to delay surgical repair or replacement. There is a risk of pulmonary edema following balloon dilation and a postcatheterization ICU bed is reserved in case complications arise. Complications include arrhythmias, cardiac perforation, and tamponade. A follow-up echocardiography is repeated later in the day or on the following day.

Figure 22.2 Changes seen with the progression of mitral stenosis (MS). Pressure in each of cardiac chambers and great vessels is indicated. In MS without pulmonary vascular disease, there is a reversible passive elevation of pulmonary vein (PV), pulmonary capillary (PC), and pulmonary artery (PA) pressures, while pulmonary vascular resistance remains normal. These elevations are secondary to an elevation of left atrial (LA) pressure, which is necessary to maintain left ventricular (LV) filling across the stenotic mitral valve. Right ventricular (RV) pressure is elevated in response to elevated PA pressure, and RV concentric hypertrophy may result. RV systolic dysfunction usually is not present. In MS with pulmonary vascular disease, the PA pressure is elevated far in excess of LA, PC, and PV pressures because of the presence of pulmonary arterial occlusive disease with elevated pulmonary vascular resistance. This results in a second stenosis at the level of the PA. This second stenosis causes dramatic elevations in RV pressure. This RV pressure elevation may result in a reduced RV stroke volume due to afterload mismatch and tricuspid regurgitation due to RV dilation. A reduction in RV stroke volume results directly in a decrease in systemic cardiac output. Similar changes would be expected over time in patients with sustained elevations in LA pressure due to mitral regurgitation. Ao, aorta; IVC, inferior vena cava; LA, left atrium; LV, left ventricle; MVA, mitral valve area; PA, pulmonary artery; PC, pulmonary capillary; PV, pulmonary vein; RA, right atrium; RV, right ventricle; SVC, superior vena cava. Reproduced from DiNardo and Zvara (2008)/with permission of John Wiley & Sons.

Anesthetic Management

Goals

- Maintain sinus rhythm when possible; control ventricular rate in atrial fibrillation.
- Maintain a slower rather than a faster heart rate.
- Maintain a normal left ventricular afterload; increases are poorly tolerated. Decreasing afterload is warranted when left ventricular systolic function is poor

and afterload is high. In this instance, preload must be maintained.
- Maintain contractility.
- When pulmonary vascular resistance is high and right ventricular systolic performance is poor, right ventricular afterload reduction will improve right ventricular and left ventricular outputs. Caution must be exercised so that excessive systemic vasodilation does not result.
- Avoid hypercarbia, hypoxemia, and acidemia, which tend to cause pulmonary

hypertension and may result in acute right ventricular decompensation.[xbl]

Pre-induction

Standard monitoring is required. For patients with severe right ventricular failure, pulmonary congestion, and systemic hypotension, efforts to improve right ventricular function with vasodilator therapy may be unsuccessful due to worsening systemic hypotension. For these patients, the addition of inotropic support is necessary. Dopamine 3–5 μg kg^{-1} min^{-1} is a good choice. Other beneficial agents include epinephrine 0.01–0.1 μg kg^{-1} min^{-1} with or without milrinone 0.5 μg kg^{-1} min^{-1} depending on the degree of systemic hypotension.

Induction and Maintenance

Adherence to the hemodynamic goals rather than using a specific agent is the most important consideration when choosing an induction and maintenance plan for anesthesia.

Hypotension may be treated initially with volume infusion and cautious use of phenylephrine. After optimization of preload and heart rate, it may be necessary to use an inotropic agent. As discussed previously, dopamine, epinephrine, and milrinone are all appropriate choices.

If surgical stimulation (skin incision, sternotomy, sternal spreading, or aortic manipulation) produces hypertension, additional doses of fentanyl (5–10 μg kg^{-1}) may be necessary. If this fails to control the hypertension, the use of additional agents will be necessary. Benzodiazepines and inhalational agents in combination with opioids will cause vasodilation in patients and reduce blood pressure. This is an ideal choice for treatment of transient elevations in peripheral vascular resistance.

Post-CPB Management

After mitral valve replacement for mitral stenosis, a small mean gradient of 2–5 mmHg usually exists across the prosthetic valve. Mechanical valves exhibit a small amount of regurgitant flow in systole. Repaired mitral valves may exhibit some residual mild regurgitation and stenosis. Transesophageal echocardiography (TEE) is an excellent method to evaluate the new valve structure and function. A full examination of the valve including color Doppler and pressure gradients is required. A dramatic improvement in left ventricular filling via the left atrium after replacement or repair is expected. As a result, preload reserve is greatly improved. This makes left ventricular afterload mismatch less likely and allows the augmentation of cardiac output via increases in preload, even when preoperative systolic dysfunction exists.

The management of right ventricular function and the pulmonary vasculature can be problematic in the post-CPB period. In all patients with elevated PAPs, there will be a dramatic reduction in PAP due to reductions in the mean left atrial pressure (LAP) and passive pulmonary congestion after valve replacement. Despite this, some patients will continue to have an elevated pulmonary vascular resistance (PVR) due to reversible (reactive pulmonary vasoconstriction) and nonreversible (morphologic changes in the pulmonary vasculature) causes. For these patients, careful management is necessary.

The left ventricular stroke volume depends on proper right ventricular function. In right ventricular failure, there is an inadequate transit of blood to the left heart and the cardiac output falls. The hallmarks of this syndrome are a high right atrial pressure (RAP) >10 mmHg) and PVR coupled with a low LAP (<5 mmHg) and cardiac index (<2.2 l min^{-1} m^{-2}). The clinician should aggressively strive to keep the PVR as low as possible by avoiding hypercarbia, hypoxemia, and acidemia, and by avoiding the use of pulmonary vasoconstrictors. If pulmonary hypertension persists despite these efforts, then active pulmonary vasodilation will be necessary. Nitroglycerin has been shown to be effective in reducing PAPs and increasing pulmonary blood flow after mitral valve replacement. Other effective pulmonary vasodilators include the inhaled agents nitric oxide (NO) and prostacyclin (PGI$_2$).

In some patients, inotropic support of the right ventricle may be necessary in addition to pulmonary vasodilation. Inotropic support without increased PVR is ideal. Epinephrine 0.01–0.1 µg kg^{-1} min^{-1}, dopamine 3–5 µg kg^{-1} min^{-1}, or dobutamine 5–10 µg kg^{-1} min^{-1} all meet this goal. Increased doses of epinephrine and dopamine may result in progressive pulmonary vasoconstriction from increased alpha-adrenergic activity. In situations where afterload reduction is deemed desirable, milrinone 0.5–0.75 µg kg^{-1} min^{-1} with or without a loading dose of 25–75 µg kg^{-1} may be added. Milrinone, a phosphodiesterase 3 inhibitor, provides some inotropic support and is a pulmonary vasodilator. Isoproterenol, a potent beta-1-agonist, can improve inotropy and induce pulmonary vasodilation; however, it is associated with an increase in heart rate, myocardial oxygen consumption, and the incidence of ventricular dysrhythmias, all of which may limit its usefulness.

In instances of refractory pulmonary hypertension and right ventricular failure after mitral valve replacement, the combination of intravenous prostaglandin E$_1$ (PGE$_1$) and norepinephrine can be effective. PGE$_1$ is a potent pulmonary and systemic vasodilator while norepinephrine is a potent inotrope, which normalizes systemic vascular resistance in this setting.

The potential for distortion of, or direct injury to, the circumflex coronary artery must be considered after mitral valve repair or replacement, given the close proximity of this artery to the posterior mitral valve annulus. This is particularly true when, in an effort to prolong the interval between prosthetic mitral valve replacements in growing children, an oversized prosthesis is placed in the mitral annulus. Compromise of flow may also occur from the placement of annuloplasty rings. TEE should be used to assess the patency of the circumflex artery. New regional wall motion abnormalities in lateral or posterior left ventricular wall segments should raise suspicion that circumflex artery flow has been compromised.

Mitral Valve Regurgitation

Introduction

Mitral valve regurgitation is much more common than mitral valve stenosis. It is commonly associated with atrioventricular septal defects.

Anatomy

Any abnormality of the mitral valve apparatus may cause mitral regurgitation, including:

- a cleft of the anterior leaflet in patients with atrioventricular septal defects
- a central jet secondary to poor central apposition of the posterior (mural) and anterior leaflets
- a structurally abnormal valve, dysplastic and retracted leaflets, abnormal papillary muscles, thick and short cords.

Physiology

Mitral regurgitation increases left atrial pressure and therefore pulmonary artery pressure. In addition, it imposes a volume load on the left ventricle and a pressure load on the right ventricle. The symptoms are similar to those of congestive heart failure.

There is a low-impedance outflow tract into the low-pressure left atrium via the incompetent mitral valve, and a high-impedance outflow tract into the high-pressure aorta via the aortic valve. The extent of regurgitation depends on the size of the mitral valve orifice, the time available for regurgitation (systole), and the pressure gradient between the left atrium and left ventricle. The area of the mitral valve orifice is determined in part by the size of the left ventricle. Dilation of the left ventricle will result in distortion and enlargement of the valve orifice. Ventricular systolic pressure, left atrial pressure, and left atrial compliance all contribute to the valve gradient.

Regurgitant flow ceases when the left ventricular and left atrial pressures equalize. The equalization of pressure will occur more rapidly when a small, noncompliant left atrium exists, because the left atrial pressure will rise more rapidly than in a large compliant atrium. An equalization of pressure also occurs more rapidly when the impedance to left ventricular ejection in the aorta is low. When aortic impedance is low, there is a larger forward stroke volume and equalization of pressure will occur quickly.

Chronic volume overloading of the left ventricle results in eccentric ventricular hypertrophy, similar to that seen in aortic regurgitation.

Myocardial oxygen consumption is altered in mitral regurgitation. There is an increase in oxygen consumption due to the large mass of myocardium that must be supplied with oxygen and the enormous volume work done by the left ventricle.

Bradycardia is detrimental in mitral regurgitation because it prolongs systole, which increases the time available for regurgitation. In addition, bradycardia prolongs diastole, allowing a large left ventricular end-diastolic volume (LVEDV) to develop. This may result in left ventricular distension, particularly in acute mitral regurgitation, in which eccentric hypertrophy and pressure–volume compensation are absent. Left ventricular distension leads to an enlargement of the mitral annulus and worsening regurgitation.

Finally, when the regurgitant fraction is large (50–60%), the total stroke volume will be large but the forward stroke volume will be low. Elevating the heart rate enhances forward flow in this situation. Efforts to increase heart rate are balanced with the increased oxygen demand and decreased oxygen supply with tachycardia. This is particularly important for patients who have mitral regurgitation secondary to papillary muscle rupture or dysfunction from ischemia.

An increased afterload is poorly tolerated by patients with mitral regurgitation because it increases the regurgitant fraction. An increased afterload tends to increase the size of the left ventricle by increasing the left ventricular end-systolic volume, followed by a compensatory increase in LVEDV. This left ventricular dilation increases the size of the mitral orifice. An increased afterload also increases the impedance to aortic ejection. This favors ejection into the left atrium via the lower-impedance outflow tract.

Surgical Management

Surgical repair is attempted in mitral regurgitation; this includes cleft closure, annuloplasty, chordal shortening, or chordal transfer.

Catheterization Laboratory Intervention

Catheter-based interventions to directly treat mitral regurgitation, such as MitraClip placement, are not currently performed in children. As with mitral stenosis, percutaneous placement of an expandable mitral valve bioprosthesis can be considered.

Anesthetic Management

Goals

- Maintain sinus rhythm when possible.
- Maintain a faster rather than a slower heart rate.
- Decrease the left ventricular afterload, as increases are poorly tolerated. Decreasing the afterload will improve cardiac output by decreasing regurgitation, but the preload must be maintained.
- Maintain contractility; there may be significant left ventricular dysfunction.
- When the pulmonary vascular resistance is high or when right ventricular systolic dysfunction exists, a reduction in right ventricular afterload will improve right ventricular, and subsequently left

ventricular, output. The concurrent systemic vasodilation will also directly reduce regurgitation.

- Avoid hypercarbia, hypoxemia, and acidemia which tend to cause pulmonary hypertension and may result in acute right ventricular decompensation.[xbl]

Premedication

For patients with MR, severe hemodynamic compromise usually is the rule. All sedatives and opioids should be given with careful observation of the fully monitored patient.

Induction and Maintenance

Patients with stable mitral regurgitation usually tolerate induction without significant hemodynamic compromise. Etomidate, ketamine, or propofol are all appropriate agents. Hypotension may be treated with vasopressors but caution is urged because in some patients, increasing afterload will increase the regurgitant volume which worsens the situation. In all patients, the heart rate and preload must be optimal. If inotropic support is required, dopamine $5–10\ \mu g\ kg^{-1}\ min^{-1}$ can be used.

Post-CPB Management

Repaired mitral valves may exhibit some residual mild regurgitation and stenosis. TEE is essential in evaluating valvular repairs.

After mitral valve replacement or repair for chronic mitral regurgitation, the ventricle is now faced with a relative pressure overload. The competent mitral valve eliminates the low-impedance outflow into the left atrium. Ejection of the stroke volume is now directed out of the high-impedance outflow tract into the aorta. This causes a substantial elevation of ventricular pressure during the isovolu-

mic contraction phase. The elimination of regurgitation by the competent valve greatly reduces the need for a large total stroke volume. Therefore, a greater proportion of total myocardial oxygen consumption goes towards the more energy-consumptive process of pressure generation to begin ejection and less towards volume ejection.

For these reasons, and particularly if poor myocardial protection is obtained during CPB and aortic cross-clamping, or if a depressed systolic function exists preoperatively, the management of these patients post CPB is challenging. The mainstays of therapy are afterload reduction and inotropic support of systolic function. The goal of vasodilator therapy is not necessarily a reduction of blood pressure; rather, it is a reduction of the impedance to left ventricular ejection with a concomitant increase in stroke volume.

The management of right ventricular function and the pulmonary vasculature can be problematic in the post-CPB period. Management of this problem is described in detail in the above section on mitral stenosis.

References and Further Reading

DiNardo, J.A. & Zvara, D.A. *Anesthesia for Cardiac Surgery*, 3rd edn. Blackwell, Massachusetts (2008).

Isaacson, E., Lucjak, C., Johnson, W. *et al.* Mitral valve surgery in neonates, infants, and children: surgical approach, outcomes, and predictors. *Semin Thorac Cardiovasc Surg* **32**, 541–550 (2020).

Maschietto, N., Prakash, A., del Nido, P. & Porras, D. Acute and short-term outcomes of percutaneous transcatheter mitral valve replacement in children. *Circulation Cardiovasc Interv* **14**, e009996 (2021).

23

Pulmonary Atresia/Intact Ventricular Septum

Introduction

Pulmonary atresia with intact ventricular septum (PA/IVS) was first described in 1783 by John Hunter, an anatomist. It is a rare form (3%) of congenital heart disease. It is rarely associated with trisomy 18 and 21.

Anatomy

Pulmonary atresia with intact ventricular septum is characterized by a lack of continuity between the right ventricle and pulmonary artery (PA) in the presence of an intact ventricular septum (IVS) (Figures 23.1 and 23.2). In 70–80% of cases, a very small patent right ventricular infundibulum is separated from the main PA by plate-like membranous atresia of the pulmonary valve (PV). The PV annulus is usually normal or slightly hypoplastic with recognizable but fused PV leaflets, while the pulmonary arteries are of normal size. The normal right ventricle is tripartite with an inflow region (tricuspid valve), a body (the trabeculated apical component), and an outflow region (infundibulum). The right ventricle tends to be hypoplastic and the size of the tricuspid valve annulus generally parallels the right ventricular cavity size.

In mild to moderate hypoplasia, the apical trabeculated component of the right ventricle is poorly developed, or even absent. With more severe degrees of hypoplasia, the infundibulum may also be absent. Occasionally,

the right ventricle is miniscule. Approximately 25% of patients have mild hypoplasia, 40% have moderate hypoplasia, and 35% have severe hypoplasia. The tricuspid valve, in addition to having a small annulus, may have abnormal morphology and function. In some cases, the valve is atretic and in others it is regurgitant. Patients with regurgitant tricuspid valves have a lower incidence of coronary artery anomalies (described below) as regurgitation through the valve decompresses the RV. A patent foramen ovale (PFO) is present and 20% of patients will have a secundum atrial septal defect (ASD).

In the presence of a small right ventricle and tricuspid valve, and particularly in the absence of significant tricuspid regurgitation, the right ventricle generates suprasystemic pressures. This elevated pressure is felt to lead to a persistence of the sinusoidal spaces that nourish the myocardium in early fetal life.

Physiology

Pulmonary atresia with intact ventricular septum is a ductal-dependent, single-ventricle physiology lesion that may be amenable to a two-ventricle repair, although in many instances patients are staged to single-ventricle palliation. There is an obligatory flow of systemic venous blood across the PFO or ASD (physiologic right-to-left [R-L] shunt). Mixed systemic venous and pulmonary venous blood is then distributed in parallel to the systemic

The Pediatric Cardiac Anesthesia Handbook, Second Edition. Viviane G. Nasr and James A. DiNardo.
© 2025 John Wiley & Sons Ltd. Published 2025 by John Wiley & Sons Ltd.

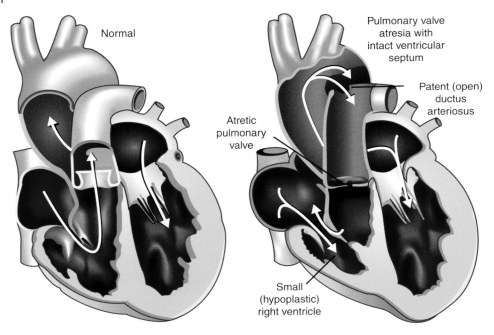

Figure 23.1 Anatomy of pulmonary atresia with intact ventricular septum (PA/IVS).

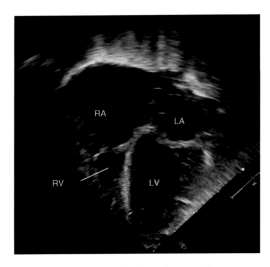

Figure 23.2 Moderately hypoplastic right ventricle in pulmonary atresia with intact ventricular septum seen from the apical four-chamber view. Note the nearly normal-sized tricuspid valve annulus. The right ventricle is about two-thirds the length of the left ventricle. LA, left atrium; LV, left ventricle; RA, right atrium; RV, right ventricle.

and pulmonary circulations from the left ventricle via the aorta and the ductus arteriosus respectively. Right ventricular pressures may be two- to three-fold the systemic pressure, and the right atrial pressure is elevated. The right ventricular filling volume in diastole is essentially equal to the volume of blood that is regurgitated back across the tricuspid valve in systole. Consequently, there is an obligatory physiologic R-L shunt at the atrial level, with complete mixing of systemic and pulmonary venous blood in the left atrium. When the ASD or PFO is restrictive, there will be a large right atrial to left atrial pressure gradient. This will result in a poor decompression of the right atrium and systemic venous congestion. Pulmonary blood flow is provided by a downstream shunt (patent ductus ateriosus; PDA). Prostaglandin E_1 is started after birth to maintain ductal patency.

The elevated RV pressure in PA/IVS is felt to lead to a persistence of the sinusoidal spaces that nourish the myocardium in early fetal life.

This elevated pressure can lead to the development of fistulous connections between the right ventricular cavity and both the left and right epicardial coronary arteries. Furthermore, coronary artery stenoses and atresia of the coronary artery ostia may be present. Retrograde coronary blood flow through these ventriculocoronary connections predisposes the coronary circulation to the development of proximal obstructive lesions from fibrous myointimal hyperplasia. As a result of these changes, the myocardium distal to any proximal coronary occlusion will be dependent on a high right ventricular pressure to provide retrograde perfusion via ventriculocoronary connections. This physiology, which is present in 10–20% of patients, is described as right ventricle-dependent coronary circulation (RVDCC), and is strictly defined by the presence of one or more of the following: (i) ventriculocoronary artery fistulas with severe obstruction of at least two major coronary arteries; (ii) complete atresia of the aortic coronary ostia; or (iii) a significant portion of the left ventricular myocardium is supplied by the right ventricle and is judged to be at risk if right ventricular decompression is performed.

It is important to point out that fistulous connections between the right ventricle and the epicardial coronary arteries in the absence of proximal coronary obstructive lesions are not necessarily a contraindication to right ventricular decompression.

Surgical and Catheter-based Therapy

Transthoracic echocardiography (TTE) is used to assess the pulmonary valve annulus size, the size and function of the tricuspid valve and right ventricle, and the size of the PDA. Although information about the coronary circulation may be obtained using TTE, cardiac catheterization is the only definitive method to delineate the coronary artery anatomy and determine whether RVDCC is present. Consequently, virtually all neonates with PA/IVS undergo cardiac catheterization.

Once the status of the coronary circulation is determined, an algorithm such as that shown in Figure 23.3 can be used to plan surgical or catheter-based interventions. Surgical therapy has two objectives: (i) the provision of sufficient pulmonary blood flow to replace the PDA; and (ii) if possible, to relieve the right ventricular outflow obstruction such that forward flow through the tricuspid valve, right ventricle, and pulmonary artery is established.

In patients with RVDCC, right ventricular decompression is contraindicated because the antegrade coronary blood flow is insufficient to prevent the development of subendocardial ischemia and infarction. These patients undergo a single-ventricle palliation which typically involves the placement of a modified Blalock–Thomas–Taussig shunt (mBTTS) during the neonatal period, followed by a bidirectional Glenn shunt (superior cavopulmonary connection) and a Fontan (total cavopulmonary connection; TCPC) procedure at the appropriate time. Recently, the percutaneous placement of a stent in the PDA has been utilized as an alternative to surgical shunt placement.

In patients with non-RVDCC, right ventricular decompression with the establishment of antegrade tricuspid valve and pulmonary valve blood flow is important to promote the right ventricular growth necessary for the consideration of biventricular repair. When there is an infundibulum in continuity with the imperforate or nearly imperforate pulmonary valve, an attempt to establish antegrade pulmonary blood flow using transcatheter radiofrequency perforation and subsequent balloon dilation of the pulmonary valve can be made at the time of initial catheterization. Alternatively, enlargement of the right ventricular outflow tract (RVOT) and a pulmonary valvotomy can be

Figure 23.3 Algorithm for surgical management of pulmonary atresia with intact ventricular septum (PA/IVS).

accomplished with a surgical transannular patch. Because the infundibulum may be very hypertrophied and the infundibular muscle usually is quite fibrotic, the incision for the transannular patch is carried well down into the body of the right ventricle. The PDA is almost always ligated at the time of the initial procedure. The presence of a dysplasic, regurgitant tricuspid valve precludes a procedure to establish antegrade pulmonary blood flow unless the valve can be repaired.

If the right ventricle is hypoplastic, patients may have to be managed with two sources of pulmonary blood flow – a systemic artery to pulmonary artery shunt (mBTTS or stented PDA) and antegrade pulmonary blood flow (RVOT perforation or transannular patch) – to provide an adequate pulmonary blood flow until a definitive decision regarding suitability for biventricular repair is made. Ultimately, the decision to pursue a biventricular repair or a 1¼ or 1½ ventricle palliation is made based on the size and function of both the tricuspid valve and right ventricle. Because decompression of the right atrium and right ventricle will occur as long

as the ASD or PFO is open, neither of the latter can be closed unless the right ventricle is capable of providing all the pulmonary blood flow without failing.

Following initial intervention, one of the following options exist depending on the presence or absence of RVDCC and the size and function of the right ventricle and tricuspid valve (Figure 23.3). In all the repairs described, the mBTTS or stented PDA, if present, is ligated. The choice of repair is based on the ability of the right ventricle to deliver a sufficient volume of blood to the left ventricle to provide adequate systemic cardiac output.

- *Fontan procedure (TCPC)*: staging to the fenestrated Fontan via a superior cavopulmonary connection (bidirectional Glenn; BDG) is reserved for patients with RVDCC or those with a severely hypoplastic right ventricle.
- *1¼ ventricle repair*: in patients with non-RVDCC and moderate to severe right ventricular hypoplasia, this repair, which consists of a BDG and an atriopulmonary connection between the roof of the right

atrium and the undersurface of the right pulmonary artery opposite the BDG anastomosis in conjunction with a right ventricular outflow patch and a fenestrated ASD (R-L "pop-off") or ASD closure, can be considered. This repair allows a small amount of superior vena cava (SVC) and inferior vena cava (IVC) blood to cross the tricuspid valve and be ejected by the right ventricle antegrade into the pulmonary bed while most of the systemic venous return is delivered directly to the pulmonary arteries.

- *1½ ventricle repair*: in patients with non-RVDCC and mild to moderate right ventricular hypoplasia, this repair, which consists of a BDG in conjunction with a right ventricular outflow patch and a fenestrated ASD (R-L "pop-off") or ASD closure, can be considered. This repair allows all or most IVC blood to cross the tricuspid valve and thus only requires that the right ventricle be capable of ejecting this IVC blood antegrade into the pulmonary arteries while SVC blood is delivered directly to the pulmonary arteries.
- *Two-ventricle repair*: in patients with non-RVDCC and mild right ventricular hypoplasia, this repair, which consists of a right ventricular outflow patch and a fenestrated ASD (R-L "pop-off")) or ASD closure, can be considered. This repair allows all, or nearly all, systemic venous blood to cross the tricuspid valve and be ejected by the right ventricle antegrade into the pulmonary bed.

In all these repairs, the fenestrated ASD can be closed at a later date in the cardiac catheterization laboratory if there is minimal R-L shunting and if right atrial hypertension is not present following temporary balloon occlusion.

Anesthetic Management

Goals

These patients are managed using the principles outlined in Chapter 28. These patients have ductal-dependent pulmonary blood flow. Patients with PA/IVS are particularly vulnerable to myocardial ischemia because, even in the absence of RVDCC, the coronary arteries are supplied in part retrograde from the body of the right ventricle. Myocardial depression is poorly tolerated not only because it may reduce pulmonary blood flow across a restrictive PDA but also because coronary blood flow may be compromised if aortic pressure and right ventricular pressure falls.

Post-CPB Management

Most of these patients are managed according to the principles described in Chapter 28 (Single-Ventricle Lesions).

Only those patients with a right ventricle large enough to require only a transannular patch will not exhibit single-ventricle physiology. For a given cardiac output and $Q_P{:}Q_S$, patients with a transannular patch and a mBTTS will have less of a volume load on the left ventricle. Following decompression of the right ventricle, PA/IVS patients are vulnerable to myocardial ischemia because, even in the absence of RVDCC, the coronary arteries are supplied in part retrograde from the body of the right ventricle.

References and Further Reading

Sukhavasi, A., McHugh-Grant, S., Glatz, A. *et al.* Pulmonary atresia with intact ventricular septum: intended strategies. *J Thorac Cardiovasc Surg* **164**, 1277–1288 (2022).

24

Tetralogy of Fallot

Introduction

Étienne Fallot described tetralogy of Fallot (TOF) in 1888. It is the most common cyanotic congenital heart defect, occurring in approximately 1 in 3500 births and accounting for 7–10% of all congenital cardiac malformations. The etiology of TOF is multifactorial. Up to 25% of patients have chromosomal abnormalities, with trisomy 21 and 22q11.2 microdeletions (DiGeorge syndrome) being the most frequent. The risk of recurrence in a family is 3%.

Anatomy

Tetralogy of Fallot is actually more accurately described as tetralogy of Fallot with pulmonary stenosis (TOF/PS) to distinguish it from TOF with pulmonary atresia (TOF/PA) and TOF with absent pulmonary valve (TOF/APV) (Figure 24.1).

Tetralogy of Fallot is characterized by a ventricular septal defect (VSD), over-riding of the aorta, right ventricular hypertrophy, and pulmonic stenosis (infundibular or subvalvular, valvular, supravalvular, or a combination) (Figure 24.2). The key malformation is underdevelopment of the right ventricular infundibulum and displacement of the infundibular septum resulting in right ventricular outflow tract (RVOT) stenosis. Patients with TOF have displacement of the infundibular septum in an anterior, superior, and leftward direction. The posterior wall of the RVOT is formed by the infundibular septum, and this abnormal displacement results in narrowing of the RVOT. In addition, this displacement of the infundibular septum creates a large malalignment VSD, with the aorta over-riding the intraventricular septum (IVS). Abnormalities in the septal and parietal attachments of the outflow tract further exacerbate the infundibular stenosis (Figure 24.3). Seventy-five percent of TOF patients will have both infundibular and valvular stenosis. A small proportion of patients will have multiple muscular VSDs.

The pulmonary valve is almost always bileaflet. At one end of the spectrum of TOF, the pulmonary valve may be mildly hypoplastic (reduced annulus size) with minimal fusion of the pulmonary valve leaflets. At the other end of the spectrum, the pulmonary annulus may be very small with near-fusion of the valve leaflets. In addition, there are varying degrees of main pulmonary artery and branch pulmonary artery hypoplasia.

The most common associated lesion, present in 25% of patients, is a right aortic arch with mirror image arch vessel branching (the innominate artery gives rise to left carotid and left subclavian, while the right carotid and right subclavian arise separately).

Physiology

Tetralogy of Fallot is a complex shunt in which a communication (VSD) and a partial obstruction to right ventricular outflow are present.

The Pediatric Cardiac Anesthesia Handbook, Second Edition. Viviane G. Nasr and James A. DiNardo.
© 2025 John Wiley & Sons Ltd. Published 2025 by John Wiley & Sons Ltd.

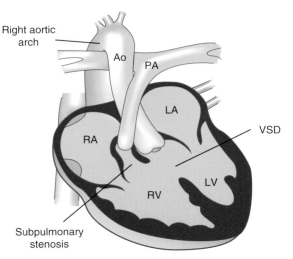

Right aortic arch

Ao

PA

LA

VSD

RA

LV

RV

Subpulmonary stenosis

Figure 24.1 Anatomy in tetralogy of Fallot. *Source:* Reproduced from DiNardo and Zvara (2008)/with permission of John Wiley & Sons.

(A)

(B)

Figure 24.2 Parasternal long-axis view. (A) Image of the large conoventricular septal defect (arrow) with the aortic valve over-riding the ventricular septum. Note the fibrous continuity between the aortic and mitral valve (arrowhead). (B) Tilting the transducer toward the left shoulder demonstrates the pulmonary valve (PV), main pulmonary artery (MPA), and proximal right pulmonary artery (RPA). Measurements of the pulmonary valve annulus and MPA are shown. AAo, ascending aorta; DAo, descending aorta; LA, left atrium; LV, left ventricle; RV, right ventricle.

In most patients with TOF, there is a fixed and a dynamic component to right ventricular outflow obstruction. The fixed component is produced by the infundibular, valvular, and supravalvular stenosis. The dynamic component (subvalvular pulmonary stenosis) is produced by variations in the caliber of the right ventricular infundibulum.

In patients with TOF, the arterial saturation is a direct reflection of pulmonary blood flow. The typical TOF patient has fixed and variable components that create severe right ventricular outflow obstruction, which produces a right-to-left (R-L) shunt and cyanosis. A small subset of TOF patients ("pink tet") have minimal obstruction to pulmonary

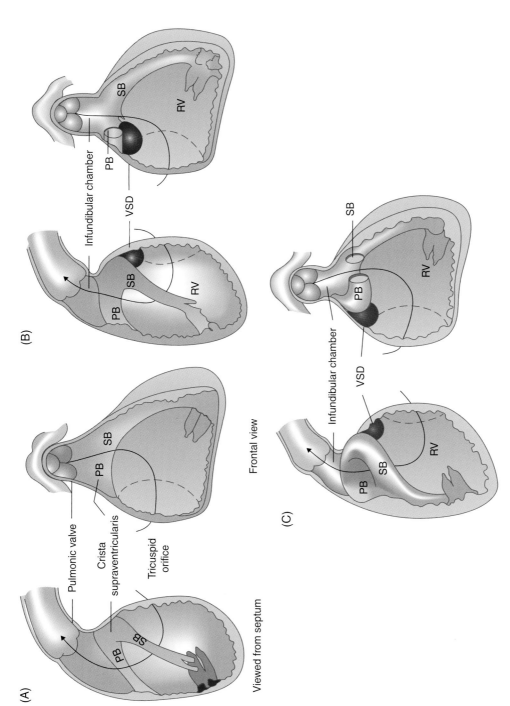

Figure 24.3 Spectrum of infundibular stenosis produced by abnormalities in septal and parietal bands of crista supraventricularis. (A) Normal anatomy of crista supraventricularis. (B) Moderate infundibular stenosis and creation of an infundibular chamber secondary to hypertrophy and anterior, superior displacement of parietal band. (C) Severe infundibular stenosis with creation of infundibular and anterior, superior displacement of both septal and parietal bands. PB, parietal band; RV, right ventricle; SB, septal band; VSD, ventricular septal defect. Source: Reproduced from DiNardo and Zvara (2008)/with permission of John Wiley & Sons.

blood flow at the right ventricular outflow and pulmonary artery level, and may have normal oxygen saturation. Some of these patients have a left-to-right (L-R) shunt with increased pulmonary blood flow and symptoms of congestive heart failure (CHF).

Hypoxic or Hypercyanotic Episodes ("Tet Spells")

The occurrence of hypoxic episodes in TOF patients may be life-threatening and should be anticipated in every patient, even those who are not normally cyanotic. Spells occur more frequently in cyanotic patients, with the peak frequency of spells between two and three months of age. The onset of spells usually prompts urgent surgical intervention, so it is not unusual for the anesthesiologist to care for an infant who is at great risk for spells during the preoperative period.

The etiology of spells is not completely understood, but infundibular spasm or constriction may play a role. Crying, defecation, feeding, fever, and awakening all can be precipitating events. Paroxysmal hyperpnea is the initial finding. There is an increase in the rate and depth of respiration, leading to increasing cyanosis and potential syncope, convulsions, or death. During a spell, the infant will appear pale and limp secondary to poor cardiac output.

Hyperpnea has several deleterious effects in maintaining and worsening a hypoxic spell. It increases oxygen consumption through the increased work of breathing. Hypoxia induces a decrease in systemic vascular resistance (SVR), which further increases the R-L shunt. Hyperpnea also lowers intrathoracic pressure and leads to an increase in systemic venous return. In the face of infundibular obstruction, this results in an increased right ventricular preload and an increase in the R-L shunt. Thus, episodes seem to be associated with events that increase oxygen demand while simultaneous decreases in PO_2 and increases in pH and $PaCO_2$ are occurring.

Under anesthesia, "Tet spells" will be heralded by a subtle, progressive decrease in end-tidal CO_2 ($ETCO_2$) that precedes a detectable decrease in SaO_2. Cardiac output will be maintained in this setting by the delivery of venous blood from the right ventricle to the aorta across the VSD.

The treatment of a "Tet spell" includes the following.

- The administration of 100% oxygen.
- Compression of the femoral arteries or placing the patient in a knee–chest position which transiently increases SVR and reduces the R-L shunt. Manual compression of the abdominal aorta or compression of the ascending aorta if the chest is open to increase impedance to ejection through the left ventricle.
- Administration of morphine sulfate 0.05–0.1 mg kg^{-1}), which sedates the patient and may have a depressant effect on respiratory drive and hyperpnea.
- Administration of 15–30 ml kg^{-1} of a crystalloid solution. An enhancing preload will increase the heart size, which may increase the diameter of the RVOT.
- Administration of sodium bicarbonate to treat the severe metabolic acidosis that occurs during a spell. Correction of the metabolic acidosis will normalize the SVR and reduce hyperpnea. Bicarbonate administration (1–2 mEq kg^{-1}) in the absence of a blood gas determination is warranted during a spell.
- Phenylephrine in relatively large doses (5–10 µg kg^{-1} intravenous as a bolus or 2–5 µg kg^{-1} min^{-1} as an infusion) increases SVR and reduces R-L shunting. In the presence of severe right ventricular outflow obstruction, phenylephrine-induced increases of pulmonary vascular resistance (PVR) will have little or no effect on increasing right ventricular outflow resistance. It is important to point out that treatment with alpha-adrenergic agents to increase the SVR does nothing to treat the underlying cause of the spell, although the decrease in unstressed venous volume induced by these agents may augment preload.

- Beta-adrenergic agonists are absolutely contraindicated. Increasing contractility will further narrow the stenotic infundibulum.
- Administration of propranolol (0.1 mg kg^{-1}) or esmolol (0.5 mg kg^{-1} followed by an infusion of 50–300 μg kg^{-1} min^{-1}) may reduce infundibular spasm by depressing contractility. In addition, slowing the heart rate may allow for improved diastolic filling (increased preload), increased heart size, and an increase in the diameter of the RVOT.
- Careful attention should be paid to mean airway pressure in intubated patients. Avoid the temptation to hyperventilate the patient, as an elevated mean airway pressure will impede right ventricular ejection and increase Zone 1 regions of the lung (ventilation, but no perfusion, physiologic dead space). This will further reduce pulmonary blood flow.
- Extracorporeal membrane oxygenation resuscitation in refractory episodes when immediate operative intervention is not possible.

Surgical Therapy

Palliative Shunts

Palliative shunt procedures increase pulmonary blood flow until definitive repair is performed. A palliative shunt can be used for patients with TOF in whom complicated surgical anatomy precludes definitive repair at the time of presentation. In addition, some institutions delay elective complete repair until 12–18 months of age, with placement of a palliative shunt if cyanosis occurs prior to that time interval.

Palliative shunt procedures involve the creation of a systemic-to-pulmonary arterial shunt, essentially a surgically created PDA. Shunt placement may distort pulmonary artery anatomy and impair subsequent growth, making definitive repair more difficult. A large shunt with a high pulmonary blood flow puts the patient at risk for development of pulmonary artery hypertension (PAH). Ideally, these surgical shunts should be mildly restrictive, simple shunts. In the presence of a proximal obstruction to pulmonary blood flow, these shunts produce a L-R shunt and an increase in pulmonary blood flow. The shunts can be summarized as follows (Figure 24.4).

- *Waterston and Potts shunts*: the Waterston shunt is a side-to-side anastomosis between the ascending aorta and the right pulmonary artery. This procedure is performed via a right thoracotomy, without cardiopulmonary bypass (CPB). The Potts shunt is a side-to-side anastomosis between the descending aorta and the left pulmonary artery. This procedure is performed via a left thoracotomy without CPB. Waterston and Potts shunts are of historic interest only. It is difficult to size the orifice of these shunts correctly. A too-small orifice will limit pulmonary blood flow, whereas a too-large orifice will create pulmonary overperfusion and congestion and predispose to the development of unilateral PAH. These shunts may produce distortion of the pulmonary artery, making subsequent definitive repair difficult. In addition, they are difficult to take down at the time of the definitive procedure.
- *Central shunt*: this shunt places a synthetic tube graft between the ascending aorta and the main or branch pulmonary artery. It is often used when prior shunt procedures have failed.
- *Blalock–Thomas–Taussig shunt (BTTS)*: as originally described, this involves the creation of an end-to-side anastomosis of the right or left subclavian artery to the ipsilateral branch pulmonary artery. Currently, a modification of this procedure known as the modified BTS (mBTTS) is used. It involves interposing a length of expanded polytetrafluoroethylene (ePTFE or Gore-Tex®) tube graft (3.5–4.0 mm in infants) between the subclavian or innominate artery and the branch pulmonary artery. These shunts are performed on the side opposite the aortic arch. This shunt can be performed with or without CPB via a thoracotomy or median sternotomy.

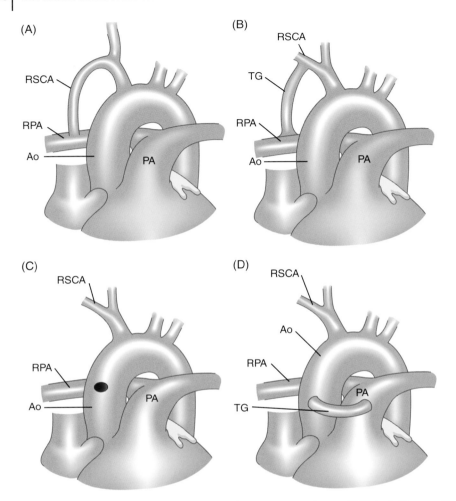

Figure 24.4 Surgically created systemic-to-pulmonary artery shunts. (A) Blalock–Thomas–Taussig shunt. (B) Modified Blalock–Thomas–Taussig shunt. (C) Waterston shunt. (D) Central shunt. Ao, aorta; PA, pulmonary artery; RPA, right pulmonary artery; RSCA, right subclavian artery; TG, tube graft. *Source:* Reproduced from DiNardo and Zvara (2008)/with permission of John Wiley & Sons.

Definitive Repair

Currently, most patients with TOF have an elective full correction between the ages of two and 10 months of age. At some centers, surgery is delayed as long as possible within this time interval, with the precise timing of repair dictated by the onset of cyanotic episodes. Definitive repair for TOF is being accomplished in neonates at some centers if a favorable anatomy is present.

Surgery is aimed at relieving the outflow obstruction by resection of hypertrophied, obstructing muscle bundles and augmentation and enlargement of the outflow tract with a pericardial patch. Unless the pulmonic annulus is near-normal size, and the pulmonary valve is only mildly stenotic, enlargement of the outflow tract involves extension of the patch across the pulmonary valve annulus and into the main pulmonary artery. Because a transannular patch creates pulmonic insufficiency, it is best avoided when possible. If stenosis of the pulmonary artery extends to the bifurcation, the pericardial patch can be extended beyond the bifurcation of the pulmonary arteries. Finally, the VSD is closed. In neonates, this is usually done through the right ventriculotomy created for the resection of RVOT obstruction and placement of the transannular patch. In infants and older children, the VSD can be closed via a transtricuspid valve approach.

An important surgical consideration for patients with TOF/PS is the occurrence of coronary artery abnormalities. Approximately 8% of patients have either the left main coronary artery or the left anterior descending artery as a branch of the right coronary artery. In these cases, a right ventriculotomy to enlarge the RVOT will endanger the left coronary artery. In such cases, an extracardiac conduit (right ventricle to main pulmonary artery) may be necessary to bypass the outflow tract obstruction and avoid injury to the coronary artery.

Catheterization Laboratory Intervention

There are two catheter-based palliation techniques available as alternatives to the surgical mBTT shunt: patent ductus arteriosus (PDA) stenting and right ventricular outflow tract (RVOT) stenting.

PDA stenting

The goal of PDA stenting is to create a nonsurgical source of pulmonary blood flow similar in quality and longevity to a mBTT shunt. Because the pulmonary blood flow is from a source more distal in the aortic arch, the risk of coronary steal imposed by the obligatory L-R physiologic shunt may be lessened. The DA in patients with duct-dependent pulmonary circulation may originate from the descending aorta, the underside of the aortic arch, the subclavian artery, the innominate artery, and the ascending aorta. Access from the femoral artery is used when the PDA arises from the proximal descending aorta, the innominate artery, the subclavian artery,

or ascending aorta. If a VSD is present, the femoral vein may be used. The carotid artery (by surgical cutdown) or axillary artery is used when the PDA arises from the underside of the aortic arch.

RVOT stenting

A bare metal stent is delivered via the femoral vein into the RVOT with the intent of establishing antegrade pulmonary blood flow. Unlike either the mBTT shunt or PDA stent, which are both L-R physiologic shunts, there is no decrease of diastolic blood pressure, no risk of diastolic coronary steal, and no additional volume load on the LV.

Adult TOF Patients

As repaired TOF patients progress towards adulthood, they may develop significant pulmonary regurgitation (PR) in the native RVOT. Patients whose repair involved placement of an RV to PA conduit can develop conduit stenosis and valve regurgitation. In both cases, intervention before end-stage right ventricular dysfunction and/or dilation occurs is often required. Balloon dilation of conduit stenosis may provide many months, if not years, of delay in the need for surgical conduit replacement. Transcatheter pulmonary valve replacement (TPVR) to treat PR in both the native RVOT and in RV to PA conduits is routinely undertaken using a variety of expandable bioprosthetic valves.

Currently, generally accepted indications for TPVR in asymptomatic patients are the following.

- RV indexed end-diastolic volume >160 ml m^2 or RV indexed end-systolic volume >80 ml m^2.
- RV end-diastolic volume >2 times of left ventricular end-diastolic volume.
- Significant RV dysfunction (RV ejection fraction <45%).
- Progressive tricuspid regurgitation in the setting of a dilated RV.
- Ventricular arrhythmias with a dilated RV.

Anesthetic Management

Goals

- Maintain heart rate, contractility, and preload to maintain cardiac output. Euvolemia is important to prevent the exacerbation of dynamic RVOT obstruction from hypovolemia and reflex increases in heart rate and contractility.
- Avoid increases in the PVR:SVR ratio. The less severe the right ventricular outflow obstructive lesions, the more important this becomes. Increases in PVR relative to SVR, and decreases in SVR relative to PVR, will increase R-L shunting, reduce pulmonary blood flow, and produce or worsen cyanosis.
- Use ventilatory measures to reduce the PVR. Care must be taken to minimize mean airway pressure so as to avoid the mechanical obstruction of pulmonary blood flow.
- Maintain or increase the SVR. This is particularly important when right ventricular outflow obstruction is severe and changes in PVR will have little or no effect on shunt magnitude and direction.
- Aggressively treat episodes of hypercyanosis.
- Maintain contractility. Depression of contractility, particularly in the face of severe right ventricular outflow obstruction, may produce right ventricular afterload mismatch and drastically reduce pulmonary blood flow. The exception to this is the patient in whom the dynamic component of infundibular obstruction is active. Reducing contractility in these patients may reduce right ventricular outflow obstruction via relaxation of the infundibulum.

The creation of surgical shunts to increase pulmonary blood flow presents the anesthesiologist with several additional management problems.

- When a thoracotomy approach is used, unilateral lung retraction will be required for surgical exposure. The resulting atelectasis may severely compromise oxygenation and CO_2 removal. Intermittent reinflation of the lung may be necessary during the operative procedure. These reinflations should be coordinated with the surgeon. For all the shunts described, the main or branch pulmonary artery will have to be partially occluded by a clamp to allow the creation of a distal anastomosis. The resulting increase in physiological dead space may compromise oxygenation and CO_2 removal, and increase the arterial–ETCO$_2$ gradient.
- Efforts to increase pulmonary blood flow by reducing PVR with ventilatory interventions and by increasing L-R shunting should be initiated before pulmonary artery occlusion.
- Partial occlusion of the aorta with a clamp will be necessary during the creation of Waterston, Potts, and central shunts. The resulting increase in left ventricular afterload may compromise systolic function.
- All the palliative shunts impose a volume load on the left ventricle. The volume load imposed on the left ventricle by these shunts parallels the increases in pulmonary flow produced. There will be progressive hypertrophy of the body and infundibulum of the right ventricle during the interval from shunt placement to definitive repair, as RVOT obstruction will not be relieved. Inotropic support may be necessary to ensure systemic and shunt perfusion after shunt creation.
- Palliative shunts are mildly restrictive simple shunts. It is important to maintain SVR and reduce PVR to maintain pulmonary blood flow in patients with surgical shunts.
- Be prepared to treat an episode of hypercyanosis.

Induction and Maintenance

Regardless of the mode of induction, aggressive volume expansion with 10–15 ml kg^{-1} of 5% albumin or normal saline should be initiated once intravenous access is obtained. This is particularly true in patients who have been nil by mouth (NPO) for a long interval prior to induction. This is the most effective first-line therapy in preventing and treating dynamic RVOT obstruction.

An intravenous induction is desirable, but most infants and children will tolerate a mask induction with sevoflurane, as there is a parallel decrease in PVR and SVR. Systemic hypotension should be avoided or treated promptly. Systemic hypotension is particularly likely to cause or increase R-L shunting when right ventricular outflow obstruction is severe, as anesthesia-induced decreases in PVR have little effect on decreasing right ventricular outflow resistance. A reduced SVR can be normalized with phenylephrine $(0.5–1.0 \, \mu g \, kg^{-1})$.

Ketamine is a useful induction agent in patients with TOF. Ketamine has been shown to cause no significant alteration in $Q_P:Q_S$ in these patients. Fentanyl or sufentanil will provide very stable induction and maintenance hemodynamics, and will blunt stimulation-induced increases in PVR. The maintenance of anesthesia with fentanyl or sufentanil, a muscle relaxant, and a benzodiazepine or inhalation agent, is appropriate.

Post-CPB Management

Goals

- Maintain heart rate (preferably sinus rhythm) at an age-appropriate rate. Cardiac output is likely to be more heart rate dependent during the post-CPB period. Atrial pacing may be necessary in the presence of junctional ectopic tachycardia (JET).
- Reduce PVR through ventilatory interventions.
- Inotropic support of the right ventricle may be necessary. Dobutamine $(5–10 \, \mu g \, kg^{-1} \, min^{-1})$ or dopamine $(5–10 \, \mu g \, kg^{-1} \, min^{-1})$ is useful in this instance because they provide potent inotropic support without increasing the PVR. Milrinone $(0.5–1.0 \, \mu g \, kg^{-1} \, min^{-1}$ following a loading dose of $50 \, \mu g \, kg^{-1})$ should be considered for its inotropic and lusitropic effects and its effect on PVR.

- In patients with right ventricular systolic or diastolic function and an atrial fenestration, a PaO_2 of 40–50 mmHg is acceptable in the presence of adequate cardiac output.
- Mean airway pressure should be minimized. During mechanical positive-pressure ventilation, the inspiratory phase increases impedance to right ventricular ejection by increasing the right ventricular afterload. As a result, the extent of this afterload elevation is directly related to mean airway pressure as determined by peak inspiratory pressure, respiratory rate (RR), and the inspiratory:expiratory (I:E) ratio.

After definitive repair for TOF, several factors may contribute to impaired right ventricular systolic and diastolic function.

- The creation of a right ventriculotomy and placement of the right ventricular outflow patch produces a segment of dyskinetic right ventricle free wall.
- Protection of the right ventricle from ischemia during aortic cross-clamping is difficult in patients with a hypertrophied right ventricle, as occurs in TOF.
- Enlargement of the RVOT with a transannular patch will create pulmonary regurgitation, which imposes a volume load on the right ventricle.
- Stenosis or hypoplasia of the distal pulmonary arteries or residual right ventricular outflow obstruction will impose a pressure load on the right ventricle.
- A residual VSD will impose a volume load on the right ventricle.

A residual VSD is likely to be very poorly tolerated in the patient with TOF, with the most likely manifestation being low cardiac output syndrome associated with elevated central venous pressure (CVP), left atrial pressure (LAP), and pulmonary artery pressure (PAP). RVOT obstruction will be completely or nearly completely eliminated post repair. PVR is likely to be low and the pulmonary vasculature very compliant. As a result, there will be potential for a large L-R intracardiac shunt with a residual VSD. This will place an acute, large-volume load on both the left and right ventricles. This is likely to be particularly poorly tolerated by the right ventricle that is concentrically hypertrophied and poorly compliant in response to the chronic pressure overload that existed preoperatively. The presence of pulmonary insufficiency will further exacerbate right ventricular dysfunction by imposing an additional volume load. Any distal pulmonary artery stenosis, high mean airway pressures, and elevated PVR will all increase the regurgitant volume and subsequent right ventricular volume load.

Following complete repair of TOF with no residual lesions and minimal intrapulmonary shunt, the SaO_2 should be 100%. In infants and small children, particularly those left with pulmonary insufficiency as the result of a transannular patch and those expected to have a restrictive right ventricular diastolic function as a result of a ventriculotomy and/or extensive right ventricular hypertrophy, the surgeon may choose to leave a "pop-off" valve by leaving the PFO open or by creating a small (3–4 mm) atrial-level fenestration. This will allow physiologic intracardiac R-L shunting, with the ability to augment systemic cardiac output at the expense of systemic oxygen saturation in the setting of right ventricular dysfunction. There will be direct delivery of some desaturated venous blood to the left atrium. In these patients, a PaO_2 of 40–50 mmHg and a SaO_2 of 70–80% are acceptable until right ventricular function improves over the course of days.

Transesophageal echocardiography (TEE) is invaluable in assessing for residual lesions, ventricular function, and the direction of shunting across the atrial fenestration. Hemodynamic and saturation data can be used to identify and quantify residual intracardiac shunts.

Postoperative Junctional Ectopic Tachycardia

Postoperative junctional ectopic tachycardia (POJET) is a transient tachyarrhythmia that occurs immediately following congenital heart surgery. The incidence of POJET following TOF repair may be as high as 20%. POJET is likely secondary to surgical trauma in the area of the atrioventricular node secondary to the retraction necessary to expose the VSD and RVOT from across the tricuspid valve.

Postoperative junctional ectopic tachycardia typically manifests with a junctional rate only slightly faster than the sinus node rate, and is the only narrow-complex tachycardia in which the atrial rate is less than the ventricular rate (A:V ratio <1:1). Much less commonly (10%), there may be retrograde activation of the atrium with inverted p-waves noted and an A:V ratio of 1:1. In either case, there is loss of AV synchrony (loss of atrial kick). At a heart rate <160–170 bpm, this arrhythmia may be well tolerated but it is unlikely to be tolerated in the presence of a restrictive diastolic function at any rate. POJET with heart rate >170 bpm is associated with hemodynamic instability and increased postoperative mortality. The vast majority of POJET is self-limited and resolves by 72 hours.

A multimodal approach to treatment of POJET is generally chosen. Neither cardioversion nor adenosine is effective. Treatment of POJET is atrial pacing at a rate slightly faster (10–20 bpm) than the junctional rate reinitiating A-V synchrony. This therapy is effective unless the junctional rate is very fast (>160–170 bpm), at which point atrial pacing at a faster rate is unlikely to improve hemodynamics because the reinitiation of A-V synchrony is offset by the reduction in diastolic filling time present at these rates.

The next most important steps in management are reducing the catecholaminergic stimuli and treating hyperthermia. This may require reducing or terminating catecholamine infusions. Hypothermia to 32–34 °C using extracorporeal cooling such as cooling blankets or ice packs is effective in many cases. Digoxin, beta-blockers, and calcium channel blockers are best avoided.

Drug treatment is very institution dependent, with some preferring procainamide as the primary treatment and others preferring amiodarone. Both drugs are administered as a continuous maintenance infusion after a loading dose. Amiodarone should be administered with caution as there is a high rate of clinically significant adverse events such as hypotension, bradycardia, and AV block, all of which are dose related. There is some evidence that perioperative infusions of magnesium sulfate or dexmedetomidine reduce the risk of POJET. Consequently, in many institutions intraoperative initiation of a low-dose dexmedetomidine infusion ($0.25-0.5\ \mu g\ kg^{-1}\ h^{-1}$) is considered in any patient at risk of POJET.

Atrial reentrant tachycardia will develop in more than 30% of patients, and high-grade ventricular arrhythmias will be seen in about 10% of cases. The overall incidence of sudden cardiac death is estimated at 0.2% per year of follow-up. The most common dysrhythmogenic mechanisms in TOF involve surgical scars and natural conduction obstacles that create narrow corridors capable of supporting macro-reentry.

Noncardiac Surgery

Patients with repaired or unrepaired TOF can present for noncardiac surgery. The preoperative assessment should include a quantitative assessment of the right and left ventricular function, pulmonary regurgitation, tricuspid regurgitation, pulmonary-to-systemic flow ratio, and an understanding of the repair and major aortopulmonary collateral arteries (MAPCAS), if present. Imaging, including echocardiography during the first decade of life and cardiac magnetic resonance starting in the second decade of life, is indicated if there is concern regarding the degree of right ventricular volume load and dysfunction and pulmonary regurgitation (PR).

Patients at high risk of ventricular tachycardia and sudden cardiac death are older, have undergone multiple cardiac operations, and have a longer QRS duration and evidence of compromised left ventricular systolic and/or diastolic dysfunction.

References and Further Reading

Barron, D.J. & Jegatheeswaran, A. How and when should tetralogy of Fallot be palliated prior to complete repair? *Semin Thorac Cardiovasc Surg Pediatric Cardiac Surg Annu* **24**, 77–84 (2021).

DiNardo, J.A. & Zvara, D.A. *Anesthesia for Cardiac Surgery*, 3rd edn. Blackwell, Massachusetts (2008).

Smith, C.A., McCracken, C., Thomas, A. *et al.* Long-term outcomes of tetralogy of Fallot. *JAMA Cardiol* **4**, 34–41 (2019).

25

Tetralogy of Fallot with Pulmonary Atresia

Anatomy

Tetralogy of Fallot with pulmonary atresia (TOF/PA) involves the features of TOF and infundibular and pulmonary valvular atresia in conjunction with varying degrees of pulmonary arterial atresia. Four groups are said to exist.

- Group 1 patients have isolated infundibular and pulmonary valve atresia with a main pulmonary artery and distal pulmonary arteries of near-normal size and architecture. In some of these patients, the main pulmonary artery (PA) may extend to the atretic infundibulum. In others, there is short segment atresia of the main PA (Figure 25.1). Patients in this group have pulmonary blood flow supplied from a patent ductus arteriosus (PDA).
- Group 2 patients have an absence of the main PA, but the PAs are in continuity and supplied by a PDA.
- Group 3 patients have severely hypoplastic native PAs; the left and right PA may not be in continuity. There are multiple aortopulmonary collateral vessels (vessels from the aorta to the PA) known as MAPCAs. A PDA may also be present. Some segments of lung may be supplied only by blood from MAPCAs, some only by the native PAs, and others by both sources (Figure 25.1).
- Group 4 patients have no native PAs and all pulmonary blood flow is derived from MAPCAs.

The anatomy of MAPCAs in TOF/PA can almost never be clearly delineated by two-dimensional echocardiography alone. Cardiac catheterization and/or magnetic resonance imaging (MRI)/magnetic resonance angiography (MRA) are necessary to delineate collateral anatomy and to determine $Q_P:Q_S$.

Physiology

Tetralogy of Fallot with pulmonary atresia is a single-ventricle physiology lesion. This lesion is generally amenable to a two-ventricle repair. TOF/PA is a complex shunt in which a communication (ventricular septal defect; VSD) and total obstruction to right ventricular outflow (pulmonary atresia) are present. This results in obligatory right-to-left (R-L) shunting across the VSD, with complete mixing of systemic and pulmonary venous blood in the left ventricle. Pulmonary blood flow is provided by a downstream simple shunt (PDA or MAPCAs). For infants, in whom the PDA provides most of the pulmonary blood flow, prostaglandin E_1 (PGE$_1$) infusion (0.01–0.05 µg kg^{-1} min^{-1}) will be necessary to ensure ductal patency.

Surgical Therapy

Surgery in Group 1 and 2 TOF/PA patients is aimed at establishing a reliable source of pulmonary blood flow in the neonatal

The Pediatric Cardiac Anesthesia Handbook, Second Edition. Viviane G. Nasr and James A. DiNardo.
© 2025 John Wiley & Sons Ltd. Published 2025 by John Wiley & Sons Ltd.

(A)
Patent ductus arteriosus
Aortopulmonary collateral
Aorta
PA
RA
SVC
RA
LV
RV
IVC

(B)
Aortopulmonary collaterals
SVC
Aorta
LA
RA
LV
IVC
RV

Figure 25.1 Anatomy of tetralogy of Fallot/pulmonary atresia. (A) TOF/PA group 1. Short-segment pulmonary atresia, with good-sized pulmonary arteries. The pulmonary arteries are in continuity and supplied by a right-sided PDA and one large MAPCA from the left subclavian artery. There is a right-sided aortic arch. (B) TOF/PA group 3. There is no main pulmonary artery. The small branch pulmonary arteries are in continuity and supplied by MAPCAs.

period, as these patients are dependent on PGE_1 to maintain a PDA and pulmonary blood flow. These patients may undergo a palliative shunt procedure (usually a modified Blalock–Taussig shunt: mBTS) or a definitive procedure. The definitive procedure would be creation of continuity between the right ventricle and the main PA via the placement of a right ventricle (RV) to PA conduit, with VSD closure generally performed via the ventriculotomy used for the proximal end of the conduit. In cases where short-segment atresia exists, it may be possible to obtain right ventricle to PA continuity with a direct anastomosis augmented with homograft material or pericardium.

Patients in Groups 3 and 4 present difficult management problems. As a rule, these patients present with univentricular physiology with a tendency for pulmonary blood flow to become excessive ($Q_P:Q_S$ >2–3:1) as the PVR drops following birth. In Group 3 patients, neonatal repair with placement of a

right ventricle to PA conduit is undertaken to place the PAs in continuity with the right ventricle in an effort to promote native PA growth. In this circumstance, the VSD is left open as a source of R-L shunting and delivery of desaturated blood to the systemic circulation, as it would be impossible for the right ventricle to deliver an adequate cardiac output to the left atrium across the hypoplastic pulmonary vascular bed. These infants then undergo multiple cardiac catheterization procedures in order to dilate and stent the hypoplastic native distal pulmonary arteries and to coil embolize MAPCAs which provide pulmonary blood flow that is competitive with blood flow supplied by native PAs.

MAPCAs that provide pulmonary blood flow to segments of lung not supplied by native PAs must be surgically unifocalized to the proximal pulmonary circulation. Unifocalization involves removal of the collateral vessel from the aorta, with subsequent reanastomosis to a RV to PA conduit or to a proximal PA branch. Although the traditional approach has been through a thoracotomy, more recently most groups have favored a central approach working through a median sternotomy. It is only when 80–90% of the pulmonary vascular bed is in direct continuity with the right ventricle that closure or fenestrated closure of the VSD can be considered. Usually, this will mean that at least 10–12 of the 18 bronchopulmonary segments are now in direct continuity with the right ventricle. As long as the VSD remains open, areas of lung that are not supplied by stenotic collaterals or native pulmonary arteries are at risk of developing the morphologic changes of PAH.

In Group 4 patient,s it is necessary to unifocalize several large collaterals to either the distal end of a conduit from the right ventricle or to a mBTS or central shunt as the initial intervention. These procedures serve to promote pulmonary vascular growth, prevent the development of pulmonary artery hypertension (PAH), and control the $Q_P:Q_S$. Following this initial procedure, Group 4 patients can often then be managed like Group 3 patients, utilizing additional catheterization and surgical interventions.

Some institutions take a more aggressive operative approach to Group 3 and 4 patients during an initial operative procedure. MAPCAs that provide pulmonary blood flow to segments of lung not supplied by native PAs are unifocalized to a right ventricle to PA conduit and MAPCAs which provide pulmonary blood flow that is competitive with blood flow supplied by native PAs are ligated. In many instances, the VSD can be closed completely or with a fenestration at the time of this initial very lengthy operation.

Anesthetic Management

These patients are managed according to the principles described in Chapter 28 (Management of single ventricle physiology, preinitial repair) (see Table 28.2). In patients who have undergone unifocalization where consideration is being given to VSD closure, it must be determined, prior to VSD closure, whether there is enough pulmonary vascular bed cross-sectional area present to allow a normal cardiac output to traverse the pulmonary bed without a PAP >25–30 mmHg. In order to determine this, a flow study is performed.

While on CPB, the unifocalized pulmonary artery is cannulated with a cannula that is the same size as that used for aortic cannulation so that full flow can be delivered to the PA. An LA vent of sufficient size to prevent LA hypertension and a postcapillary source of PAP elevation is placed. CPB flow (systemic flow) is reduced to an index of 1.0 while flow to the PA is increased to 125% of a normal cardiac output (indexed flow of 3 l min^{-1} m^{-2}) in increments of 0.5 l min^{-1} m^{-2}. The goal of the flow study is to evaluate the performance of the unifocalized pulmonary artery bed with 3 l min^{-1} m^{-2} flow passing through it. During the study, since the systemic flow is only ~50% normal, the patient will likely be hypotensive. At each stepwise flow rate through the PA, the PAP is reassessed by direct measurement with a separate transducer. If the PAP is <25–30 mmHg at 3 l min^{-1} m^{-2}), then the VSD may be closed.

While the protocol may vary by institution, ventilation is managed during the flow study as follows.

- Suction out lungs.
- Reexpand/recruit alveoli.
- Patient is not rewarmed.
- No inotropes.
- Ensure surgeons have suctioned blood/fluid from the pleural spaces.
- PEEP 5, tidal volume 7 ml kg^{-1}, FiO$_2$ 1.0.
- No nitric oxide or additional anesthetic gases during this time.

Post-CPB Management

The management issues in patients with Type 1 and 2 TOF/PA who have undergone definitive repair with a RV to PA conduit and

VSD closure are similar to those encountered in the care of the patient who has undergone repair for TOF/PS. A few differences merit discussion. These TOF/PA patients will not have pulmonary insufficiency due to the presence of a competent valve in the conduit. The placement of a conduit will, however, require a larger right ventriculotomy and potential for significant right ventricular free wall hypokinesis and dyskinesis.

The management issues in patients with Type 3 and 4 TOF/PA who have undergone a palliative aortopulmonary shunt and unifocalization without VSD closure will be similar to those described for patients with single-ventricle physiology. Management of those patients with a right ventricle to PA conduit placement and unifocalization without VSD closure will be similar to patients with a large, nonrestrictive VSD. In either case, significant run-off from the aorta, high pulmonary blood flow, and a large ventricular volume load will be present if there are a large number of non-unifocalized MAPCAs. In these patients, in the cardiac catheterization laboratory, post-operative embolization of MAPCAs responsible for redundant pulmonary blood flow may be necessary.

References and Further Reading

Barron, D.J. & Botha, P. Approaches to pulmonary atresia with major aortopulmonary collateral arteries. *Semin Thorac Cardiovasc Surg Pediatric Cardiac Surg Annu* **21**, 64–74 (2018).

Ganigara, M., Sagiv, E., Buddhe, S., Bhat, A. & Chikkabyrappa, S.M. Tetralogy of Fallot with pulmonary atresia: anatomy, physiology, imaging, and perioperative management. *Semin Cardiothorac Vasc Anesthesia* **25**, 208–217 (2021).

26

Tetralogy of Fallot with Absent Pulmonary Valve

Anatomy

Tetralogy of Fallot with absent pulmonary valve (TOF/APV) is a rare form of congenital heart disease, occurring in approximately 2–6% of patients with TOF (Figure 26.1). These patients have all the components of TOF with pulmonary stenosis (PS), with the exception that the pulmonary valve is severely dysplastic, rendering it both regurgitant and stenotic. *In utero*, free to-and-fro flow between the pulmonary artery and the right ventricle results in right ventricular dilation, dilation of the main and branch pulmonary arteries, and changes in the structure of the intrapulmonary segmental vasculature. At birth, in the most severe form, this results in extrinsic compression of the distal trachea and proximal bronchi by aneurysmal pulmonary arteries, often with associated development of tracheobronchomalacia.

The anatomy of the segmental pulmonary arteries is abnormal, with a single segmental artery replaced by an intertwined network of vessels. The compression of intrapulmonary bronchi from these distended and highly pulsatile vessels results in air trapping and lung hyperinflation, with an alveolar gas exchange pattern similar to that seen in obstructive lung disease. In the most severe instances, right ventricular dilation may result in compression of the left ventricle.

An interesting feature of TOF/APV is that the ductus arteriosus is almost invariably absent. It is postulated that the combination of a patent ductus, severe pulmonary regurgitation, and a large ventricular septal defect (VSD) is simply incompatible with survival, as it will result in massive aortopulmonary shunting and biventricular volume overload.

Physiology

Patients with TOF/APV present with a wide spectrum of pathophysiology. At one end of the spectrum, where pulmonary regurgitation is mild and dilation of the pulmonary arteries is largely absent, patients have a clinical picture similar to those with TOF and PS. At the other end of the spectrum, symptoms of both large and small airway obstruction define the clinical picture. Children with significant airway pathology present in infancy with severe respiratory symptoms, and often require mechanical ventilation carefully managed to minimize air trapping and hyperinflation. These patients often benefit from ventilation in the prone position as it can reduce extrinsic airway compression. Such patients require immediate surgical intervention. Children with less severe airway pathology can undergo semielective surgical repair similar to that scheduled for patients with TOF and PS.

Surgical Therapy

Surgical therapy involves a reduction of the size of the dilated main and branch pulmonary arteries, VSD closure, and the creation of a

The Pediatric Cardiac Anesthesia Handbook, Second Edition. Viviane G. Nasr and James A. DiNardo.
© 2025 John Wiley & Sons Ltd. Published 2025 by John Wiley & Sons Ltd.

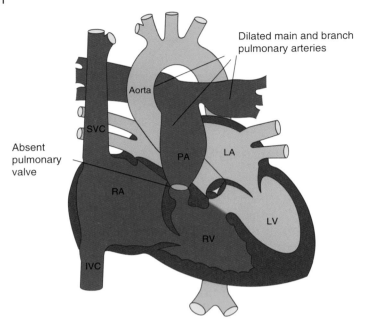

Figure 26.1 Tetralogy of Fallot with absent pulmonary valve with aneurysmal dilation of the pulmonary arteries.

competent pulmonary valve. The elimination of pulmonary regurgitation will reduce the pulsatility of the segmental arteries, and thereby reduce the amount of intrapulmonary bronchial compression. A number of surgical strategies employing one or more of the following are utilized: (i) replacement of the main pulmonary artery with a valved homograft; (ii) surgical reduction of the dilated branch pulmonary arteries, both proximal and distal to the hilum of the lungs; (iii) creation of a monocusp valve in the surgically reduced main pulmonary artery; and (iv) translocation of the pulmonary arteries anterior to the aorta (Lecompte maneuver) to reduce bronchial compression. In some instances, concomitant tracheobronchopexy or tracheoplasty may be performed to correct airway obstruction.

Anesthetic Management

Patients without respiratory pathophysiology are managed according to the principles outlined in Chapter 24 on TOF.

In patients with respiratory pathophysiology, the challenge is to provide adequate alveolar ventilation, given the constraints imposed by proximal and distal airway obstruction.

Post-CPB Management

These patients are managed from a hemodynamic perspective according to the principles outlined in Chapter 24 on TOF. A marked improvement in ventilation should occur following surgical repair, but complete resolution is unlikely secondary to the tracheobronchomalacia that may persist for weeks or months after repair.

References and Further Reading

Chow, O.S., Hoganson, D., Kaza, A. *et al.* Early infant symptomatic patients with tetralogy of Fallot with absent pulmonary valve:

pulmonary artery management and airway stabilization. *Ann Thorac Surg* **110**, 1644–1650 (2020).

Jochman, J.D., Atkinson, D.B., Quinonez, L.G. & Brown, M.L. Twenty years of anesthetic and perioperative management of patients with tetralogy of Fallot with absent pulmonary valve. *J Cardiothorac Vasc Anesth* **31**, 918–921 (2017).

27

Transposition of the Great Arteries

Introduction

Transposition of the great arteries (TGA) accounts for 7–8% of all congenital heart defects, with a prevalence of 0.2 per 1000 live births and a male preponderance of 3:1. Sibling recurrence rates of 0.27% and 2% have been noted.

Anatomy

In TGA there is concordance of the atrioventricular connections associated with discordance of the ventriculoarterial connections (Figure 27.1). The most common manifestation of this anatomy occurs in patients with [S,D,D] segmental anatomy. That is, there is atrial situs solitus, D-loop ventricles, and D-loop great arteries. A right-sided right atrium connects via a right-sided tricuspid valve and right ventricle to a right-sided and anterior aorta. A left-sided left atrium connects via a left-sided mitral valve and left ventricle to a left-sided and posterior pulmonary artery. As a result, there is fibrous continuity between the mitral and pulmonic valves, with lack of fibrous continuity between the tricuspid and aortic valves (conus). This anatomy is most commonly referred to as D-TGA. In D-TGA, the combination of atrioventricular concordance (right atrium to right ventricle; left atrium to left ventricle) and ventriculoarterial discordance (right ventricle to aorta; left ventricle to pulmonary artery) produces a parallel rather than a normal series circulation (See Chapter 2, Figure 2.2).

The coronary arteries in D-TGA arise from the aortic sinuses that face the pulmonary artery. In normally related vessels, these sinuses are located on the anterior portion of the aorta, while in D-TGA they are located posteriorly. In the majority of D-TGA patients (70%), the right sinus is the origin of the right coronary artery, whereas the left sinus is the origin of the left main coronary artery. In the remainder of cases, there is considerable variability (Figure 27.2).

In patients with D-TGA, the most commonly associated cardiac anomalies are a persistent patent foramen ovale (PFO), patent ductus arteriosus (PDA), ventricular septal defect (VSD), and subpulmonic stenosis or left ventricular outflow tract (LVOT) obstruction. Approximately 50% of patients with D-TGA will present with a PDA. The foramen ovale is almost always patent, but a true secundum atrial septal defect (ASD) exists in only about 5% of patients. Although angiographically detectable VSDs may occur in 30–40% of patients, only about one-third of these defects are hemodynamically significant. Thus, for practical purposes, 75% of patients have an intact ventricular septum (IVS). LVOT obstruction is present in about 30% of patients with VSD, and is most often due to an extensive subpulmonary fibromuscular

The Pediatric Cardiac Anesthesia Handbook, Second Edition. Viviane G. Nasr and James A. DiNardo.
© 2025 John Wiley & Sons Ltd. Published 2025 by John Wiley & Sons Ltd.

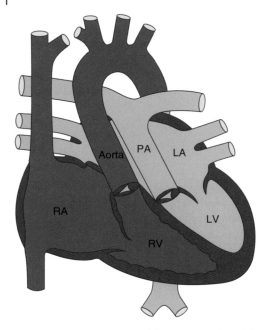

Figure 27.1 Transposition of the great arteries with intact ventricular septum. RA, right atria; RV, right ventricle; LA, left atria; LV, left ventricle; PA, pulmonary arteries.

ring or posterior malposition of the outlet portion of the ventricular septum. Only 5% of patients with IVS have significant LVOT obstruction. In these patients, there is a dynamic obstruction of the LVOT during systole due to a leftward bulging of the ventricular septum and anterior movement of the anterior mitral valve leaflet. The septal shift necessary to produce this obstruction is uncommon in neonates due to the presence of an elevated pulmonary vascular resistance (PVR). Valvular pulmonary stenosis is rare in patients with TGA.

Other, less commonly seen lesions are tricuspid or mitral regurgitation (4% of each) and a coarctation of the aorta (5%).

Bronchopulmonary collateral vessels (aorta to pulmonary artery proximal to the pulmonary capillaries) are visible angiographically in 30% of patients with D-TGA. The larger and more extensive collaterals generally involve the right lung. These collaterals provide a site for intercirculatory mixing and have been implicated in the accelerated development of pulmonary hypertension.

Physiology

D-TGA produces two parallel circulations with recirculation of systemic and pulmonary venous blood. Survival depends on one or more communications between the two circuits to allow intercirculatory mixing. The sites available for intercirculatory mixing in D-TGA can be intracardiac (PFO, ASD, VSD) or extracardiac (PDA, bronchopulmonary collaterals). Several factors affect the amount of intercirculatory mixing. The number, size, and position of anatomic communications are important. One large, nonrestrictive communication will provide better mixing than two or three restrictive communications. Reduced ventricular compliance and elevated systemic vascular resistance (SVR) and PVR tend to reduce intercirculatory mixing by impeding flow across the anatomic communications. The position of the communication is also important. Poor mixing occurs even with large anterior muscular VSDs due to their unfavorable position.

Patients with pulmonary stenosis will have a low pulmonary blood flow and may be hypoxemic, despite a relatively large intercirculatory communication. Patients with a high pulmonary blood flow, particularly those with a VSD in whom systemic pressures are transmitted to the pulmonary vasculature, are at risk of developing pulmonary arterial hypertension (PAH). In the presence of a good-sized intercirculatory communication, these patients will initially not be hypoxemic. However, the progressive development of PAH will eventually reduce pulmonary blood flow and produce hypoxemia. Finally, all patients with TGA and increased pulmonary blood flow will have a large volume load imposed on the left atrium and left ventricle.

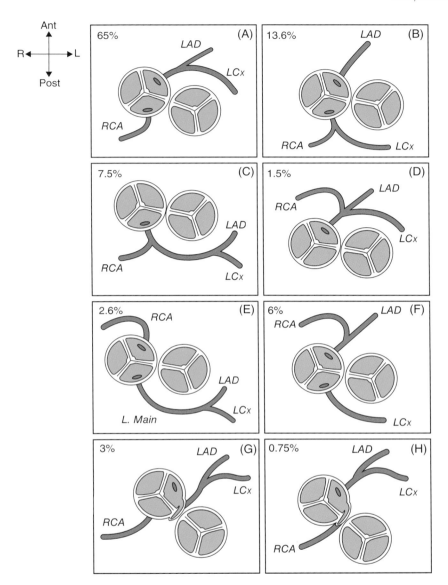

Figure 27.2 Most common coronary artery patterns in transposition of the great arteries and their percentages in patients with TGA. The aorta is anterior and rightward to the pulmonary artery. (A) Normal coronary anatomy. (B) LCX from RCA and LAD coming from sinus 1. (C) Single coronary coming from sinus 2. (D) Single coronary coming from sinus 1. (E) Inverted origins RCA coming from sinus 1 and LCA coming from sinus 2. (F) LAD and RCA coming from sinus 1 and LCx coming from sinus 2. (G) Intramural LCA with origin of LCA and RCA both from sinus 2 and intramural course of LCA. (H) Intramural RCA with origin of RCA and LCA from sinus 1 and intramural course of RCA. Sinus 1 is the left or anterior facing sinus. Sinus 2 is the right or posterior facing sinus. LAD, left anterior descending; LCA, left coronary artery; LCx, left circumflex; RCA, right coronary artery.

Four clinical subsets based on anatomy, pulmonary blood flow, and intercirculatory mixing can be used to characterize patients with D-TGA. These are summarized in Table 27.1.

In TGA with VSD, some intercirculatory mixing occurs at the ventricular level, but there is predominantly anatomic right-to-left (R-L) shunting (effective pulmonary blood

Table 27.1 Characterization of patients with D-TGA based on anatomy, pulmonary blood flow, and intercirculatory mixing.

Anatomy	Pulmonary blood flow	Intercirculatory mixing
D-TGA with IVS	Increased	Small
D-TGA with IVS; nonrestrictive atrial septum or PDA	Increased	Large
D-TGA with VSD	Increased	Large
D-TGA with VSD and LVOT obstruction	Reduced	Small
D-TGA with PAH	Reduced	Small

flow) at the VSD (RV-LV-PA) and PDA (RV-AO-PA) and anatomic left-to-right (L-R) shunting (effective systemic blood flow) at the PFO or ASD (LA-RA-RV-AO). In TGA with IVS the anatomic mixing sites are usually a PDA and a PFO.

The dynamics of intercirculatory mixing in TGA/IVS are complex. In the absence of other anatomic mixing sites, shunting at the atrial level is ultimately determined by the size of the atrial communication and the cyclical pressure variations between the left and right atria. The volume and compliance of the atria, ventricles, and vascular beds in each circuit, as well as heart rate and phase of respiration, influence this relationship. Shunting is from the right atrium to the left atrium during diastole as the result of the reduced ventricular and vascular compliance of the systemic circuit. In systole, shunting is from the left atrium to the right atrium, primarily because of the large volume of blood returning to the left atrium as a result of the high volume of recirculated pulmonary blood flow.

The direction of shunting across the PDA largely depends on the PVR and the size of the intraatrial communication. When the PVR is low and the intraatrial communication is nonrestrictive, shunting is predominantly from the aorta to the pulmonary artery via the PDA (effective pulmonary blood flow) and almost exclusively from the left to right atrium across the atrial septum (effective systemic blood flow). When PVR is elevated, shunting across the PDA is likely to be bidirectional,

which would in turn encourage bidirectional shunting across the atrial septum. When the PVR is high and the pulmonary artery pressure (PAP) exceeds aortic pressure, shunting at the PDA will be predominantly from the pulmonary artery to the aorta. This will create reverse differential cyanosis.

Reverse differential cyanosis is a finding unique to D-TGA/IVS with elevated PVR or aortic arch obstruction. In this physiology, the preductal arterial saturation is lower than the postductal arterial saturation. This is usually the result of a restrictive atrial communication producing left atrial hypertension and elevated pulmonary artery pressures, and is associated with low effective blood flows (poor mixing) and hypoxemia. A balloon atrial septostomy (BAS) can be life saving in this setting. Decompression of the left atrium promotes mixing at the atrial level and also reduces PVR and PAP promoting mixing at the PDA.

Neonates with D-TGA/IVS and a restrictive PDA and atrial septum will be hypoxemic (arterial saturation $\leq 60\%$) within the first day of life. A proportion of these patients will have severely reduced effective pulmonary and systemic blood flows resulting in a PaO_2 <20 mmHg, hypercarbia, and an evolving metabolic acidosis secondary to the poor tissue oxygen delivery. Prostaglandin E_1 (PGE_1; maintenance dose 0.01–0.05 $\mu g \, kg^{-1} \, min^{-1}$) is routinely administered to dilate and maintain the patency of the ductus arteriosus. This will be effective in increasing effective pulmonary and systemic blood flows, and in improving PaO_2 and tissue oxygen delivery if PVR is less than SVR and there is a nonrestrictive or minimally restrictive atrial septal communication.

At some centers, all neonates stabilized on PGE_1 alone will undergo a BAS to enlarge the atrial septal communication so that PGE_1 can be stopped and surgery scheduled on a semielective basis. PGE_1 infusion is associated with apnea, pyrexia, fluid retention, and platelet dysfunction. Recent investigations linking BAS to subsequent embolic neurologic injury must be considered in the risk–benefit analysis of nonemergent BAS.

If PGE_1 does not improve tissue oxygen delivery, then an emergent BAS is performed in the catheterization laboratory utilizing angiography, or in the intensive care unit utilizing echocardiography. These patients require tracheal intubation and mechanical ventilation. This allows a reduction of PVR via the induction of a respiratory alkalosis and elimination of pulmonary V/Q mismatch. Sedation and muscle relaxation reduce oxygen consumption, thereby increasing mixed venous O_2 saturation. For a given amount of intercirculatory mixing and total systemic blood flow, an increase in systemic venous or pulmonary venous saturation will result in an increase in arterial saturation.

In rare instances, the combination of PGE_1, a BAS, and mechanical ventilation with sedation and muscle relaxation may be ineffective. In this circumstance, extracorporeal membrane oxygenation (ECMO; either venoarterial or venovenous) support to improve tissue oxygenation and to reverse end-organ insult and lactic acidosis prior to surgery is indicated.

Surgical Therapy

Anatomic Repair or the Arterial (Jatene) Switch Procedure

The arterial switch operation (ASO) anatomically corrects the discordant ventriculoarterial connections. After repair, the right ventricle is connected to the pulmonary artery and the left ventricle is connected to the aorta. Clinical success with the ASO

(as summarized in Figure 27.3) was achieved in 1975. In brief, the pulmonary artery and aorta are transected distal to their respective valves. The coronary arteries are initially explanted from the ascending aorta with 3–4 mm of surrounding tissue. The explant sites are repaired with either pericardium or synthetic material. The coronary arteries are reimplanted into the proximal pulmonary artery (neoaorta), and the great arteries are then switched with the distal pulmonary artery brought anterior (Lecompte maneuver) to be reanastomosed to the old proximal aorta (right ventricular outflow), and the distal aorta reanastomosed to the old proximal pulmonary artery (left ventricular outflow).

Most patients with D-TGA have a coronary anatomy that is suitable for coronary reimplantation. Patients with certain types of coronary anatomy (inverted coronaries, single right coronary artery) are at risk for postoperative myocardial ischemia and death because reimplantation can result in distortion of the coronary ostia or narrowing of the artery itself. The emergence of two parallel coronary arteries above, but in contact with, the posterior valve commissure or the intramural origin of the coronaries also presents a technical challenge. These patients may require resuspension of the neopulmonary valve after the coronaries and a surrounding tissue cuff have been excised.

In order for the ASO to be successful, the original pulmonary (left) ventricle must have sufficient mass to be capable of becoming the systemic ventricle. Patient selection and the timing of the surgical procedure are important variables in determining the success of this procedure. Two-dimensional echocardiography is used to noninvasively assess the left ventricle:right ventricle pressure ratio and to determine the extent to which the left ventricular mass has regressed.

The ASO was originally described in patients with D-TGA and a large VSD or large PDA. In these patients, the pulmonary (left) ventricle remains exposed to systemic pressures and the left ventricular mass remains sufficient to support the systemic

(A) (B) (C) (D)

Figure 27.3 Arterial switch operation (ASO). (A) The aorta is transected and the left and right coronary arteries are excised using either (A) a button of aortic wall or (B) a segment of aortic wall extending from the rim of the aorta. (B) An equivalent segment of pulmonary arterial wall (previously marked) is excised, and the coronary arteries are sutured to the pulmonary artery. (C) The distal pulmonary artery is brought anterior to the ascending aorta, and the proximal pulmonary artery is anastomosed to the distal aorta. (D) The sites of coronary artery are repaired using either (A) a patch of Gore-Tex® or (B) a segment of pericardium. Finally, the proximal aorta is sutured to the distal pulmonary artery. *Source:* Reproduced with permission from Casteneda *et al.* (1984)/with permission of Elsevier.

circulation. For such patients, the ASO must be performed within the first 2–3 months of life to prevent intractable congestive heart failure (CHF) or irreversible pulmonary arterial hypertension. In these patients, the ASO is generally performed within the first few weeks of life. Closure of the VSD is preferentially performed transatrially through the tricuspid valve. It is desirable to avoid approaching a VSD through the right ventricle

because an incision in the ventricle may contribute substantially to postoperative right ventricular dysfunction.

In patients with D-TGA and IVS, there is progressive reduction in left ventricular mass as the physiologic pulmonary hypertension present at birth resolves progressively over the first days after birth. Adequate left ventricular mass to support the systemic circulation exists in these patients for only the first

2–3 months after birth. In patients with D-TGA and IVS, the ASO can be performed primarily or as the second phase of a staged procedure. A primary ASO is generally suitable for D-TGA and IVS patients within the first two months of life and is usually performed within the first week of life.

The two-stage repair for D-TGA with IVS is used for neonates in whom there has been significant regression of left ventricular mass. These are generally neonates in whom surgery cannot be performed during the first several weeks of life secondary to prematurity, sepsis, low birth weight (<1.5 kg), or late referral. The left ventricle is prepared to accept the systemic workload by placement of a pulmonary artery band. In addition, an aortopulmonary shunt with entry to the pulmonary artery distal to the band is necessary to prevent hypoxemia. The band must be tight enough to increase pressure in the pulmonary (left) ventricle to approximately one-half to two-thirds that in the systemic (right) ventricle. This will increase the afterload sufficiently to prevent any regression of left ventricular mass. However, if the band is too tight, there may be left ventricular decompensation secondary to afterload mismatch.

Generally, a rapid two-stage repair is performed. The ASO is performed as early as one week after preparatory pulmonary artery banding, often during the same hospitalization. This approach is based on the fact that a doubling of left ventricular mass is seen after one week of pulmonary artery banding. The staged procedure is complicated by the fact that placement of the pulmonary artery band to the proper tightness is not an easy task, and that the pulmonary artery band and systemic to pulmonary artery shunt may result in distortion of the pulmonary artery, making the definite ASO difficult.

The ASO is generally not performed on patients in whom mechanical LVOT obstruction (subpulmonic stenosis) exists. Correction of the LVOT obstruction is difficult, and without its complete correction these patients will be left with aortic or subaortic stenosis. On the other hand, patients with dynamic LVOT obstruction have been shown to have no gradient across the LVOT after the ASO.

Intraatrial Physiologic Repair: Mustard and Senning Procedures

Both the Mustard and Senning procedures (Figure 27.4) are atrial switch procedures that surgically create discordant atrioventricular connections in the presence of the preexisting discordant ventriculoarterial connections. Therefore, after repair, systemic venous blood is routed to the left ventricle, which is in continuity with the pulmonary artery. Likewise, pulmonary venous blood is routed to the right ventricle, which is in continuity with the aorta. This arrangement results in a physiologic but not anatomic correction of D-TGA. Following these procedures, the right

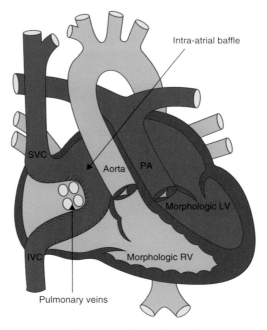

Figure 27.4 The Mustard procedure redirects pulmonary and systemic venous return via an intraatrial baffle after excision of the interatrial septum. The baffle is made from pericardium or synthetic material. Note the trabeculated right ventricle and smooth inner wall of the left ventricle. SVC, superior vena cava; IVC, inferior vena cava; RV, right ventricle; LV, left ventricle; PA, pulmonary artery.

ventricle remains the systemic ventricle and the tricuspid valve remains the systemic atrioventricular valve.

The Mustard procedure redirects pulmonary and systemic venous return via an intraatrial baffle after excision of the intraatrial septum. The baffle is made from pericardium or synthetic material. In the Senning procedure, autologous tissue from the right atrial wall and intraatrial septum is used in place of pericardium or synthetic material. Following both procedures, pulmonary venous blood is directed over the top of the baffle to cross the tricuspid valve, while systemic venous blood is directed beneath the baffle to cross the mitral valve.

Long-term exposure of the right ventricle and tricuspid valve to systemic pressure results in progressive right ventricular dysfunction. Both systemic and pulmonary venous obstruction may occur as the result of these procedures. The incidence of dysrhythmias after these procedures is high: 64% of patients have dysrhythmias, 28% of which are serious (bradycardia, sick sinus syndrome, atrial flutter). Because the Senning procedure uses autologous atrial tissue, some believe that it is superior to the Mustard procedure in preserving atrial contractility and optimizing atrial growth potential.

Rastelli, Lecompte, and Nikaidoh Procedures

The ASO is generally not performed on patients with significant anatomic and fixed LVOT obstruction (subpulmonic stenosis; patients with dynamic LVOT obstruction are likely to have no gradient across the LVOT after the ASO). Correction of some types and severities of anatomic LVOT obstruction is possible, and these patients are also potential candidates for ASO. For patients with D-TGA, VSD, and severe anatomic LVOT obstruction (subpulmonary stenosis), a Lecompte, Nikaidoh, or Rastelli procedure is performed (Figure 27.5).

With the Rastelli procedure, the VSD is closed via a right ventriculotomy with a patch that directs left ventricular blood

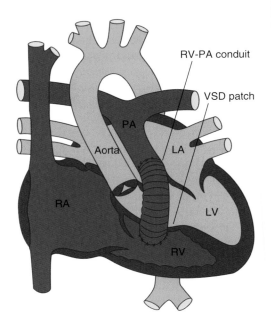

Figure 27.5 Rastelli procedure. The VSD is closed via a right ventriculotomy with a patch that directs left ventricular blood through the aorta. The proximal pulmonary artery is ligated and a valved conduit is placed from the right ventriculotomy to the pulmonary artery, thereby bypassing the subpulmonic stenosis. RV-PA, right ventricle–pulmonary artery conduit; VSD, ventricular septal defect; RA, right atria; RV, right ventricle; LA, left atria; LV, left ventricle.

through the aorta. The proximal pulmonary artery is ligated and a valved conduit is placed from the right ventriculotomy to the pulmonary artery, thereby bypassing the subpulmonic stenosis. LVOT obstruction may result from the nonanatomic pathway created between the left ventricle and the aorta. Balloon dilations and eventual replacement of the valved right ventricle–pulmonary artery conduit are usually necessary because of conduit calcification leading to stenosis and because the patient outgrows the conduit. Conduit balloon dilation in turn may cause conduit regurgitation.

The Lecompte and Nikaidoh procedures are performed to create a more anatomic, less tortuous pathway between the left ventricle and aorta, thereby potentially reducing the incidence of reintervention to treat LVOT obstruction. The Lecompte or REV (*Reparation a L'etage Ventriculaire*) procedure involves enlargement of the VSD prior to patch closure to direct left ventricular flow to the aorta. The pulmonary artery is transected just above the valve and the proximal stump is ligated. The Lecompte maneuver to bring the pulmonary artery anterior to the aorta is performed. The distal pulmonary artery segment, augmented with autologous pericardium, is reanastomosed to the right ventriculotomy site, creating a right ventricle to pulmonary artery continuity. The pulmonary artery segment may be fitted with an autologous pericardial monocusp valve to reduce the severity of pulmonary insufficiency.

The Nikaidoh procedure involves translocation of the root of the aorta posteriorly to overlie the left ventricle, closure of the VSD, and translocation of the pulmonary artery anteriorly (Lecompte maneuver) prior to creating right ventricle to pulmonary artery continuity.

Anesthetic Management

Goals

- Maintain heart rate, contractility, and preload to maintain cardiac output. Decreases in cardiac output decrease systemic venous saturation with a resultant decrease in arterial saturation.
- Maintain ductal patency with PGE_1 (0.01–0.05 µg kg^{-1} min^{-1}) in ductal-dependent patients.
- Avoid increases in PVR relative to SVR. Increases in PVR will decrease pulmonary blood flow and reduce intercirculatory mixing. For patients with PAH, ventilatory interventions should be used to reduce PVR. For patients with LVOT obstruction that is not severe, ventilatory interventions to reduce PVR increase pulmonary blood flow and intercirculatory mixing.
- Reductions in SVR relative to PVR should be avoided. Decreased SVR increases recirculation of systemic venous blood and decreases arterial saturation.

Induction and Maintenance

In prostaglandin-dependent neonates, the PGE_1 infusion should be continued until cardiopulmonary bypass (CPB) to assure an adequate intercirculatory mixing. The increased pulmonary blood flow will limit the cardiac reserve of these patients, and the immature myocardium will be sensitive to anesthetic-induced myocardial depression.

In the absence of intravenous access in infants older than 6–8 months, oral premedication should be considered to facilitate intravenous placement. Midazolam (1.0 mg kg^{-1}) with/without oral ketamine (5–7 mg kg^{-1}) is useful in this circumstance. Older, better-compensated children, such as those presenting for a Rastelli repair with a functioning systemic to pulmonary artery shunt, may require a substantial oral premedication.

An inhalational induction or an intramuscular ketamine induction followed by placement of an intravenous line and conversion to a high-dose fentanyl technique may be suitable for these patients. A similar approach may be taken for older children with subpulmonic stenosis. A high-dose fentanyl technique is useful in blunting the stress-induced increases in PVR that are so detrimental to these patients.

Hypercarbia, acidosis, and hypoxemia further increase PVR and should be avoided because of the limited myocardial reserve of neonates and infants. This is particularly true in neonates with TGV and IVS, where systemic oxygen delivery is tenuous, and in infants with TGV and VSD, in whom left ventricular volume overload is present. In addition, reactive increases in PVR are commonly seen in the immature pulmonary vasculature and may severely compromise pulmonary blood flow.

Post-CPB Management

Goals

- Maintain heart rate (preferably sinus rhythm) at an age-appropriate rate. Cardiac output is likely to be more heart rate dependent during the post-CPB period. For patients having undergone atrial baffle procedures, antidysrhythmic therapy or pacing may be necessary.

- Myocardial ischemia after coronary reimplantation should be treated aggressively and prompt an immediate reevaluation of the anastomoses and the possibility of external compression.
- Reductions in aortic and pulmonary artery pressures may be necessary to help prevent suture line bleeding after the ASO.
- Systemic ventricular (right ventricle after atrial baffle procedures and left ventricle after arterial switch procedures) dysfunction may necessitate inotropic and vasodilator therapy to terminate CPB. Dobutamine (5–10 μg kg^{-1} min^{-1}), dopamine (5–10 μg kg^{-1} min^{-1}), or epinephrine (0.05–0.1 μg kg^{-1} min^{-1}) are useful. Milrinone (0.5–1.0 μg kg^{-1} min^{-1} following a loading dose of 25–50 μg kg^{-1}) may be added if the SVR is high. Milrinone has direct SVR- and PVR-reducing effects in addition to weak inotropic and lusitrophic properties.

After atrial baffle repairs, there may be pulmonary and systemic venous obstruction. Systemic venous obstruction will produce systemic venous congestion and a low right atrial pressure. Pulmonary venous obstruction may result in pulmonary venous and postcapillary PH, pulmonary edema, and hypoxemia. Efforts to reduce SVR will reduce the right ventricular afterload and help prevent tricuspid regurgitation. Therapy for atrial dysrhythmias also may be necessary. Transesophageal echocardiography (TEE) will prove useful in ruling out pulmonary and systemic venous obstruction. In addition, large baffle leaks that may require surgical revision will be detected.

After the arterial switch procedure, there may be extensive bleeding from the aortic and pulmonary suture lines. Myocardial ischemia following reimplantation of the coronary arteries is a potential problem following the ASO. In some circumstances, the ischemia is transient secondary to coronary air emboli. TEE is very useful to assure adequate removal of air from the left atrium and ventricle prior to the termination of CPB. It is also useful in assessing the patency of the reimplanted coronary arteries. Maintenance of high perfusion pressures on CPB after aortic cross-clamp removal will facilitate the distal migration of air emboli. In other instances, kinking of the reimplanted artery or compromise of the implanted coronary ostia may require immediate surgical intervention. External compression of the coronaries by clot or surgical hemostatic packing material should also be considered. Pharmacologic intervention with traditional therapies to improve the balance of myocardial oxygen demand and delivery such as nitroglycerin and beta-blockade is never a long-term alternative to prompt surgical revision of the appropriate anastomosis.

Despite comprehensive preoperative evaluation, the left ventricle of patients undergoing an ASO may be marginal in its ability to support the systemic circulation in the post-CPB period. This may occur as the result of myocardial ischemia, inadequate left ventricular mass, poor protection of the left ventricle during aortic cross-clamping, or a combination of these variables. TEE is useful in identifying and continuously evaluating both global and regional left ventricular systolic dysfunction. It also detects mitral regurgitation, which may occur secondary to papillary muscle dysfunction or dilation of the mitral valve annulus. Inotropic support of the left ventricle and afterload reduction may be necessary to terminate CPB. Initial inotropic support is accomplished with dopamine, and in rare instances where left ventricular failure is severe, epinephrine may be added.

A unique cycle of left ventricular dilation initiating and exacerbating myocardial ischemia exists in patients having undergone the arterial switch. Myocardial ischemia, afterload mismatch, or overzealous volume infusion can result in left ventricular distension and left atrial hypertension. This will be particularly likely if there is mitral insufficiency from either papillary muscle dysfunction or dilation of the mitral valve annulus. Left ventricular distension may result in tension on and kinking of the coronary reanastomosis sites. In addition, left atrial hypertension produces elevations in PAP and distension of the pulmonary artery. Since the Lecompte maneuver (see Figure 27.3) brings the distal pulmonary artery anterior to the ascending aorta, distension of the pulmonary artery may actually compress or place tension on the coronary ostia. The resulting myocardial ischemia produces further left ventricular dilation, progressive elevations in left atrial and pulmonary artery pressures, and continuing compromise of coronary blood flow.

Noncardiac Surgery

Patients presenting for noncardiac surgery should be investigated for the type of repair, and evaluated for ventricular and valvular function, and possible arrhythmias or sinus node dysfunction.

Congenitally Corrected Transposition of the Great Vessels

Introduction

Congenitally corrected transposition of the great vessels (C-TGV) is a lesion that may go undetected for decades, or it may manifest in the neonatal period depending on the other associated cardiac lesions. Traditional surgical therapy for this lesion has less than optimal long-term results. Fortunately, recent advances in surgical therapy offer new options for patients with C-TGV.

Anatomy

Congenitally corrected transposition of the great vessels refers specifically to the anatomic circumstance wherein there is

discordance of the atrioventricular connections associated with discordance of the ventriculoarterial connections. The most common manifestation (94%) of this physiology occurs in patients with [S,L,L] segmental anatomy; that is, there is atrial situs solitus, L-loop ventricles, and L-loop great arteries. A right-sided right atrium connects via a right-sided mitral valve and a left ventricle to a right-sided pulmonary artery. A left-sided left atrium connects via a left-sided tricuspid valve and a right ventricle to a left-sided aorta (Figure 27.6). Although these patients have a series circulation, there is a high incidence of associated cardiac abnormalities that are of clinical importance. In addition, the morphologic right ventricle functions as the systemic arterial ventricle. A VSD is present in 70% of patients. The VSD is typically a large subpulmonary perimembranous defect. LVOT obstruction (pulmonary atresia, pulmonary and subpulmonary stenosis) occurs in 56% of patients, and is always associated with a VSD. Subpulmonary obstruction may be the result of a posterior deviation of the conal septal

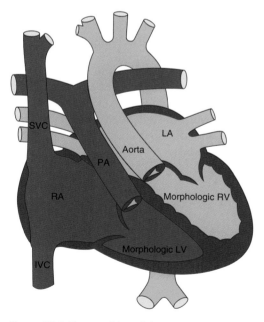

Figure 27.6 Transposition of the great arteries with ventricular inversion, intact ventricular septum, and left aortic arch.

portion of the VSD towards the left ventricle free wall or atrioventricular (AV) valve tissue. Isolated pulmonary valve stenosis is rare.

Abnormalities of the left-sided systemic valve (tricuspid valve) are intrinsic to this lesion, although functional consequences are limited to about 50% of patients. The valve is said to be Ebstein-like, with tethering of the septal and posterior leaflets to the posterior wall of the right ventricle by short, thickened chordae. Unlike Ebstein anomaly, there is rarely apical displacement of the valve leaflets with subsequent atrialization of the right ventricle, nor is there associated tricuspid stenosis.

Disturbances of AV conduction (primarily AV block) are common in patients with [S,L,L] anatomy, with the incidence of spontaneous complete heart block approximately 2% per year for each patient. The position of the AV node is abnormal; it is located anteriorly, superiorly between the orifice of the right atrial appendage and the mitral valve annulus rather than in the apex of the triangle of Koch. As a result, the nonbranching portion of the AV conduction bundle has an elongated, tenuous course just under the right, anterior facing leaflet of the pulmonary valve. AV block is felt to be the result of fibrosis of the junction between the AV node and the AV conduction bundle.

Coronary artery anatomy in C-TGV is consistently inverted. The right-sided coronary artery gives rise to the LAD and circumflex arteries, while the left-sided coronary has the course and distribution of a normal right coronary artery.

Physiology

In C-TGV or physiologically corrected TGV, the combination of atrioventricular discordance (RA to LV; LA to RV) and ventriculoarterial discordance (RV to aorta; LV to pulmonary artery) produces a "normal" series circulation wherein blood circulates physiologically. Patients with associated VSD will have a physiology identical to that of patients with normal segmental anatomy and VSD, while those with VSD and LVOT obstruction will have a physiology identical to that of patients with normal segmental anatomy and VSD with pulmonary or subpulmonary stenosis.

Surgical Management

Traditional Repair for C-TGV

Traditional repair for C-TGV involves the surgical treatment of associated lesions in the context of a physiologic repair (morphologic right ventricle as systemic ventricle). As such, this repair can involve any or all of the following: (i) pacemaker placement for heart block; (ii) VSD closure; (iii) the creation of a morphologic left ventricle to pulmonary artery connection in the setting of pulmonary atresia or severe pulmonary stenosis; (iv) tricuspid valve repair or replacement for severe tricuspid insufficiency.

Heart block may complicate VSD closure because the conduction system travels along the septum of the right-sided morphologic left ventricle (pulmonary ventricle). To avoid compromise of the conduction system, the sutures for closure of the VSD must be placed on the right ventricle (systemic ventricle) side of the septum. This can be accomplished with exposure across the aortic valve so as to avoid a ventriculotomy in the systemic (right) ventricle. Bypass of pulmonary atresia or severe pulmonary stenosis with a conduit from the anatomic left ventricle to the pulmonary artery is also problematic. The left ventriculotomy and proximal portion of the conduit must be positioned so as to avoid the papillary muscle attachments of the mitral valve and the major coronary arteries.

Double Switch Procedure and Atrial Switch-Rastelli Procedures

The double switch procedure was first performed in 1989, and is applied to patients with C-TGV with or without VSD who do not have significant LVOT (pulmonary arterial) obstruction. It consists of an atrial-level switch (Mustard or Senning) in combination

Figure 27.7 Double switch. It consists of an atrial-level switch (Mustard or Senning) in combination with an ASO.

with an ASO (Figure 27.7). The atrial switch-Rastelli procedure was first reported in 1990 and is applied to patients with C-TGV with a VSD and significant LVOT (pulmonary arterial) obstruction. It consists of an atrial-level switch (Mustard or Senning) in combination with a Rastelli procedure. As such, it is commonly referred to as a Mustard–Rastelli or Senning–Rastelli procedure.

These procedures produce an anatomic repair; that is, atrioventricular and ventriculoarterial concordance with the morphologic mitral valve and left ventricle as the systemic AV valve and ventricle. Like the ASO, the success of these procedures is dependent on retention of a sufficient left ventricular mass to support the systemic circulation. These procedures are performed with hypothermic CPB and aortic cross-clamping with cardioplegic arrest.

Both of these procedures have also been applied to patients with C-TGV who have undergone previous traditional repair and as a result are experiencing tricuspid regurgitation, right ventricular dysfunction, and heart block. The decision-making process regarding the timing of surgery, necessary preparatory procedures, and selection of patients for these procedures is complex and controversial, and is currently evolving at many centers. Briefly, the issues which must be considered in the decision-making process are summarized below.

Candidates for a double switch should have a systolic morphologic left ventricular pressure that is at least 70% of systemic systolic pressure (morphologic right ventricular systolic pressure). Adolescent candidates should probably have systolic morphologic left ventricular pressure that is 90–100% of systemic systolic pressure. Mild valvular pulmonary stenosis or dynamic pulmonary stenosis is not a contraindication to the procedure as long as only minimal LVOT obstruction exists at the end of the procedure. The presence of these lesions preoperatively may confer some benefit by stimulating retention of left ventricular mass.

The timing of surgery for a double switch procedure is dictated by the severity of CHF, which in turn is determined by the size of the VSD and/or presence of tricuspid regurgitation (TR). The larger the VSD, the more likely it is that the left ventricle will retain its mass; however, it is also more likely that CHF and ultimately PAH will develop. The double switch operation in the first three months of life is recommended for patients with severe CHF. Because dextrocardia in association with [S,L,L] anatomy complicates surgical exposure for the completion of a Mustard or Senning procedure, a pulmonary artery band (PAB) may be considered to control pulmonary blood flow and CHF, and to promote the retention of left ventricular mass until the child is older and larger. Patients without CHF (no VSD or restrictive VSD, no TR) may be followed and before evidence of right ventricular failure or tricuspid regurgitation develops, undergo placement of a PAB with the intention of increasing left ventricular mass so that a subsequent double switch can be performed following retraining of the left ventricle. The appropriate interval necessary to retrain the left ventricle in this older subset of patients has not been firmly established, but on average it is of the order of 19 months. It can be expected that some patients will require more than one PAB, and that some will fail to have adequate accumulation of left ventricular mass to go on to a double switch.

Candidates for the atrial switch-Rastelli procedure must be free of significant PAH and have a nonrestrictive VSD committed to the aorta, so that patch tunnel closure of the VSD will create left ventricle to aortic continuity. The timing of surgery for an atrial switch-Rastelli procedure is dictated by the severity of the limitation of pulmonary blood flow. In neonates with pulmonary atresia or severe pulmonary stenosis, a systemic to pulmonary artery shunt (such as a modified Blalock–Taussig shunt) is placed. When the child outgrows the shunt (at 6–18 months of age), an atrial switch-Rastelli procedure is performed. In neonates with milder pulmonary stenosis, the atrial switch-Rastelli procedure can be deferred until cyanosis progresses. In patients where the limitation of pulmonary blood flow is such that Q_P:Q_S <2:1, the procedure may be delayed but should be performed prior to development of right ventricular failure, tricuspid regurgitation, or increased PVR.

References and Further Reading

Casteneda, A.R., Norwood, W.I., Jonas, R.A., *et al*. Transposition of the great arteries and intact ventricular septum: anatomical repair in the neonate. *Ann Thorac Surg* **38**, 438–443 (1984).

Fricke, T.A., Buratto, E., Weintraub, R. *et al*. Long-term outcomes of the arterial switch operation. *J Thorac Cardiovasc Surg* **163**, 212–219 (2021).

Marathe, S.P., Chavez, M., Schultz, A. *et al*. Contemporary outcomes of the double switch operation for congenitally corrected transposition of the great arteries. *J Thorac Cardiovasc Surg* **164**, 1980–1990 (2022).

28

Single-ventricle Lesions

Introduction

Single-ventricle lesions can be amenable to a two-ventricle repair or require a staged approach to a Fontan procedure (Figure 28.1). Single-ventricle lesions amenable to two-ventricle repair include truncus arteriosus, severe neonatal aortic stenosis, interrupted aortic arch, and tetralogy of Fallot (TOF) with pulmonary atresia. Other single-ventricle lesions such as tricuspid atresia and hypoplastic left heart syndrome require a staged approach to the Fontan procedure. Pulmonary atresia with intact ventricular septum (PA/IVS) is an example of a single-ventricle lesion that is occasionally amenable to a two-ventricle repair.

There are three phases in the single-ventricle pathway: the initial physiology; the superior cavopulmonary shunt (generally a bidirectional Glenn [BDG] shunt); and the completed Fontan procedure that creates a total cavopulmonary connection (TCPC). During each of these phases three physiologic goals must be achieved.

- There must be a reliable source of an appropriate quantity of pulmonary blood flow. The appropriate quantity is the quantity that is sufficient to prevent hypoxemia but not so large as to cause pulmonary arterial hypertension (PAH). The presence of PAH is a contraindication to completion of the Fontan procedure.
- There must be unobstructed delivery of pulmonary venous blood to the systemic ventricle.
- There must be an unobstructed pathway from the systemic ventricle to all segments of the aorta.

Physiology and Initial Procedures

The initial palliative procedures described here are applicable to any patient with single-ventricle physiology.

Initial Procedures to Optimize Pulmonary Arterial Blood Flow

The following describes the initial approach to optimize pulmonary blood in patients with single-ventricle physiology.

- Patients with ductal-dependent pulmonary blood flow will require stabilization with prostaglandin E_1 (PGE_1), followed by placement of a surgical aortopulmonary shunt. In most cases a modified Blalock-Thomas-Taussig shunt (mBTTS) will be placed and the patent ductus arteriosus (PDA) ligated. A superior cavopulmonary shunt (bidirectional Glenn) cannot be used in the neonatal period as the pulmonary vascular resistance (PVR) is elevated and supraphysiologic superior vena cava (SVC) pressure would be necessary to provide adequate pulmonary blood flow. More than 70% of patients with tricuspid atresia have ductal-dependent pulmonary blood flow and require a shunt in the newborn period.

The Pediatric Cardiac Anesthesia Handbook, Second Edition. Viviane G. Nasr and James A. DiNardo.
© 2025 John Wiley & Sons Ltd. Published 2025 by John Wiley & Sons Ltd.

(A)   (B)   or   (C)

(D)   (E)

Figure 28.1 Sequence of repairs for hypoplastic left heart syndrome. (A) Hypoplastic left heart. (B) Initial repair with a Damus–Kaye–Stansel repair and a Blalock-Thomas-Taussig shunt. (C) Initial repair with a Damus–Kaye–Stansel repair and a right ventricle to pulmonary artery graft. (D) Bidirectional Glenn procedure. (E) Lateral Fontan with a fenestration. *Source:* Reproduced from DiNardo and Zvara (2008)/with permission of John Wiley & Sons.

- Patients with unrestricted pulmonary blood flow are at risk for compromise of systemic oxygen delivery due to high pulmonary blood flow in the setting of fixed cardiac output and, ultimately, for the development of PAH. These patients need restriction of pulmonary blood flow.
  - In patients with high pulmonary blood flow and significant intracardiac sources of pulmonary blood flow (type 1C or 2C tricuspid atresia; see Table 28.1), the PDA can close and appropriately limit pulmonary blood flow. More commonly, it will be necessary to mechanically restrict pulmonary blood flow and reduce Q_P:Q_S and the volume load on the systemic ventricle by banding the pulmonary artery. The main pulmonary artery is constricted with a circumferential band. This reduces pulmonary blood flow and distal pulmonary artery pressure by the creation of a restrictive lesion. Banding is most effective when the pulmonary artery pressure (PAP) distal to the band is reduced to one-third or one-half of systemic blood pressure.

Pulmonary artery banding may cause distortion of the main pulmonary artery. In addition, distortion of the branch pulmonary arteries may be caused by migration of the band distally. This distortion may complicate or preclude definitive repair. Pulmonary artery banding is accomplished via a thoracotomy or a median sternotomy, without cardiopulmonary bypass (CPB). An excessively tight pulmonary artery band will severely reduce pulmonary blood flow and expose the ventricle to a high afterload. Pulse oximetry has proved useful during pulmonary artery banding because arterial oxygen desaturation precedes hypotension and bradycardia when banding is excessive. Transesophageal echocardiography (TEE) is valuable in assessing ventricular function during pulmonary artery banding. Ventricular distension may require loosening of the band or initiation of inotropic support. TEE or epicardial echocardiography also allows the pressure gradient across the band to be determined. This will help in determining the tightness of the band. Pulmonary

Table 28.1 Classification of tricuspid atresia and sources of aortic and pulmonary blood flows.

Type of tricuspid atresia	Frequency (%)	Pulmonary blood flow (amount)	Aortic blood flow pathway	Pulmonary blood flow pathway
Type 1	**70**			
1A: TA, NRGA, PA	10	Decreased	LV	PDA, MAPCAs
1B: TA, NRGA, restrictive VSD, PS	50	Decreased	LV	LV through VSD to RV
1C: TA, NRGA, nonrestrictive VSD, no PS	10	No change or Increased	LV	LV through VSD to RV
Type 2	**30**			
2A: TA, D-TGA, nonrestrictive VSD, PA	2	Decreased	LV through VSD to RV	PDA, MAPCAs
2B: TA, D-TGA, nonrestrictive VSD, PS	8	No change or decreased	LV through VSD to RV	LV
2C: TA, D-TGA, restrictive VSD, no PS	20	Increased	LV through VSD to RV	LV
Type 3	**<1**			
3A: TA, D-loop ventricles, L-TGA, subpulmonic stenosis		Decreased	LV	LV through VSD to RV
3B: TA, L-loop ventricles, L-MGA, subaortic stenosis		Increased	LV through VSD to RV	LV

TA, tricuspid atresia; NRGA, normally related great arteries; PA, pulmonary atresia; LV, left ventricle; PDA, patent ductus arteriosus; MAPCAs, major aortopulmonary collaterals; VSD, ventricular septal defect; RV, right ventricle; PS, pulmonary stenosis; TGA, transposition of the great arteries; MGA, malposition of the great arteries

artery banding is contraindicated in patients where the aortic blood flow is derived from a restrictive intracardiac pathway from the systemic ventricle, or where this pathway is likely to become restrictive once the ventricular volume load is reduced by a pulmonary artery band. These patients require a Damus–Kaye–Stansel (DKS) procedure (see below) to provide an unobstructed pathway to the aorta from the systemic ventricle.

- An alternative to PA banding is percutaneous placement of bilateral, internal PA flow restrictors in the proximal branch pulmonary arteries in the cardiac catherization laboratory. These flow restrictors are microvascular plugs with six of the eight PTFE cells removed.

- The treatment of patients with high pulmonary blood flow due to major aortopulmonary collateral arteries (MAPCAs) is discussed in Chapter 25.
- Rarely, the combination of a restrictive ventricular septal defect (VSD) and mild pulmonary stenosis (type 1B or 3A tricuspid atresia) can result in the appropriate quantity of pulmonary blood flow without intervention.

Initial Procedures to Optimize Pulmonary Venous Blood Flow

In instances where pulmonary venous blood must cross the atrial septum to reach the systemic ventricle, the atrial septum must be nonrestrictive. Creating a nonrestrictive atrial septum may occur in the cardiac catheterization laboratory using a Rashkind–Miller balloon atrial septostomy. In some cases the septum may be so thick as to require the placement of a stent. A surgical atrial septectomy to create a nonrestrictive atrial septum (common atrium) can also be performed at the time of initial palliation in procedures that require CPB.

Initial Procedures to Optimize Systemic Blood Flow

When the pathway to the aorta from the systemic ventricle is obstructed (type 2C or 3B tricuspid atresia), or when the left ventricle and proximal/transverse aorta are hypoplastic (as with hypoplastic left heart syndrome [HLHS]), a DKS procedure alone or in conjunction with an aortic arch reconstruction (as with HLHS) can be used. The pulmonary artery is transected just proximal to its bifurcation, and the proximal end of the pulmonary artery is reanastomosed end to side or side to side to the ascending aorta. This provides systemic ventricle to aortic continuity (left ventricle to proximal pulmonary artery to aorta in type 3B tricuspid atresia; right ventricle to proximal pulmonary artery to aorta in HLHS). In the neonatal period, pulmonary blood flow is then supplied to the oversewn end of the main pulmonary artery by a mBTTS in patients with type 3B tricuspid atresia, or a mBTTS or right ventricle to pulmonary artery conduit in patients with HLHS.

Management of Single-ventricle Physiology

The primary goal in the management of patients with single-ventricle physiology is the optimization of systemic oxygen delivery and perfusion pressure. This is necessary if end-organ (myocardial, renal, hepatic, splanchnic) dysfunction and failure are to be prevented. This goal is achieved by balancing the systemic and pulmonary circulations. The term "balanced circulation" is used

because both laboratory and clinical investigations have demonstrated that maximal systemic oxygen delivery (the product of systemic oxygen content and systemic blood flow) is achieved for a given single-ventricle output when $Q_P:Q_S$ is at or just below 1:1. Increases in $Q_P:Q_S$ in excess of 1:1 are associated with a progressive decrease in systemic oxygen delivery, because the subsequent increase in systemic oxygen content is more than offset by the progressive decrease in systemic blood flow. Decreases in $Q_P:Q_S$ just below 1:1 are associated with a precipitous decrease in systemic oxygen delivery because the subsequent increase in systemic blood flow is more than offset by the dramatic decrease in systemic oxygen content.

Since $Q_P:Q_S$ is not a readily measurable parameter in a clinical setting, SaO_2 is commonly used as a surrogate method of assessing the extent to which a balanced circulation exists. An arterial saturation of 75–80% is felt to be indicative of a balanced circulation. It is important to note, however, that an arterial saturation of 75–80% is indicative of a $Q_P:Q_S$ at or near 1:1 only if the pulmonary venous saturation is 95–100% and the mixed venous saturation is 50–55%. In fact, based on these assumptions, the equation used to calculate $Q_P:Q_S$ in patients with univentricular physiology ($SaO_2 - SmvO_2)/(SpvO_2 - SaO_2$) can be simplified to: $25/(95 - SaO_2)$. In this simplified equation, $SpvO_2$ is assumed to be 95% and the A-V O_2 saturation difference is assumed to be 25%. Use of this simplified equation requires that the FiO_2 be at or near 0.21 in order that the dissolved O_2 content of the pulmonary venous blood can be ignored and an $SpvO_2$ of 95% used. Unfortunately, an arterial saturation of 75–80% can exist at the extremes of $Q_P:Q_S$, depending on pulmonary and systemic venous saturation. Specifically, in the presence of a high $Q_P:Q_S$ it is possible to have inadequate systemic oxygen delivery (systemic venous desaturation, a wide Sa-vO$_2$ difference, metabolic acidosis) in the presence of what is considered to be an adequate arterial saturation of 75–80%. In addition, clinically unrecognized episodes of pulmonary venous desaturation (SpvO$_2$ <90%) further confound assessment of Q$_P$:Q$_S$ based on SaO$_2$.

Mathematic modeling of univentricular physiology reveals that systemic O$_2$ delivery (CaO$_2$•Q$_p$) is a complex function of cardiac output (CO), pulmonary venous O$_2$ content (CpvO$_2$), systemic O$_2$ consumption (CVO$_2$), and Q$_p$:Q$_s$ described by the equation:

$$CaO_2 \times Q_s = \frac{CO \times CpvO_2}{1 + Q_p/Q_s} - \frac{CVO_2}{Q_p/Q_s}$$

Given the complex relationships of the multiple variables that determine Q$_p$:Q$_s$ and O$_2$ delivery in patients with univentricular physiology, it is not surprising that neither SaO$_2$ nor the equation 25/(95 − SaO$_2$) reliably predicts Q$_p$:Q$_s$.

In fact, SaO$_2$ correlates poorly with Q$_p$:Q$_s$ and the measurement of SpvO$_2$ and SsvcO$_2$ substantially improves estimation of Q$_p$:Q$_s$. Regression analysis demonstrates that SaO$_2$ accounts for 8% of the error in estimating Q$_p$:Q$_s$ while SsvcO$_2$ and SpvO$_2$ contribute 48% and 44% respectively. Figure 28.2 illustrates the effect of CO (450 versus 300 ml min^{-1} kg^{-1}) on O$_2$ delivery, SvO$_2$, SaO$_2$, and Sa-vO$_2$ as Q$_p$:Q$_s$ varies with SpvO$_2$ = 95% and O$_2$ consumption = 9 ml min^{-1} kg^{-1}. It is clear that while SaO$_2$ remains satisfactory over a wide range of Q$_p$:Q$_s$, SvO$_2$ decreases precipitously outside a narrow range of Q$_p$:Q$_s$ near 1.0. Furthermore, Sa-vO$_2$ increases dramatically once Q$_p$:Q$_s$ >1.0. It is also clear that a higher CO allows maintenance of satisfactory O$_2$ delivery and SsvcO$_2$ over a wider range of Q$_p$:Q$_s$.

Any combination of variables which produces a SsvcO$_2$ <30% is likely to result in the development of anaerobic metabolism. A modification of the O$_2$ delivery equation can be used to take this into account, where a threshold level of capillary saturation (Sat$_{Thresh}$) is defined. Any contributions to O$_2$ delivery by saturations below this threshold are ignored, as they do not provide physiologically useful oxygen delivery. As a result, a new term "useful O$_2$ delivery to the body" defined as D(u)O$_2$ = [(CaO$_2$)(1 − Sat$_{Thresh}$)]

(Q$_S$) is utilized rather than the traditional O$_2$ delivery DO$_2$ = (CaO$_2$)(Q$_S$). A realistic Sat$_{Thresh}$ would be 30–35%.

Ω is the oxygen excess factor calculated as SaO$_2$/(Sa-vO$_2$); it is the inverse of the oxygen extraction ratio. A direct linear relationship between Ω and O$_2$ delivery exists. This direct linear relationship is independent of SpvO$_2$ and CO but the slope of this relationship increases as O$_2$ consumption increases. Nonetheless, interventions to improve systemic O$_2$ delivery will be associated with an increase in measured Ω. This is a clinically useful parameter as it can be obtained with a systemic saturation from an arterial blood gas or a pulse oximeter and an SVC saturation obtained from a venous blood gas drawn from a central venous catheter positioned just at or above the SVC/RA junction.

These patients are at risk for subendocardial ischemia because volume overload increases the ventricular end-diastolic volume and pressure, and because the run-off of blood into the lower-resistance pulmonary circuit reduces aortic diastolic blood pressure. Under these conditions, a small increase in heart rate may reduce subendocardial perfusion enough to induce ischemia and ventricular fibrillation.

Anesthetic Management, Preinitial Repair

Goals

- A continuous infusion of PGE$_1$ is used to maintain ductal patency in patients with ductal-dependent blood flow (either systemic or pulmonary). PGE$_1$ can be discontinued in any patient determined by echocardiogram to have a reliable nonductal source of systemic or pulmonary blood flow. Ductal patency generally produces unrestrictive pulmonary blood flow.
- A target PaO$_2$ of 40–45 mmHg and a SaO$_2$ of 70–80% are reasonable, and likely to be associated with adequate systemic O$_2$ delivery.

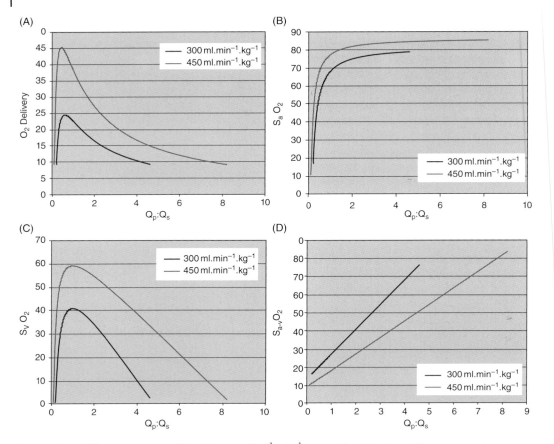

Figure 28.2 (A) Systemic oxygen (O_2) delivery (ml kg^{-1} min^{-1}) versus Qp:Qs for two different systemic ventricular outputs (300 ml kg^{-1} min^{-1} and 450 ml kg^{-1} min^{-1}) in single-ventricle physiology. Oxygen consumption is assumed to be 9 ml kg^{-1} min^{-1} and SpVo$_2$ = 95%. It is clear that systemic oxygen delivery peaks just below a Qp:Qs of 1:1 and declines rapidly above or below this narrow peak. (B) SaO$_2$ versus Qp:Qs for two different systemic ventricular outputs (300 ml kg^{-1} min^{-1} and 450 ml kg^{-1} min^{-1}) in single-ventricle physiology. Oxygen consumption is assumed to be 9 ml kg^{-1} min^{-1} and SpVo$_2$ = 95%. It is clear that SaO$_2$ remains at or near 80% over a wide range of Qp:Qs and consequently is a very poor surrogate measure of Qp:Qs. (C) SvO$_2$ versus Qp:Qs for two different systemic ventricular outputs (300 ml kg^{-1} min^{-1} and 450 ml kg^{-1} min^{-1}) in single-ventricle physiology. Oxygen consumption is assumed to be 9 ml kg^{-1} min^{-1} and SpVo$_2$ = 95%. SvO$_2$ decreases precipitously outside a narrow range of Qp:Qs near 1.0. (D) Sa-vO$_2$ versus Qp:Qs for two different systemic ventricular outputs (300 ml kg^{-1} min^{-1} and 450 ml kg^{-1} min^{-1}) in single-ventricle physiology. Oxygen consumption is assumed to be 9 ml kg^{-1} min^{-1} and SpVo$_2$ = 95%. Sa-vO$_2$ increases linearly as Qp:Qs increases with the slope of the increase decreased by increased systemic ventricular output.

- In single-ventricle patients with unrestricted pulmonary blood flow, the control and manipulation of PVR and subsequently of Q$_P$:Q$_S$ are accomplished most reliably through ventilatory interventions. Clinically, both hypercarbia in combination with a 21% FiO$_2$ to achieve a pH of 7.30–7.35 and normocarbia in combination with a 17% FiO$_2$ (inspired N$_2$) can be utilized to increase PVR and reduce Q$_P$:Q$_S$. Both strategies reduce Q$_P$:Q$_S$ to a comparable degree versus baseline (21% FiO$_2$ and normocarbia) but hypercarbia results in a better systemic O$_2$ delivery (as determined by a narrower A-V O$_2$ saturation difference and a higher SaO$_2$/(Sa-vO$_2$)), a higher mean arterial pressure, and a higher cerebral O_2 saturation (as determined by near-infra-red spectrometry).

- Hypercarbia ($PaCO_2$ of 45–55 mmHg) can be reliably obtained via alveolar hypoventilation or via increased inspired CO_2 (3% $FiCO_2$). Hypercarbia can be obtained utilizing hypoventilation without the use of inspired CO_2. Care is taken to assure adequate tidal volumes with maintenance of functional residual capacity (FRC) and avoidance of atelectasis so as not to induce intrapulmonary shunting and V/Q mismatch resulting in inadvertent hypoxemia. An appropriate degree of hypercarbia can be obtained with a tidal volume of 8–12 ml kg^{-1}, a positive end-expiratory pressure (PEEP) of 3–5 cmH_2O, and a respiratory rate of 4–8 breaths per minute. Additional PEEP and larger tidal volumes can be used to mechanically limit excessive pulmonary blood flow. The lower rates are required as the infant cools and the metabolic rate decreases.
- Avoid a high FiO_2 unless the PaO_2 <35–40 mmHg and intrapulmonary V/Q mismatch is suspected.
- Because ventilatory interventions are incapable of reducing $Q_P:Q_S$ much below 2:1, an increased cardiac output is often necessary to ensure adequate systemic oxygen delivery and coronary perfusion pressure in these patients. The ability to recruit stroke volume with preload augmentation is very limited in patients with volume-overloaded ventricles. An increasing heart rate >140–150 bpm has the potential of initiating myocardial ischemia in patients with aortic diastolic blood pressures in the range of 20–30 mmHg. This is a particular risk in patients with HLHS. Inotropic support may be necessary; dopamine in doses of 3–5 μg kg^{-1} min^{-1} is usually sufficient to accomplish these goals.
- Once the chest is open, the surgeon can mechanically limit pulmonary blood flow and reduce $Q_P:Q_S$ by placing a vessel loop around a pulmonary artery (usually the right). This will often dramatically improve hemodynamics. The end-tidal (ET) CO_2 will fall as the $ETCO_2–PaCO_2$ gradient increases. It is not appropriate to decrease minute ventilation at this time; in fact, it may need to be increased slightly. A small increase in FiO_2 may also be necessary.
- Infants with single-ventricle physiology who arrive in the operating room unintubated from the intensive care unit require special attention. These patients may clinically have a balanced circulation, but this occurs in the setting of several factors that increase PVR, including low lung volumes, increased interstitial lung water, and hypoxic pulmonary vasoconstriction. Following induction, intubation, and mechanical lung expansion, these patients may have a precipitous drop in PVR and an immediate compromise of systemic circulation. Despite this, denitrogenation with 100% O_2 is recommended prior to laryngoscopy and tracheal intubation so as to prevent hypoxemia during this interval. Once the airway is secured, the FiO_2 can be reduced.

Induction and Maintenance

These patients have a tenuous cardiovascular status with limited cardiovascular reserve. Ventricular fibrillation can be seen in association with light anesthesia or during routine maneuvers, such as opening the pericardium. Many of them arrive in the operating room intubated and receiving inotropic support and PGE_1. In the absence of an accurate prenatal diagnosis, some neonates initially present in shock or following cardiopulmonary resuscitation. These neonates usually require one or more days of medical stabilization prior to surgery.

An intravenous induction using a high-dose synthetic narcotic technique in combination with a muscle relaxant is recommended. A benzodiazepine (usually midazolam) can be added as tolerated. Inhalation agents are generally poorly tolerated. Rocuronium is normally utilized and well tolerated.

Post-CPB Management, Postinitial Repair

Goals

After the initial repair, single-ventricle physiology persists and the same principles described for pre-CPB management hold true, with a few notable exceptions.

1) After CPB, it is not uncommon for a high PVR to result in reduced pulmonary blood flow and hypoxemia.
2) The mBTTS or RV-PA conduit may be too large or too small for prevailing physiologic conditions.
3) Ventricular dysfunction may exist due to the long CPB and DHCA or regional low-flow perfusion intervals that are necessary to complete these complicated repairs.
4) Myocardial and tissue edema may be significant, precluding chest closure.
5) Bleeding from long arterial suture lines may be significant.
6) Inhaled pulmonary vasodilators such as NO may be necessary to improve SaO_2 or reduce the transpulmonary gradient in this patient population. This is particularly true in the subgroup of patients who have repair of partially obstructed pulmonary venous drainage at the time of their initial repair.

Management of the four clinical scenarios present after initial repair, and the appropriate interventions necessary, are summarized in Table 28.2.

The agents chosen for inotropic support are institution dependent. Dopamine 5–10 $\mu g\ kg^{-1}\ min^{-1}$, epinephrine 0.01–0.1 $\mu g\ kg^{-1}\ min^{-1}$, and epinephrine in combination with milrinone 0.5–1.0 $\mu g\ kg^{-1}\ min^{-1}$ are all reasonable choices. Institutional preference determines which agents are used when afterload reduction is undertaken. Typically sodium nitroprusside and/or milrinone are administered. Use of these agents should be targeted to a goal SVR and not empirically delivered. Immediately prior to termination of CPB, the SVR should be calculated as follows: [(MAP-CVP)/CPB flow]. The target SVR should be 10–15 iWU. At a CPB flow around 3 l $min^{-1}\ m^{-2}$ this will result in a MAP of 40–50 mmHg. The 3 l $min^{-1}\ m^{-2}$ on CPB represents systemic blood flow. Assuming a conservative post-CPB $Q_P{:}Q_S$ of 1:1, this will require the right ventricle to generate a total output of 6 l $min^{-1}\ m^{-2}.$ If the perfusionist is flowing 3 l $min^{-1}\ m^{-2}$ and the MAP is 20–30 mmHg prior to termination of CPB, it makes little sense to administer an empiric loading dose of milrinone on CPB and be forced to infuse either norepinephrine or vasopressin post CPB to treat iatrogenically low SVR and hypotension.

See Chapter 11 for a more detailed explanation of the treatment of SVR in single-ventricle patients.

Single-ventricle Pathway, Superior Cavopulmonary Shunt or Bidirectional Glenn

The BDG (Figure 28.1D) directs systemic venous blood from the SVC directly to the pulmonary circulation. The BDG is normally undertaken at 3–6 months of age, at which point the PVR has decreased such that the pulmonary blood flow can be provided with systemic venous pressure as the driving pressure. Patients who have outgrown their PA band, RV-PA conduit, or mBTS and have a low SaO_2, and patients who are not tolerating the additional volume on their ventricle with a loose PA band or large mBTS will be staged to a BDG earlier in this interval.

The original Glenn shunt involved an end-to-side anastomosis of the cranial end of the transected SVC to the distal end of the transected right pulmonary artery (RPA). Both the proximal SVC and RPA were oversewn. This procedure was performed through a right thoracotomy, without CPB. Currently, the bidirectional Glenn

Table 28.2 Management of single-ventricle physiology.

Clinical presentation	Physiology	Management
SaO_2 75–80%	**Balanced flow**	No intervention
$Sa-vO_2$ 25–30%	$Q_P:Q_S$ = 0.7–1.5:1	
BP >60/30 mmHg		
SaO_2 >85–90%	**High pulmonary blood flow**	*Raise PVR:*
$Sa-vO_2$ 35–40%	$Q_P:Q_S$ >2–3:1	Controlled hypoventilation
BP <60/30	*Causes:*	Mild acidosis
Diastolic BP <15–25 mmHg with mBTS; likely higher with RV-PA conduit	Low PVR	Low Fio_2 (0.17–0.19); compromises cerebral O_2 delivery
	Large MBTTS or RV-PA conduit	*Increase systemic O_2 delivery:*
	Residual arch obstruction	Afterload reduction
	High SVR	Inotropic support
		Hematocrit >40%
		Surgical intervention:
		Clip MBTTS or RV-PA conduit
		Revise arch reconstruction
SaO_2 <65–75%	**Low pulmonary blood flow**	*Lower PVR:*
$Sa-vO_2$ 25–30%; but SvO_2 likely less than critical value of 30%	$Q_P:Q_S$ <0.7:1	Controlled hyperventilation
	Causes:	Alkalosis
BP >70/40 mmHg	High PVR	Sedation/paralysis
Diastolic BP >40 mmHg	Small mBTTS or RV-PA conduit	Aggressively treat atelectasis (pulmonary venous desaturation)
	Pulmonary venous desaturation with underestimation of actual $Q_P:Q_S$	
		Consider NO
		Increase systemic O_2 delivery:
		Inotropic support
		Surgical intervention:
		Revise MBTTS or RV-PA conduit
SaO_2 <70–75%	**Low cardiac output**	*Minimize O_2 consumption:*
$Sa-vO_2$ 35–40% and SvO_2 likely less than critical value of 30%	*Causes:*	Sedation/paralysis
	Ventricular dysfunction	Inotropic support/afterload reduction
BP <60/30 mmHg	• Myocardial ischemia	

(Continued)

Table 28.2 (Continued)

Clinical presentation	Physiology	Management
	• Depressed contractility	
	• Afterload mismatch (residual arch obstruction)	*Surgical intervention:*
	• AV valve regurgitation	Repair AV valve
		Revise arch
		Consider mechanical support:
		• Postcardiotomy support
		• Bridge-to-transplantation

AV, atrioventricular; BP, blood pressure; mBTTS, modified Blalock–Thomas–Taussig shunt; PVR, pulmonary vascular resistance; RV-PA, right ventricle-pulmonary artery; SVR, systemic vascular resistance.

is used in which the cranial end of the transected SVC is anastomosed end to side to the RPA (which is in continuity with the main and left PAs) and the cardiac end of the SVC is oversewn. This creates SVC continuity with both the left and right pulmonary arteries, and bidirectional pulmonary blood flow. The main PA is oversewn if it is not atretic. Unless the IVC is interrupted with azygous continuation, the azygous vein is ligated so that the SVC does not decompress retrograde to the IVC, thereby reducing the quantity of blood delivered to the PAs. This procedure is performed on CPB through a median sternotomy. The previous aortopulmonary shunt is ligated or the PA band taken down.

Normally, all upper-extremity and cerebral venous drainages reach the SVC. In some patients with congenital heart disease (particularly those with heterotaxy syndrome), there may be bilateral SVCs that are not in continuity via a connecting vein. In this case, a bilateral BDG must be performed with one SVC anastomosed end to side to the RPA and the other SVC anastomosed end to side to the LPA. LPA-RPA continuity is maintained.

The differences between an aortopulmonary shunt and a BDG are summarized in Figure 28.3. The most obvious difference between the two is that, for a given cardiac output, SaO_2, $SpvO_2$, and SvO_2, the volume load on the systemic ventricle will be twice as

large with an aortopulmonary shunt as it is with a BDG. Effective pulmonary blood flows in the aortopulmonary shunt and BDG circulations are equal. However, in the aortopulmonary shunt circulation there is recirculated pulmonary blood (physiologic L-R shunt), while in the BDG circulation there is no recirculated pulmonary blood flow. As a result, a child with a BDG will have the same SaO_2 as a child with an aortopulmonary shunt, but with a significant reduction in the volume load on the systemic ventricle.

The determination of Qp:Qs in patients with BDG deserves some discussion. In BDG physiology, systemic cardiac output (Qs) is the sum of pulmonary venous flow (Qp) and IVC flow (Qivc):

$$Qs = Qp + Qivc$$

$$Qivc = Qs - Qp$$

Oxygen delivery is the product of flow (Q) and oxygen content (C); therefore, systemic oxygen delivery is the sum of pulmonary venous oxygen delivery and IVC oxygen delivery:

$$Qs \cdot CaO_2 = Qp \cdot CpvO_2 + Qivc \cdot CivcO_2$$

$$Qs \cdot CaO_2 = Qp \cdot CpvO_2 + (Qs - Qp) \cdot CivcO_2$$

$$Qs \cdot CaO_2 = Qp \cdot CpvO_2 + Qs \cdot CivcO_2 - Qp \cdot CivcO_2$$

(A)

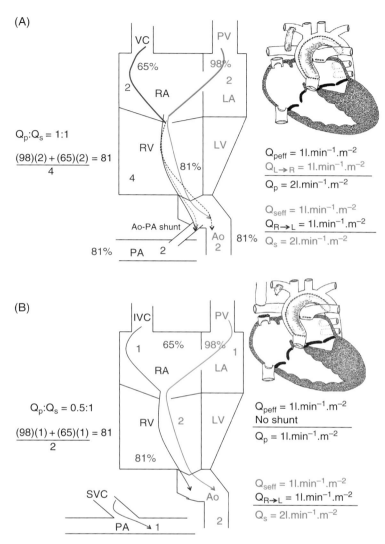

$Q_p:Q_s = 1:1$

$$\frac{(98)(2) + (65)(2)}{4} = 81$$

$Q_{peff} = 1l.min^{-1}.m^{-2}$
$Q_{L\to R} = 1l.min^{-1}.m^{-2}$
_____
$Q_p = 2l.min^{-1}.m^{-2}$

$Q_{seff} = 1l.min^{-1}.m^{-2}$
$Q_{R\to L} = 1l.min^{-1}.m^{-2}$
_____
$Q_s = 2l.min^{-1}.m^{-2}$

(B)

$Q_p:Q_s = 0.5:1$

$$\frac{(98)(1) + (65)(1)}{2} = 81$$

$Q_{peff} = 1l.min^{-1}.m^{-2}$
No shunt
_____
$Q_p = 1l.min^{-1}.m^{-2}$

$Q_{seff} = 1l.min^{-1}.m^{-2}$
$Q_{R\to L} = 1l.min^{-1}.m^{-2}$
_____
$Q_s = 2l.min^{-1}.m^{-2}$

Figure 28.3 (A) Depiction of saturations and blood flows in a neonate with HLHS palliated with a Damus–Kaye–Stansel (DKS) anastomosis, aortic arch reconstruction and coarctectomy, atrial septectomy, and an aortopulmonary shunt. Complete mixing occurs at the atrial level. The right ventricle (RV) is volume overloaded in this parallel circulation to provide both systemic and pulmonary blood flow. Q_S and Q_P are 2 l min^{-1} m^{-2} and the arterial saturation is 81% ($Q_P:Q_S = 1:1$.) (B) Depiction of saturations and blood flows in the same patient now palliated with a bidirectional superior cavopulmonary shunt. Complete mixing occurs at the atrial level. The RV is not volume overloaded in this series circulation. Q_S is 2 l min^{-1} m^{-2}, and Q_P is 1 l min^{-1} m^{-2}; $Q_P:Q_S = 0.5:1.0$. Nonetheless, cardiac output and arterial saturation are identical to the patient palliated with the aortopulmonary shunt. This is because arterial saturation in complete mixing is determined by the relative volumes and saturations of systemic and pulmonary venous blood. In this instance, Q_S and the volume of systemic venous blood reaching the right atrium (RA) are not equal because half of Q_S has been diverted to become pulmonary venous blood. As a result, $Q_P:Q_S$ is deceptive here. Ao, aorta; IVC, inferior vena cava; LA, left atrium; LV, left ventricle; PA, pulmonary artery; RA, right atrium; RV, right ventricle; SVC, superior vena cava. Effective blood flows are shown as solid lines and shunted blood flows are shown as dotted lines.

$$Qs \cdot \left(CaO_2 - CivcO_2\right)$$
$$= Qp \cdot \left(CpvO_2 - CivcO_2\right)$$

$$Qp / Qs = \left(CaO_2 - CivcO_2\right)$$
$$/ \left(CpvO_2 - CivcO_2\right)$$

Content (C) can be simplified to the measured saturation (Sat) if a low FiO_2 is utilized because the contribution of O_2 dissolved in blood to C ($PaO_2 \cdot 0.0031$) can be ignored. If the hemoglobin concentration (Hb) in g dl^{-1} is known then C = Sat $\cdot$ [Hb] $\cdot$ 1.39 where [Hb] $\cdot$ 1.39 is a constant. Then:

$$Qp / Qs = \left(SaO_2 - SivcO_2\right)$$
$$/ \left(SpvO_2 - SivcO_2\right)$$

Obviously, this approach requires sampling of IVC blood. In actual practice, it is assumed that $SsvcO_2$ and $SivcO_2$ are equal, and thus:

$$Qp / Qs = \left(SaO_2 - SsvcO_2\right)$$
$$/ \left(SpvO_2 - SsvcO_2\right)$$

Modifications of the BDG have been devised to potentially simplify the conversion to a Fontan. The hemi-Fontan refers specifically to a procedure in which an atriopulmonary anastomosis is constructed between the dome of the right atrium at the RA/SVC junction and the inferior surface of the right pulmonary artery. A Gore-Tex* baffle or dam is used to supplement the central pulmonary artery area and to isolate the cavopulmonary connection from the right atrium. Another modification (incorrectly called a hemi-Fontan) involves the creation of a double cavopulmonary anastomosis, where the cranial end of the divided SVC is anastomosed to the superior surface of the right pulmonary artery. The cardiac end of the divided SVC is anastomosed to the inferior surface of the right PA. The internal orifice of the cardiac end of the superior vena cava is closed with a Gore-Tex patch (Figure 28.4).

A further modification of the BDG is the Super Glenn, a procedure wherein a mBTTS or central shunt is used to augment PBF to

Figure 28.4 The anatomy of a double cavopulmonary anastomosis with internal patch closure of the cardiac end of the SVC anastomosis. Both the cardiac and cephalic portions of the superior vena cava are in continuity with the right pulmonary artery.

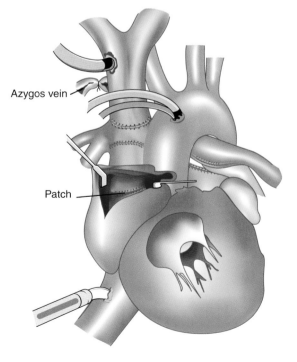

Azygos vein

Patch

the contralateral lung and a restrictive connection (either externally with a band or internally with a fenestrated intraluminal patch) is placed between the shunted lung and the lung supplied by the SVC. This limits the rise in SVC pressure while still providing hepatic venous blood to the lung supplied by the SVC. The shunt size and restriction are constructed to limit the mean PA pressures in the shunted lung to the mid-20s mmHg. This strategy allows for contralateral PA growth and regression of any associated pulmonary arterial collaterals or pulmonary arteriovenous malformations (PAVMs) while limiting the rise in SVC pressure and the associated complications. Using this strategy, patients with pulmonary vascular disease and elevated PVR secondary to unilateral lung disease and patients with pulmonary vein stenosis have been successfully palliated (Figure 28.5).

Anesthetic Management, Presuperior Cavopulmonary Shunt

Goals

The principles outlined above on management of single-ventricle physiology after the initial repair apply (see Table 28.2). By the age of 3–6 months, when these infants present for their cavopulmonary shunt, they have generally grown and gained weight such that their $Q_P:Q_S$ is likely to be 1.0–1.5:1. As a result, these patients are much less prone to compromise of systemic O_2 delivery by an excess of pulmonary blood flow.

Induction and Maintenance

An IV induction is preferred in these patients. Vascular access may be difficult, as many of these patients have prolonged intensive care unit (ICU) stays after their initial repair. In addition, many are tolerant to opioids and benzodiazepines following their ICU stay. This should be considered if premedication is planned prior to IV placement.

Figure 28.5 The Super Glenn procedure consists of a superior cavopulmonary anastomosis to the right pulmonary artery, an additional source of pulmonary blood flow to the left pulmonary artery, which in this case is a modified Blalock–Thomas–Taussig shunt, and an intraluminal fenestrated intrapulmonary septation between the bidirectional Glenn and the modified Blalock–Thomas–Taussig shunt. In addition, there is fenestrated atrial septation. *Source:* Reproduced from Roche Rodriguez & DiNardo (2022)/with permission of Elsevier.

Post-CPB Management, Postsuperior Cavopulmonary Shunt

Goals

Maintain heart rate, contractility, and preload to maintain cardiac output. Decreases in cardiac output will reduce IVC saturation. In BDG physiology, where there is mixing of IVC and pulmonary venous blood in a common atrium, this will reduce arterial saturation.

- Low $PpvO_2$ saturation will produce a low SaO_2. Maneuvers to reduce V/Q mismatch and intrapulmonary shunt should be undertaken. A high FiO_2 may be necessary in the presence of significant V/Q mismatch.

- Normocarbia or mild hypercarbia (40–45 mmHg) should be maintained. The mean airway pressure should be kept at the minimal compatible with delivery of an adequate tidal volume and lung expansion. A high mean airway pressure will mechanically limit the nonpulsatile pulmonary blood flow. This can usually be accomplished with a relatively large tidal volume (10–12 ml kg^{-1}), slow respiratory rates (10–15 breaths per min), and short inspiratory times (I:E of 1:3 or 1:4). PEEP should be used with caution.
- A central line placed in the internal jugular (IJ) vein will measure SVC pressure, which equals mPAP following a BDG. A surgically placed atrial line will measure common atrial pressure. The TPG (mPAP – common atrial pressure) is usually <10 mmHg, with appropriate ventilation. A mPAP of 12–18 mmHg is usually seen in the presence of good systemic ventricular function.
- Inotropic support of the systemic ventricle may be necessary due to ventricular dysfunction induced by chronic volume overload and CPB. Dopamine (3–5 µg kg^{-1} min^{-1}) is useful. Milrinone (0.5–1.0 µg kg^{-1} min^{-1}) may be useful for those patients who have high SVR and hypertension.
- Inhaled pulmonary vasodilators such as NO generally do not improve SaO$_2$ or reduce the transpulmonary gradient in this patient population. The exception to this may be the subgroup of patients who have repair of partially obstructed pulmonary venous drainage at the time of their BDG.
- The most likely cause of a low SaO$_2$ following a BDG is low cardiac output with a low IVC saturation. TEE will help to delineate the cause (ventricular dysfunction, hypovolemia, AV valve dysfunction). If a low SaO$_2$ persists despite optimization of the ventricular function, consideration should be given to causes of reduced pulmonary blood flow, such as a stenotic anastomosis or the presence of decompressing venous collaterals from the SVC to the IVC.

These patients will have a SaO$_2$ of 75–80%, similar to that prior to their BDG (Figure 28.6). The Q$_P$:Q$_S$ ranges from 0.5:1 to 0.7:1 and as a result there will be an acute reduction in volume load on the systemic ventricle. There is an acute increase in SVC pressure and presumably in ICP. The volume load reduction and elevated SVC pressure are believed to contribute to the initial systemic hypertension and postoperative irritability commonly seen in these patients. The majority of pulmonary blood flow will be supplied via venous blood from the brain; this is the largest contributor to venous drainage from the upper body. Hyperventilation and hypocarbia, while beneficial in reducing PVR, will also reduce cerebral blood flow and cerebral venous drainage. Maintaining normocarbia or mild hypercarbia following BDG has been shown to provide maximal Q$_P$:Q$_S$ and SaO$_2$. These patients tend to have a large ETCO$_2$–PaCO$_2$ gradient due to an increased physiologic dead space. An increased portion of the lung in these patients is ventilated but not perfused due to the low pulmonary artery driving pressure (SVC pressure).

Attention is focused on the transpulmonary gradient (TPG) that, in normal patients, is defined as the mPAP–LAP. In BDG patients, the mPAP = SVC pressure. In BDG patients, the equivalent of a LAP or pulmonary venous atrial pressure is the common atrial pressure. A common atrium exists in these patients because the atrial septectomy creates a nonrestrictive communication between the left and right atria.

Definitive Repair: The Fontan Procedure or Total Cavopulmonary Connection

Fontan Physiology

The Fontan procedure is generally performed in staged patients at the age of 2–3 years. As a child with a BDG grows, the BDG becomes progressively less efficient in providing pulmonary blood flow. The ratio of venous return from the SVC:IVC changes from 50:50

Figure 28.6 A hydraulic schematic of the Fontan circulation in which the systemic and pulmonary resistance beds are arranged in series. The single ventricle is represented as a pump that moves blood from a high-compliance, high-capacitance, low-pressure venous reservoir into a low-compliance, low-capacitance, high-pressure arterial reservoir. Blood return to the venous reservoir is gradient driven across a single resistance, the systemic vascular resistance (SVR). Unlike a two-ventricle circulation, blood return to the pump (ventricular preload) is gradient driven from the venous reservoir across two interposed resistances: the pulmonary vascular resistance (PVR) and the resistance across the cavopulmonary connection (not shown separately here but incorporated in PVR). There are two mechanisms whereby the driving pressure in the venous reservoir can be increased to increase ventricular preload: increase the volume of the venous reservoir by expanding the blood volume or reduce venous capacitance. Unique to the Fontan circulation is the fact that increases in venous reservoir pressure simultaneously increase preload and afterload to the single ventricle because all resistances and pressures are in series. All the energy necessary to provide sufficient gradients for flow in the presence of elevated venous pressure is supplied by the single ventricle. *Source:* Reproduced from Jolley et al. (2015)/with permission of International Anesthesia Research Society.

at three months to the adult value of 30:70 at 3–4 years of age. In addition, the child becomes ambulatory with the large muscle groups of the lower body returning deoxygenated blood to the heart. Furthermore, deprivation of the lungs of blood return from the splanchnic bed through the liver is associated with the development of pulmonary arteriovenous shunting similar to that seen in end-stage liver disease.

Fontan physiology is a series ("normal") circulation that can be described as follows.

- There is one ventricle with sufficient diastolic, systolic, and atrioventricular valve function to support systemic circulation. This ventricle must in turn:
  - be in unobstructed continuity with the aorta, and
  - be in unobstructed continuity with pulmonary venous blood.
- There is unobstructed delivery of systemic venous blood to the pulmonary circulation (total cavopulmonary continuity).

In the absence of any residual physiologic intracardiac or intrapulmonary R-L shunting, these patients should have a normal SaO_2. It is often stated that pulmonary blood flow is passive. In fact, it is gradient driven (systemic venous pressure > mean pulmonary artery pressure > pulmonary venous atrial pressure). The systemic ventricle generates the energy necessary to create this pressure gradient and provide flow through the pulmonary capillary bed because the systemic vascular bed and pulmonary vascular bed are in continuity without an intervening atria and ventricle to provide a reservoir and pumping capacity. As a result, the single ventricle in a series Fontan circulation is faced with higher afterload than the systemic ventricle in a two-ventricle series circulation. In addition, preload to the single ventricle is relatively low compared to a normal ventricle due to the fact that the systemic venous pressure and not the right ventricle is the energy source for volume delivery to the systemic ventricle (Figures 28.6 and 28.7).

The Fontan procedure was first performed in 1968 and was applied to patients with tricuspid atresia. The original operation included a Glenn shunt, which drained the SVC directly into the distal right pulmonary artery. The proximal end of the right pulmonary artery

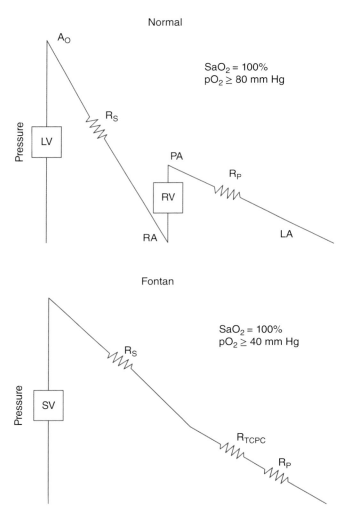

Figure 28.7 The normal and Fontan circulation demonstrating a single-ventricle driving flow across three resistances in series: systemic (R_S), total cavopulmonary connection (R_{TCPC}), and pulmonary (R_P). In a normal, two-ventricle circulation, each ventricle drives flow across one resistance. *Source:* Reproduced from Jolley et al. (2015)/with permission of International Anesthesia Research Society.

was joined to the right atrial appendage via an aortic valve homograft, and a pulmonary valve homograft valve was placed at the IVC-RA junction. The main pulmonary artery was ligated and the ASD was closed. Subsequently, creation of the Glenn shunt and placement of homograft valves at the RA-PA and IVC-RA junctions were eliminated, resulting in the creation of a direct atriopulmonary connection.

Since then, many modifications have been described. Despite the modifications, the goal of the procedure remains the same: to provide delivery of all systemic venous blood directly to the pulmonary arteries without the benefit of the reservoir or pumping capability of a ventricle. This requires total cavopulmonary continuity either directly or via the system venous atrium. Currently, the most commonly performed procedures are the lateral tunnel and extracardiac Fontan (Figure 28.8). The lateral tunnel procedure avoids incorporating any substantial volume of atrium in the cavopulmonary pathway, while the extracardiac procedure does not

incorporate any atrium. These procedures are referred to as total cavopulmonary connections. Over time, in atriopulmonary connections, an elevated systemic venous pressure leads to atrial dilatation. The atrium often expands to a volume as large as 300–500 ml. This is a source of stasis and a nidus for atrial arrhythmias. In theory, the extracardiac procedure may offer additional protection from development of atrial arrhythmias due to a lack of suture lines in atrium.

Traditionally cited contraindications to the Fontan procedure include early infancy, PVR >4 Wood units m^{-2}, severe pulmonary artery hypoplasia, an ejection fraction (EF) <25–30%, and a ventricular diastolic pressure >25 mmHg. The majority of lesions felt in the past to be relative contraindications to the Fontan procedure, such as AV valve regurgitation/stenosis or focally narrowed or distorted pulmonary arteries, can now be corrected at the time of the Fontan procedure.

Use of the staged single-ventricle pathway results in reduced morbidity and mortality compared to the acute transition from

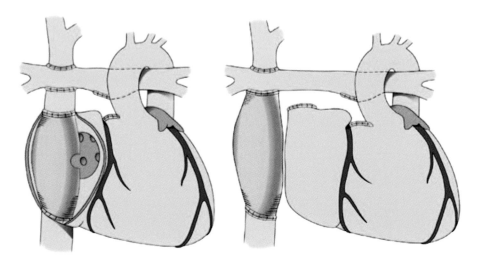

Figure 28.8 Fontan procedure. Illustrations of a fenestrated lateral tunnel (intraatrial baffle) Fontan (left) and an unfenestrated extracardiac Fontan (right). Both place the inferior vena cava and superior vena cava in continuity with the pulmonary arteries, a complete cavopulmonary connection, with no interposed ventricle. The fenestration allows a "pop off" of blood from the systemic venous circulation to the pulmonary venous (common) atrium when baffle pressures are elevated. This allows cardiac output to be maintained in the presence of elevated resistance across the cavopulmonary connection and the pulmonary vascular bed in exchange for lower systemic arterial saturation.

single-ventricle to Fontan physiology. As previously described, the staged pathway makes use of a bidirectional cavopulmonary shunt procedure before the Fontan procedure. Use of the cavopulmonary shunt at 3–6 months of age allows an early reduction in the volume overload that accompanies univentricular physiology. This allows the systemic ventricular volume load to be reduced to normal, and allows remodeling of the ventricle at lower end-diastolic volume.

An acute reduction of systemic ventricular volume in the univentricular heart results in impaired ventricular compliance because the wall thickness does not regress as quickly as ventricular volume. The result is impaired ventricular diastolic function and elevated end-diastolic pressure. This will impede pulmonary venous return, which is a liability in the Fontan procedure because it will subsequently reduce pulmonary blood flow. A low cardiac output state will result because systemic ventricular output can only equal the quantity of blood that transverses the pulmonary vascular bed. The impaired ventricular diastolic function that accompanies acute ventricular volume reduction is better tolerated in BDG or hemi-Fontan physiology than in Fontan physiology. When there is impairment of pulmonary venous return after the BDG or hemi-Fontan, blood from the IVC will continue to provide systemic ventricular filling and cardiac output at a lower pressure than that required to traverse the pulmonary bed.

A risk of the staged procedures is the development of pulmonary arteriovenous malformations, which are the result of diversion of hepatic venous blood flow to another capillary bed (systemic) before delivery to the pulmonary capillary bed as occurs in the bidirectional cavopulmonary shunts. This is generally not a problem when the BDG is eventually converted to a Fontan.

Fenestrated Fontan

With Fontan physiology, increased impedance to systemic venous blood flow across the pulmonary capillary bed will result in decreased delivery of blood to the pulmonary venous atrium, systemic ventricle and aorta, producing a low cardiac output state with a normal or near-normal SaO_2. This increased impedance is not uncommon in the initial days and weeks following Fontan surgery. Attempts to increase cardiac output by increasing systemic venous pressure may result in the development of refractory pleural effusions and ascites. In many institutions, a 4 mm hole or fenestration is intentionally left in the cavopulmonary pathway or baffle. This allows systemic venous blood to "pop off" into the pulmonary venous atrium and, ultimately, into the systemic ventricle and aorta. This physiologic R-L shunt allows the maintenance of systemic cardiac output at the expense of SaO_2. The fenestration can be easily closed in the cardiac catheterization laboratory with an occlusion device at a later date following the demonstration of adequate hemodynamics, gas exchange, and cardiac output, by using a balloon occlusion of the fenestration.

Anesthetic Management, Pre-Fontan

Goals

The principles outlined in the section on management of BDG physiology after CPB generally apply here. At the age of 2–3 years, patients with a superior cavopulmonary shunt (BDG) generally have a stable cardiovascular system with a SaO_2 of 75–80%, unless there are significant decompressing venous collateral vessels from the SVC to either the IVC or pulmonary venous system. These are usually addressed by coil occlusion in the cardiac catheterization laboratory prior to the Fontan. While these patients will tolerate an inhalation induction from a cardiovascular standpoint, it should be recognized that several factors might make a pure inhalation induction difficult.

- Venous congestion of the head and tongue due to a relatively high SVC pressure.

- Coughing, breath-holding, or any other cause of high intrathoracic pressure will cause almost complete cessation of pulmonary blood flow. Almost immediate arterial hypoxemia will occur.
- With a $Q_P:Q_S$ of 0.5–0.7:1, the speed of an inhalation induction will be slow.

Induction and Maintenance

Consideration should be given to premedication, as these patients and their families generally have had multiple hospital exposures for check-ups and procedures. In addition, many of these patients are tolerant to opioids and benzodiazepines following neonatal and subsequent exposure. This should be considered if premedication is planned prior to IV placement.

Post-CPB Management, Post-Fontan Procedure

Goals

Maintain heart rate, contractility, and preload to maintain cardiac output. In Fontan patients with a fenestration or intrapulmonary shunt, decreases in cardiac output will reduce SvO_2 and SaO_2. SvO_2 can be easily determined using a sample drawn from a central venous catheter.

- Low $PpvO_2$ saturation will produce a low SaO_2. Maneuvers to reduce V/Q mismatch and intrapulmonary shunt should be undertaken. A high FiO_2 may be necessary in the presence of significant V/Q mismatch.
- Ventilation and acid–base management should be optimized to keep the PVR low. The mean airway pressure should be kept at the minimum compatible with the delivery of an adequate minute ventilation and lung expansion. A high mean airway pressure will mechanically limit the non-pulsatile pulmonary blood flow. This can usually be accomplished with a relatively large tidal volume (10–12 ml kg^{-1}), slow respiratory rates (10–15 breaths per min), and short inspiratory times (I:E of 1:3 or 1:4). PEEP should be used with caution.
- A central line placed in the IJ will measure caval (baffle) pressure, which equals mPAP following a Fontan. A surgically placed atrial line will measure common atrial pressure. The TPG (mPAP – common atrial pressure) is usually <10 mmHg with appropriate ventilation. A mPAP of 15–18 mmHg is usually seen in the presence of good systemic ventricular function.
- Inotropic support of the systemic ventricle may be necessary due to ventricular dysfunction induced by chronic volume overload and CPB. Dopamine (3–5 μg kg^{-1} min^{-1}) or epinephrine (0.01–0.1 μg kg^{-1} min^{-1}) are useful. Milrinone (0.5–1.0 μg kg^{-1} min^{-1}) is useful for those patients who have a high SVR and afterload/contractility mismatch.
- Inhaled pulmonary vasodilators such as NO generally do not improve SaO_2 or reduce the transpulmonary gradient in this patient population. The exception to this may be the subgroup of patients who have repair of partially obstructed pulmonary venous drainage at the time of their Fontan.
- Fontan patients are exceedingly vulnerable to decreases in intravascular volume and to acute increases in venous capacitance (venodilation causing an increased unstressed venous volume) such as those caused by the direct effects of anesthetic and vasodilator agents, or by a diminished central sympathetic output. Acute increases in venous capacitance and/or compliance can result in lower pulmonary perfusion pressures and subsequently lower ventricular filling pressures, resulting in low cardiac output.
- Hydrostatic pulmonary edema in BDG and Fontan patients is unusual because the driving pressure for pulmonary blood flow is limited by systemic venous pressure. Nonetheless, pulmonary lymphatic drainage is impaired in these patients due to the high central venous pressure present and this contributes to accumulation of lung water.

The management goals following the Fontan procedure are summarized in Table 28.3.

Table 28.3 Management of Fontan physiology.

Physiology	Clinical presentation	Management
Low pulmonary blood flow and inadequate preload delivery to systemic (common) atrium TPG >10 mmHg *Causes:* Baffle obstruction Pulmonary artery obstruction Pulmonary vein obstruction Premature baffle fenestration closure	**No fenestration or premature fenestration closure** SaO$_2$ 95–100% Sa-vO$_2$ > 35–40% Baffle pressure >20 mmHg Common atrial pressure <10 mmHg Hypotension Tachycardia Poor distal perfusion Metabolic acidosis **Fenestration patent or baffle leak present** SaO$_2$ 75–80% Sa-vO$_2$ >35–40% Baffle pressure >20 mmHg Common atrial pressure <10 mmHg Hypotension Tachycardia Poor distal perfusion Metabolic acidosis	Volume replacement to keep baffle pressure stable Reduce PVR Correct acidosis Inotropic support Afterload reduction Consider catheterization intervention to open or create baffle fenestration
Systemic ventricular dysfunction TPG = 5–10 mmHg *Causes:* Systolic dysfunction Diastolic dysfunction AV valve regurgitation/stenosis Loss of AV synchrony Afterload/contractility mismatch	**No fenestration or premature fenestration closure** SaO$_2$ 85–90% Sa-vO$_2$ >35–40% Baffle pressure >20 mmHg Common atrial pressure >15 mmHg Pulmonary edema Hypotension Tachycardia Poor distal perfusion Metabolic acidosis **Fenestration patent or baffle leak present** SaO$_2$ 70–75% Sa-vO$_2$ >35–40% Baffle pressure >20 mmHg Common atrial pressure >15 mmHg Pulmonary edema Hypotension Tachycardia Poor distal perfusion Metabolic acidosis	Volume replacement to keep baffle pressure stable Correct acidosis PEEP may be cautiously used for pulmonary edema Inotropic support Afterload reduction Provide AV synchrony (antiarrhythmics/pacing) Mechanical support (postcardiotomy support or bridge to transplantation) Surgical intervention (takedown to BDG)

AV, atrioventricular; BDG, bidirectional Glenn procedure; PVR, pulmonary vascular resistance; TPG, transpulmonary pressure gradient.

$$Q_{peff} = 1.6l.min^{-1}.m^{-2}$$
No shunt
$$Q_p = 1.6l.min^{-1}.m^{-2}$$

$$Q_{seff} = 1.6l.min^{-1}.m^{-2}$$
$$Q_{R \to L} = 0.4l.min^{-1}.m^{-2}$$
$$Q_s = 2l.min^{-1}.m^{-2}$$

$$Q_p:Q_s = 0.8:1$$

$$\frac{(98)(1.6) + (65)(0.4)}{2} = 91$$

Figure 28.9 Fenestrated Fontan procedure. Systemic and pulmonary saturations and blood flows. Effective blood flows are shown as solid lines and shunted flows as dotted lines.

The systemic and pulmonary blood flow in a Fontan circulation is shown in Figure 28.9.

As with a BDG patient, attention is focused on the transpulmonary gradient (TPG). In Fontan patients the mPAP = CVP. A central venous pressure in a Fontan patient will measure pressure in the caval portion of the cavopulmonary connection, and is commonly called a baffle pressure. As with a BDG patient, in Fontan patients the equivalent of a LAP is the common atrial pressure. In Fontan patients the pressure in the cavopulmonary connection can be obtained via a percutaneously placed central venous catheter or a surgically placed transthoracic baffle catheter. The common atrial pressure is obtained via a surgically placed transthoracic catheter. Thus in patients with a Fontan, the TPG = CVP − common atrial pressure.

Low pulmonary blood flow produces low cardiac output in this series circulation. The systemic ventricle can only pump the volume of blood that is delivered to it across the pulmonary vascular bed. This differs from the situation after superior cavopulmonary shunts because, in these patients, there is a source of blood supply to the systemic ventricle that does not cross the pulmonary bed. It should be emphasized that in a Fontan patient, low cardiac output will not result in a low SaO_2 unless there are significant sources of intrapulmonary or intracardiac (fenestration,

baffle leak) physiologic R-L shunting. When low cardiac output is due to ventricular dysfunction, common (pulmonary venous) atrial hypertension will lead to the accumulation of lung water and physiologic R-L intrapulmonary shunting. This situation is analogous to a normal patient with series circulation and no intracardiac lesions. Low cardiac output in a normal patient will result in a low SaO_2 only if a significant quantity of intrapulmonary R-L shunt exists and a low cardiac output produces a low SvO_2. The presence of a fenestration or baffle leak will exacerbate this SaO_2 decrease in the Fontan patient.

It is commonly stated that early tracheal extubation and spontaneous ventilation enhance pulmonary gas exchange and hemodynamics in Fontan patients. It must be emphasized that low lung volumes, hypercarbia, and hypoxemia will negate any advantage obtained by spontaneous ventilation.

Noncardiac Surgery

Noncardiac surgery for patients following Stage 1 is discussed in Chapter 29.

For Glenn and Fontan patients, the systemic ventricular preload is dependent on pulmonary blood flow. As previously discussed, decreases in intravascular volume such as those associated with prolonged fasting periods should be avoided. Anesthetic agents should be chosen and administered with recognition of the vulnerability of these patients to acute increases in venous capacitance. A preinduction fluid bolus of 10–15 ml kg^{-1} and titration of a drug that decreases venous capacitance (low-dose dopamine) may be beneficial. Factors that increase PVR (e.g., acidosis, atelectasis, hypoxia, severe hypercapnia, hypothermia) need to be controlled, and corrected if needed.

References and Further Reading

DiNardo, J.A. & Zvara, D.A. *Anesthesia for Cardiac Surgery*, 3rd edn. Blackwell, Massachusetts (2008).

Hsia, T.-Y., Conover, T., Figliola, R. & Investigators, for the M. of C.H.A. (MOCHA). Computational modeling to support surgical decision making in single ventricle physiology. *Semin Thorac Cardiovasc Surg Pediatric Cardiac Surg Annu* **23**, 2–10 (2020).

Jolley, M., Colan, S.D., Rhodes, J. & DiNardo, J. Fontan physiology revisited. *Anesth Analg* **121**, 172–182 (2015).

Roche Rodriguez, M. & DiNardo, J.A. Biventricular repair as an alternative to single-ventricle palliation in a child with hypoplastic left heart structures: what the anesthesiologist should know. *J Cardiothorac Vasc Anesth* **36**(10), 3927–3938 (2022).

Salim, M.A., Case, C., Sade, R. *et al.* Pulmonary/systemic flow ratio in children after cavopulmonary anastomosis. *J Am Coll Cardiol* **25**, 735–738 (1995).

29

Hypoplastic Left Heart Syndrome

Introduction

Hypoplastic left heart syndrome (HLHS) occurs in approximately 1 in 10,000 live births, and is one of the more common complex congenital heart defects. About 40 years ago, comfort care was often the only option offered to parents but over the past few decades a staged surgical approach to repair/palliation of this lesion – the single-ventricle pathway (SVP) – has been developed. It usually involves a first stage repair within a few days after birth, either in form of a classic Norwood procedure with a modified Blalock-Thomas-Taussig shunt or the alternative, a right ventricle to pulmonary artery Sano shunt. Following Stage 1 repair, HLHS patients proceed to Stage 2 – the bidirectional Glenn at age 3–8 months followed by the completion of the single-ventricle palliation with the Fontan procedure at 2–5 years of age.

During the first years after introduction of the SVP, less than 30% of patients survived. However, as perioperative management – including anesthetic, surgical and postoperative care – improved, survival rates increased and many patients will now reach adolescence and adulthood. Studies have shown that the survival rate after Stage 1 increased from 68% in 2002 to more than 80% in 2009. In a subset of infants with mitral stenosis, aortic stenosis, and a suitable left ventricular volume and mass, a staged biventricular repair may be feasible.

Anatomy

Patients with HLHS have hypoplasia of all left-heart structures. (Figure 29.1). In the most severe form, mitral and aortic atresia with hypoplasia of the left atrium, left ventricle, ascending aorta, and aortic arch (including coarctation) are present. Distal aortic blood flow occurs via the patent ductus arteriosus (PDA). Proximal aortic blood flow and coronary blood flow occur by retrograde filling of a tiny ascending aorta via the PDA (Figure 29.2). This unique variation of single-ventricle physiology in HLHS patients puts them at increased risk for the development of myocardial ischemia.

Physiology

Hypoplastic left heart syndrome is ductal-dependent single-ventricle physiology lesion. These patients are staged to a Fontan procedure. HLHS is a complex shunt with complete obstruction to outflow. There is a communication (atrial septal defect [ASD] or patent foramen ovale [PFO]) and a complete or near-complete obstruction to left atrial outflow (mitral atresia or severe mitral stenosis) and left ventricular outflow (aortic atresia or severe aortic stenosis). This results in an obligatory left-to-right (L-R) shunt at the atrial level, with complete mixing of systemic and pulmonary venous blood in the right atrium and right

The Pediatric Cardiac Anesthesia Handbook, Second Edition. Viviane G. Nasr and James A. DiNardo.
© 2025 John Wiley & Sons Ltd. Published 2025 by John Wiley & Sons Ltd.

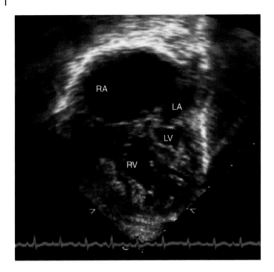

Figure 29.1 An apical four-chamber view of hypoplastic left heart syndrome (HLHS). The left-sided structures are small and incapable of contributing to systemic output. LA, left atrium; LV, left ventricle; RA, right atrium; RV, right ventricle.

atrium, pulmonary venous congestion, and pulmonary hypertension.

These patients need emergency decompression of the left atrium (pulmonary venous chamber) and medical stabilization prior to surgery. This usually requires transatrial stent placement in the cardiac catheterization laboratory because of the thickness of the intraatrial septum. The survival of these patients *in utero* is dependent on the presence of a levoatrial cardinal vein decompressing the left atrium to the systemic venous circulation.

Systemic blood flow is provided by a simple downstream shunt (PDA). The shunt at the level of the PDA is a dependent shunt with net systemic and pulmonary blood flow that is determined by the ratio of systemic to pulmonary vascular resistance. A low pulmonary vascular resistance (PVR) relative to systemic vascular resistance (SVR) will allow diastolic run-off of blood into the pulmonary circuit, compromising systemic perfusion. Flows to the ascending aorta, coronary arteries, and arch vessels are supplied entirely (aortic atresia) or almost entirely (severe mitral and

ventricle. When the ASD or foramen ovale is restrictive, there will be a large left atrial-to-right atrial pressure gradient. This will result in poor decompression of the left

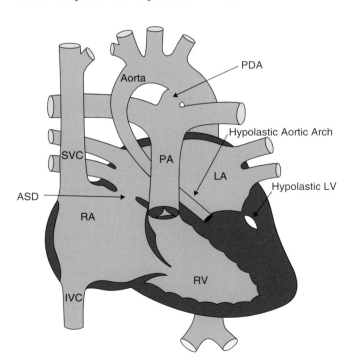

Figure 29.2 Anatomy of the hypoplastic left heart syndrome. There is severe mitral stenosis/atresia, hypoplasia of the ascending aorta and transverse aortic arch. Pulmonary and systemic blood flows are both delivered via the right ventricle. Aortic blood flow is provided via a large ductus arteriosus. There is antegrade flow from the patent ductus arteriosus (PDA) to the descending aorta, and retrograde flow to the proximal aortic arch and cerebral circulation. The coronaries are perfused retrograde via the tiny aorta.

aortic stenosis) retrograde from the PDA. Flow to the descending aorta is antegrade from the PDA. Closure of the PDA in infants with HLHS terminates coronary and systemic blood flow, and results in immediate cardio-vascular collapse. Prostaglandin E_1 therapy is life saving for these patients.

Surgical Therapy

Patients with HLHS are staged along the single-ventricle pathway to a Fontan proce-dure (see Figure 28.1). The initial procedure utilizing a modified Blalock–Thomas–Taussig shunt (mBTTS) is commonly referred to as a Norwood stage 1 (see Figure 28.3). The initial procedure utilizing a right ventricle to pulmonary artery conduit is commonly referred to as a modified Norwood stage 1 or Sano procedure. The surgical intervention must incorporate procedures to meet the objective necessary at each stage in the single-ventricle pathway.

- A Damus–Kaye–Stansel (DKS) anastomo-sis in conjunction with an aortic arch reconstruction/coarctation repair utilizing homograft or pericardial tissue is neces-sary to provide an unobstructed systemic ventricle-to-aortic connection.
- An atrial septectomy is performed to allow unobstructed delivery of pulmonary venous blood from the left atrium to the systemic right ventricle via the right atrium.
- A mBTTS (usually 3.5 mm Gore-Tex* con-duit) or right ventricle to pulmonary artery conduit (Sano shunt) is created to provide pulmonary blood flow.
- With a mBTTS, blood is distributed to the pulmonary circulation after it has entered the systemic arterial tree (from the innominate artery to the pulmonary artery), while with a Sano conduit, blood is distributed to the pulmonary circula-tion before it has entered the systemic arterial tree (from the right ventricle to the pulmonary artery, much like a double-outlet right ventricle). As a result,

for a given cardiac output and Q_P:Q_S, the pulse pressure is wider and the aortic diastolic blood pressure lower in patients with a mBTTS. The higher diastolic blood pressure obtained with the Sano shunt may provide better cerebral, coronary, and splanchnic perfusion.

- The Sano shunt requires the creation of a small right ventriculotomy. The right ven-tricle is the systemic ventricle, and the long-term functional consequences of this ventriculotomy are unknown.
- The Sano conduit is traditionally valveless, resulting in some pulmonary insufficiency. The volume load on the right ventricle is small and probably offset by the fact that Sano shunt patients have a slightly lower Q_P:Q_S and volume load than mBTTS patients. More recently, surgeons have been utilizing valved Sano shunts to mini-mize regurgitation. The proximal end of the conduit is a calibrated ringed Gore-Tex graft which is dunked into the RV while the distal end, inserted into the main pulmo-nary artery, is a piece of cryopreserved femoral vein with a valve.

Following Stage 1 repair, HLHS patients pro-ceed to what is often called Stage 2 – a supe-rior cavopulmonary connection (BDG or hemi-Fontan) – at the age of 3–6 months, and then on to the Fontan procedure at 1–2 years of age. Patients with a right ventricle to pulmonary artery conduit generally have their superior cavopulmonary connection at an earlier age than children with a mBTTS as they have a lower Q_P:Q_S and tend to "out-grow" their shunt sooner.

Anesthetic Management

Goals

Patients with HLHS have ductal-dependent systemic blood flow and are particularly vulnerable to myocardial ischemia because the coronary arteries are supplied retrograde from the PDA down a segment of hypoplastic ascending aorta (often 1–2 mm in diameter). These patients are managed according to the principles described in Table 28.2. Subsequent management for the superior cavopulmonary shunt and Fontan procedure is described in later portions of the section on the Management of Single-Ventricle Physiology.

Post-CPB Management

There are a few subtle differences in the management of patients with a mBTTS as opposed to a Sano right ventricle to pulmonary artery conduit in the initial postoperative period.

- In patients with a mBTTS, a high SVR tends to increase $Q_P:Q_S$, increase aortic diastolic run-off, and promote pulmonary overcirculation with compromise of systemic O_2 delivery.
- High SVR is less disadvantageous to a patient with a Sano right ventricle to pulmonary artery conduit because pulmonary blood flow is derived from the right ventricle prior to distribution to the arterial circulation, and because of the inherent high resistance through the long right ventricle to pulmonary artery conduit. In these patients, aggressive afterload reduction and a reduced right ventricular pressure may result in a low $Q_P:Q_S$ and hypoxemia.

Biventricular Repair

It is now well recognized that there is a wide spectrum of hypoplasia of left-heart structures inherent in the diagnosis of HLHS. Patients with mild left ventricular hypoplasia, mitral stenosis, and aortic stenosis are good candidates for a biventricular repair, while patients with severe left ventricular hypoplasia with aortic and mitral atresia continue to be managed with SVP, as described above. However, a subset of HLHS patients are described as having a "borderline" left ventricle; that is, a sufficient left ventricular volume

and adequate mitral and aortic valve function to be considered candidates for a staged approach to a biventricular repair.

The "Borderline" Left Heart

There is no strict definition of a "borderline" left heart. This designation is made based on data regarding left ventricle, mitral valve, and aortic valve size and function, and the extent of endocardial fibroelastosis (EFE) as delineated by magnetic resonance imaging (MRI), echocardiography, and cardiac catheterization. MRI is the preferred imaging modality to quantify EFE and left ventricular volumes in patients with borderline left-heart structures. The anatomic features defining borderline left heart include aortic and mitral valve stenosis, coarctation, small left ventricular cavity volume, globular or elongated and apex forming left ventricle, ventricular restriction caused by the presence of EFE, and Z scores for left-heart structures between −5 and −0.5.

The Left Heart Rehabilitation

Left heart rehabilitation consists of a variety of interventions to relieve inflow and/or outflow tract obstructions, either by catheter-based balloon dilation of the aortic valve or surgical repair of coarctation of the aorta and EFE resection. These interventions are based on the concept that the myocardium in infants and children can potentially grow. In fact, the growth potential of the left ventricle has been demonstrated in neonates. Balloon dilation of critical aortic stenosis in neonates with associated left ventricular hypoplasia is associated with near-normalization of left ventricular dimensions.

Staged Left Ventricular Recruitment

A "staged left ventricular recruitment" strategy is applied for patients at high risk of failure with primary biventricular repair. Persistent left atrial hypertension, pulmonary edema, and pulmonary hypertension may occur despite relief of anatomic obstructions in patients with EFE and impaired systolic and diastolic myocardial function.

Candidates for the staged left ventricular recruitment are patients with left ventricular Z scores between −5 and −0.5, and usually include those with unbalanced AV canal defects, variants of HLHS, and Shone complex.

This strategy is designed to improve blood flow and loading conditions for the left ventricle in an effort to stimulate flow- and load-mediated growth. The circulation is initially supported via the SVP with a Stage 1 procedure, followed by superior cavopulmonary anastomosis, while the left heart is rehabilitated.

Surgical techniques for rehabilitation of the left ventricle include: (i) endocardial fibroelastosis resection, which involves removal of the noncompliant, restrictive, membrane-like lining of the left ventricle by sharp dissection; (ii) mitral valvuloplasty; (iii) redistribution of the atrioventricular valve in an unbalanced canal; (iv) aortic valvuloplasty; (v) atrial septal defect restriction; and occasionally (vi) the creation of an additional source of pulmonary blood flow (aortopulmonary shunt, right ventricle-pulmonary artery conduit, or Super Glenn) in order to further augment left ventricular preload. Left-heart dimension Z-scores increase significantly over time after the left ventricular recruitment strategy, whereas they decline after traditional SVP.

Biventricular Conversion

The term "biventricular conversion" is used for patients who initially underwent SVP palliations and are later "surgically converted" to a biventricular circulation with the goal of avoiding the previously described long-term complications associated with SVP. Typical candidates are SVP patients with characteristics such as tricuspid regurgitation, right ventricular dysfunction, genetic syndromes, noncardiac comorbidities, and elevated PVR historically associated with poor outcomes. The biventricular conversion procedure following staged SVP and staged left ventricular recruitment includes: (i) takedown of the aortopulmonary anastomosis; (ii) reestablishment of separate left and right ventricles; and (iii) establishment of separate outflow tracts from the left and right ventricles.

Noncardiac Surgery

Stage I patients present for noncardiac surgeries including, but not limited to, laparoscopic gastrostomy, peripherally inserted central catheter (PICC) line or central venous line placement, imaging studies, or airway evaluations. Preoperative echocardiography is important for risk assessment. The presence of tricuspid (systemic atrioventricular valve) regurgitation, reduced right ventricular function, aortic arch obstruction, and stenosis of the right ventricle-pulmonary artery conduit or mBTTS all contribute to the risk of perioperative hemodynamic instability. The judicious use of inotropic support may be necessary to maintain systemic oxygen delivery. There should be a low threshold to employ invasive blood pressure monitoring. Laparoscopic procedures are increasingly being utilized, and it is important to recognize the effects of abdominal insufflation of CO_2 on both hemodynamics and the reliability of end-tidal CO_2 as a surrogate measure of $PaCO_2$

Extubation in the operating room is possible, but a postoperative intensive care unit bed should always be available in case postoperative ventilatory or hemodynamic support is necessary.

References and Further Reading

Davies, S.J., DiNardo, J.A., Emani, S.M. & Brown, M.L. A review of biventricular repair for the congenital cardiac anesthesiologist. *Semin Cardiothorac Vasc Anesthesia* **27**, 51–63 (2023).

Rodríguez, M.R. & DiNardo, J.A. Biventricular repair as an alternative to single ventricle palliation in the child with hypoplastic left heart structures: what the anesthesiologist should know. *J Cardiothorac Vasc Anesth* **36**, 3927–3938 (2022).

Zaleski, K.L., Valencia, E., Matte, G.S., Kaza, A.K. & Nasr, V.G. How we would treat our own hypoplastic left heart syndrome neonate for stage 1 surgery. *J Cardiothorac Vasc Anesth* **37**, 504–512 (2023).

30

Interrupted Aortic Arch

Introduction

Interrupted aortic arch (IAA) is a complete interruption of the aorta, and is a relatively rare disorder constituting approximately 1% of congenital heart lesions. Some 50% of patients with IAA have 22q11 microdeletions.

Anatomy

Interrupted aortic arch is classified into three types (A, B, and C) depending on the site of aortic interruption.

- *Type A*: the arch is interrupted distal to the left subclavian artery at the level of the aortic isthmus (similar to very severe coarctation). This type comprises 15% of IAAs (Figures 30.1 and 30.2).
- *Type B*: the arch is interrupted between the left common carotid and left subclavian arteries. The origin of the right subclavian artery is commonly aberrant, arising from the descending aorta distal to the interruption. This is the most common presentation of IAA and comprises 80% of all IAAs (Figures 30.3 and 30.4).
- *Type C*: the arch is interrupted between the innominate and the left common carotid artery. This is the least common presentation of IAA and comprises 5% of all IAAs (Figure 30.5).

In all cases the aorta distal to the interruption is supplied by the ductus arteriosus. In the setting of two ventricles, there is invariably a large conoventricular septal defect with posterior malalignment (deviation) of the conal septum. IAA is commonly associated with left ventricular outflow tract obstruction (LVOTO). This is due to combinations of hypoplasia of the aortic annulus and subaortic area, the posterior deviation of the conal septum into the LVOT, and the presence of a bicuspid aortic valve due to commissural fusion. It is possible that the increased risk of LVOTO in type B associated with an aberrant right subclavian artery occurs because of the increased antegrade blood flow that must pass through the ductus arteriosus during fetal development to supply the aberrant artery, resulting in less antegrade flow through the LVOT and ascending aorta, with subsequent hypoplasia. IAA can also occur in conjunction with single-ventricle lesions, truncus arteriosus, aortopulmonary window, and double-outlet right ventricle.

Physiology

Interrupted aortic arch is a ductal-dependent lesion, and is a complex shunt with complete obstruction to aortic outflow at the level of the interruption. A simple downstream shunt

The Pediatric Cardiac Anesthesia Handbook, Second Edition. Viviane G. Nasr and James A. DiNardo.
© 2025 John Wiley & Sons Ltd. Published 2025 by John Wiley & Sons Ltd.

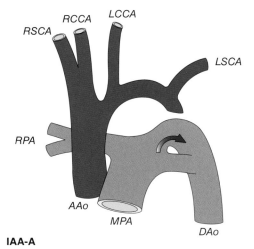

IAA-A

Figure 30.1 Type A interrupted aortic arch. The interruption is distal to the left subclavian artery (LSCA). The descending aorta (DAo) is supplied via the arterial duct. The ascending aorta (AAo) gives rise to all brachiocephalic arteries. LCCA, left common carotid artery; MPA, main pulmonary artery; RCCA, right common carotid artery; RPA, right pulmonary artery; RSCA, right subclavian artery. *Source:* Reproduced from Marek et al. (2009)/ with permission of John Wiley & Sons.

Figure 30.2 Type A interrupted left aortic arch distal to the left subclavian artery (LSA). The descendent aorta (DAO) is supplied via the arterial duct (arrow). AOA, aortic arch; LCAR, left carotid artery; LSA, left subclavian artery; PA, pulmonary trunk.

(patent ductus arteriosus; PDA) provides aortic flow distal to the interruption. Flow to the aorta proximal to the obstruction is supplied by the left ventricle. In addition, there is a simple shunt (ventricular septal defect; VSD) and there may be fixed obstruction due to LVOTO. There is a physiologic left-to-right (L-R) shunt at the level of the VSD. In the presence of significant LVOTO, there may be a compromise of proximal aortic perfusion due to a large L-R shunt. There is predominantly a physiologic right-to-left (R-L) shunt at the level of the PDA. As a result, there will be differential cyanosis with a lower SaO_2 in the lower body and arch vessels distal to the interruption than in the arch vessels proximal to the interruption. The oxygen saturation difference between right upper and lower extremities is described in Table 30.1.

The shunt at the level of the PDA is a dependent shunt with net systemic and pulmonary blood flow determined by the ratio of systemic to pulmonary vascular resistance (PVR). A low PVR relative to systemic vascular resistance (SVR) will allow diastolic run-off of blood into the pulmonary circuit (increased physiologic L-R shunting at the PDA). A unique feature of IAA is that the diastolic hypotension associated with diastolic run-off of blood into the pulmonary arteries occurs only in the aorta distal to the interruption. The diastolic blood pressure will be lower and the pulse pressure wider in the distal compared to the proximal aorta. Consequently, coronary perfusion is preserved while splanchnic perfusion is potentially compromised. Closure of the PDA in infants with IAA terminates the distal aortic flow, severely compromising splanchnic perfusion, and usually results in immediate cardiovascular collapse. Prostaglandin E_1 (PGE_1) therapy is life saving for these patients.

Surgical Management

The surgical repair is performed as a one-stage repair in the neonatal period via a median sternotomy. The repair involves direct arch reanastomosis, and augmentation of the arch

IAA-B

IAA-B + aberrant RSA

Figure 30.3 Type B interrupted aortic arch, in which the interruption is between the left carotid artery (LCCA) and left subclavian artery (LSCA). The descending aorta (DAo) and LSCA are supplied via the arterial duct (arrow) and brachiocephalic trunk (RCCA, RSCA), and the LCCA is supplied from the ascending aorta (AO). Also shown is a type B interruption with an aberrant RSCA with its origin off the descending aorta. LPA, left pulmonary artery; PA, pulmonary trunk; RCCA, right common carotid artery; RPA, right pulmonary artery; RSCA, right subclavian artery; PDA, patent ductus arteriosus. *Source:* Reproduced from Marek et al. (2009)/with permission of John Wiley & Sons.

Figure 30.4 Type B interrupted aortic arch. (A) 2D imaging from a leftward-oriented high right parasternal view. (B) Color Doppler flow indicates the flow within the left carotid (LCAR) and left subclavian arteries (LSA). Note the long-segment discontinuity (arrow) between the left carotid and left subclavian arteries (LSA). PDA, patent ductus arteriosus; RPA, right pulmonary artery.

with graft material is commonly necessary. In order to reduce tension on the arch anastomosis, it may be necessary to divide and ligate the left subclavian artery during the repair of type B lesions. In addition, it may be necessary to divide and ligate an aberrant right subclavian artery, if present, to reduce tension on the descending aortic portion of the anastomosis.

Arterial cannulation for cardiopulmonary bypass (CPB) must be modified to provide

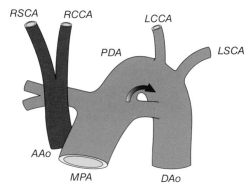

IAA-C

Figure 30.5 Type C interrupted aortic arch, in which the interruption is between the right common carotid artery (RCCA) and left common carotid artery (LCCA). The descending aorta (DAo), LCCA, and left subclavian artery (LSCA) are supplied by the arterial duct (arrow). The ascending aorta (AAo) supplies only the right subclavian artery (RSCA) and right carotid artery (RCCA). MPA, pulmonary trunk; PDA, patent ductus arteriosus. *Source:* Reproduced from Marek et al. (2009)/with permission of John Wiley & Sons.

Table 30.1 Anatomy and oxygen saturation in IAA.

Classification	Anatomy	Oxygen saturation
Type A	Isthmus: distal to the left subclavian artery	Both upper extremities (UE) > lower extremities (LE)
Type B	Distal arch: distal to the origin of the left common carotid artery	Right UE > left UE and LE
Type C	Proximal arch: proximal to the origin of the left common carotid artery	Right UE > left UE and LE

total body perfusion. Both the ascending aorta and pulmonary artery are cannulated and connected with a Y-connector to the arterial line of the CPB circuit. Tourniquets are then placed around the right and left pulmonary arteries, ensuring perfusion of the distal aorta via the ductus arteriosus. This allows total body perfusion and hypothermia to be achieved. The procedure can then be carried out under deep hypothermic circulatory arrest or with regional cerebral perfusion.

Additional intracardiac defects (VSD, ASD) are also repaired at the time of surgery. When LVOTO is severe, additional procedures are necessary in addition to IAA repair. One approach is to perform a Ross/Konno procedure (Ross procedure in conjunction with patch enlargement of the aortic annulus and LVOT in the area of the interventricular septum). Alternatively, a Yasui (Norwood/Rastelli) procedure can be performed. This approach involves closing the VSD by baffling it to the pulmonary annulus, performing a Damus–Kaye–Stansel anastomosis (proximal pulmonary artery to aorta), and recreating right ventricle to pulmonary artery continuity with a conduit.

Catheterization Laboratory Intervention

Hybrid palliation, utilizing either bilateral pulmonary artery banding or percutaneous placement of bilateral internal branch pulmonary artery flow restrictors in conjunction with ductus arteriosus stenting, is a palliative management option utilized in order to delay definitive surgical repair beyond the neonatal period.

Anesthetic Management

Goals

Maintain heart rate, contractility, and preload to maintain cardiac output.

- Continuation of PGE_1 therapy ($0.01–0.05$ µg kg^{-1} min^{-1}) to maintain ductal patency is necessary.
- A reduction in the PVR:SVR ratio should be avoided as this will increase pulmonary blood flow and compromise somatic oxygen delivery.
- Avoid increases in SVR.

Arterial monitoring sites must be chosen carefully. The right radial artery pressure will reflect distal aortic pressure in the presence of an aberrant right subclavian artery. If the left subclavian artery is divided and ligated during repair, a left radial arterial line will be of little use post repair. Ideally, the arterial line should be in the right arm. The surgeon may also request that a femoral arterial catheter be placed to assess the adequacy of the repair by way of comparison of proximal and distal blood pressures. At a minimum, a pulse oximeter probe and a non invasive blood pressure (NIBP) cuff should be applied to a lower extremity. A pulse oximeter probe should also be placed on the right hand. The use of cerebral near-infra-red spectroscopy (NIRS) may be helpful in assessing the adequacy of cerebral blood flow, while flank NIRS may be used to indirectly assess somatic blood flow.

Induction and Maintenance

Neonates and infants presenting for IAA repair are PGE_1 dependent with pulmonary congestion and potentially compromised distal perfusion. A technique using high-dose fentanyl in combination with a benzodiazepine, or a low inspired concentration of an inhalation agent is well tolerated by these patients.

Post-CPB Management

Determining whether there is a residual arch obstruction is a priority following the termination of CPB. This requires use of transesophageal or epicardial echocardiography and/or accurate simultaneous measurements of both upper and lower aortic blood pressures, obtained with either percutaneously or surgically placed catheters. A significant gradient may necessitate surgical revision. Bleeding from the arch suture lines may be significant. Residual LVOTO may produce left ventricular contractility/afterload mismatch. An elevated PVR due to left atrial hypertension, and reactive pulmonary vasoreactivity due to high $Q_P:Q_S$ preoperatively, may also result in right ventricular contractility/afterload mismatch. In addition, the long CPB and deep hypothermic circulatory arrest/regional cerebral perfusion times necessary to complete this procedure may further compromise left ventricular and right ventricular functions and produce myocardial edema.

Goals

Maintain heart rate (preferably sinus rhythm) at an age-appropriate value. Cardiac output is likely to be more heart rate dependent during the post-CPB period.

- Reduce PVR when necessary through ventilatory interventions.
- Inotropic support of the left and right ventricles may be necessary for the reasons addressed previously. Dopamine $5-10$ µg kg^{-1} min^{-1} or epinephrine $0.01-0.1$ µg kg^{-1} min^{-1} are useful in this instance because they provide potent inotropic support without increasing the PVR. Milrinone ($0.5-1.0$ µg kg^{-1} min^{-1}) should be considered for its PVR-reducing effect, recognizing that it has weak inotropic and lusitrophic properties and is a potent reducer of SVR.

References and Further Reading

Kanter, K.R. The Yasui operation. *Oper Techn Thorac Cardiovasc Surg* **15**, 206–222 (2010).

LaPar, D.J. & Baird, C.W. Surgical considerations in interrupted aortic arch. *Semin Cardiothorac Vasc Anesth* **22**, 278–284 (2018).

Marek, J., Fenton, M. & Khambadkone, S. Aortic arch anomalies: coarctation of the aorta and interrupted aortic arch. In: Lai, W.W., Mertens, L.L., Cohen, M.S. & Geva, T. (eds) *Echocardiography in Pediatric and Congenital Heart Disease: From Fetus to Adult*. John Wiley & Sons, Chichester (2009).

31

Vascular Rings

Introduction

A vascular ring is a rare disorder making up less than 1% of congenital cardiac lesions. It results from persistence or failure of regression of embryonic structures of the aortic arch during fetal development (see Chapter 1).

Anatomy

Vascular rings can be complete rings encircling both trachea and esophagus (e.g., double aortic arch and right aortic arch with a left ligamentum arteriosum), and incomplete rings that compress the trachea and esophagus (pulmonary artery sling and innominate artery compression syndrome) (Figures 31.1–31.6). There is increased recognition that acquired tracheobronchial malacia (TBM) occurs in the airway with normally developed cartilages as the result of extrinsic compression by vascular rings, pulmonary slings, or aberrant subclavian arteries. Multidetector computed tomography with contrast and direct, three-phase dynamic, rigid tracheobronchoscopy are the diagnostic techniques of choice in the evaluation of TBM. This combination of tests demonstrates the complex relationships of vascular and nonvascular structures (systemic, pulmonary arteries and veins, the heart, the tracheobronchial tree, and thorax), allowing a three-dimensional reconstruction and precise anatomic delineation.

The different types of vascular anomalies associated with airway compression are detailed in Table 31.1. It is important to be familiar with mirror-image branching of the aortic arch vessels as this term appears frequently in discussion of these lesions. A right aortic arch is characterized by the aortic arch coursing to the right of the trachea. Mirror-image branching of the aortic arch vessels occurs in conjunction with a right aortic arch and is characterized by the brachiocephalic trunk (innominate artery) giving rise to the left subclavian and left carotid arteries.

Physiology

Patients with vascular rings may present with wheezing, stridor, respiratory distress, aspiration, and cyanotic or apneic episodes. Patients with esophageal compression can present with dysphagia, feeding difficulties, and failure to thrive.

The association of cardiac defects and vascular tracheobronchial compression is important, since delayed diagnosis and treatment can significantly increase morbidity and mortality.

Surgical Management

The surgical approach to most vascular rings is via a left posterolateral thoracotomy. However, a right or left arch with a right ligamentum arteriosum will necessitate a

The Pediatric Cardiac Anesthesia Handbook, Second Edition. Viviane G. Nasr and James A. DiNardo.
© 2025 John Wiley & Sons Ltd. Published 2025 by John Wiley & Sons Ltd.

Figure 31.1 Double aortic arch. The ring encircling the trachea and esophagus comprises the right and left aortic arches and the ductal ligament.
Source: Reproduced from Powell (2016)/with permission of Springer Nature.

Figure 31.3 Right aortic arch with mirror-image branching and a left ductal ligament. The ring encircling the trachea and esophagus comprises the right aortic arch, retroesophageal ductal diverticulum, and left-sided ductal ligament.
Source: Reproduced from Powell (2016)/with permission of Springer Nature.

Figure 31.2 Right aortic arch with mirror-image branching and an aberrant origin of the left subclavian artery. The ring encircling the trachea and esophagus comprises the right aortic arch, base of the left subclavian artery (diverticulum of Kommerell), and the left-sided ductal ligament.
Source: Reproduced from Powell (2016)/with permission of Springer Nature.

right thoracotomy. A sternotomy is indicated when an intracardiac defect exists and cardiac surgical repair is planned. Surgical options for TBM include aortopexy and/or bronchopexy, tracheal resection and end-to-end anastomosis or slide tracheoplasty, and placement of either absorbable or permanent external splints and/or internal stents. In patients with a right aortic arch and an aberrant left subclavian artery, dilation of the descending aorta at the origin of an aberrant subclavian artery due to persistence of the dorsal fourth aortic arch (Kommeral diverticulum) may be present. Resection of the diverticulum and reimplantation of the left subclavian artery onto the left carotid may be necessary to avoid sacrificing the left subclavian artery. The recurrent laryngeal nerve (RLN) is at risk of injury during all vascular ring repairs.

Figure 31.4 Right aortic arch with mirror-image branching, left descending aorta, and left ductal ligament. The ring encircling the trachea and esophagus comprises the right aortic arch, retroesophageal right-sided dorsal aorta, and left-sided ductal ligament. Here, unlike the typical right aortic arch, where the aorta descends to the right of the spine for some distance before gradually crossing to the left of the spine at the level of the diaphragm, the descending aorta is positioned leftward within the thorax. *Source:* Reproduced from Powell (2016)/with permission of Springer Nature.

Catheterization Laboratory Intervention

Cardiac catheterization and angiography are rarely performed given the superior imaging capabilities of CT and MRI. A cardiac catheterization may be necessary to define associated intracardiac defects.

Anesthetic Management

Ventilation and securing the airway are critical. Therefore, it is important to understand the cause, degree, and location of airway compromise. Communication with the surgical team regarding the need for controlled versus spontaneous ventilation, the need for

Figure 31.5 Left aortic arch with normal branching, right descending aorta, and right ductal ligament. The ring encircling the trachea and esophagus comprises the left aortic arch, retroesophageal left-sided dorsal aorta, and right-sided ductal ligament. *Source:* Reproduced from Powell (2016)/ with permission of Springer Nature.

Figure 31.6 Left pulmonary artery sling. The left pulmonary artery arises aberrantly from the proximal right pulmonary artery and courses posterior to the trachea and anterior to the esophagus toward the left hilum. *Source:* Reproduced from Powell (2016)/with permission of Springer Nature.

preoperative bronchoscopy, and single-lung ventilation is a must. Optimal positioning of the endotracheal tube may require

Table 31.1 Classification of vascular anomalies associated with airway and/or esophageal compression. *Source:* Kussman et al. (2004)/with permission of John Wiley & Sons.

I) Double aortic arch
II) Right aortic arch
    Aberrant left subclavian artery with left ligamentum arteriosum
    Mirror-image branching with right (retroesophageal) ligamentum arteriosum
III) Left aortic arch
    Aberrant right subclavian artery with right ligamentum arteriosum
    Right descending aorta and right ligamentum arteriosum
    Aberrant right subclavian artery with left ligamentum arteriosum
IV) Anomalous innominate artery
V) Cervical aortic arch
VI) Pulmonary artery sling

---

bronchoscopy when tracheal narrowing is present. If intraoperative nerve moniting is to be used to prevent RLN injury, there must be a discussion regarding the use and timing of administration of neuromuscular blocking agents. In cases with significant airway narrowing, an induction technique that confirms the ability to ventilate with positive pressure without air trapping prior to administration of neuromuscular blocking agents may be prudent. In addition, the possibility that the otolaryngology team and rigid bronchoscopy may be needed to secure the airway should be considered.

The direct, three-phase dynamic, rigid tracheobronchoscopy procedure is summarized as follows.

- The first phase of the rigid bronchoscopy is performed with the patient taking spontaneous, shallow breaths, allowing for evaluation of static compression of the trachea and bronchi.
- In the second phase of bronchoscopy, vigorous breathing or coughing is initiated by stimulating the airway with a fine wire or small 3F ureteral catheter to assess maximum dynamic motion and collapse during expiration

- In the final phase of bronchoscopy, all secretions are removed and the airway is examined while the patient is deeply anesthetized and the airway distended to 40 cmH$_2$O (30 cmH$_2$O in neonates) to dilate the trachea. The airway is carefully evaluated for structure and anatomy, and the posterior membrane is evaluated for tracheal diverticulum.

It is important to remember that successful repair of the ring may not immediately relieve airway obstruction. Residual anatomic obstruction and dynamic obstruction related to tracheobronchial malacia may be observed immediately on extubation or postoperatively following surgical repair.

References and Further Reading

Choi, S., Lawlor, C., Rahbar, R. & Jennings, R. Diagnosis, classification, and management of pediatric tracheobronchomalacia. *JAMA Otolaryngol Head Neck Surg* **145**, 265–275 (2019).

Dodge-Khatami, A., Tulevski, I.I., Hitchcock, J.F., Mol, B.A.J.M. de & Bennink, G.B.W.E. Vascular rings and pulmonary arterial sling: from respiratory collapse to surgical cure, with emphasis on judicious imaging in the hi-tech era. *Cardiol Young* **12**, 96–104 (2002).

Kussman, B.D., Geva, T. & McGowan, F. Jr. Cardiovascular causes of airway compression. *Pediatr Anaesth* **14**, 60–74 (2004).

Powell, A.J. Vascular rings and slings. In: Lai, W.W., Mertens, L.L., Cohen, M.S. & Geva, T. (eds) *Echocardiography in Pediatric and Congenital Heart Disease: From Fetus to Adult*, 2nd edn. John Wiley & Sons, Chichester (2016).

Priya, S., Thomas, R., Nagpal, P., Sharma, A. & Steigner, M. Congenital anomalies of the aortic arch. *Cardiovasc Diagnosis Ther* **8**, S26–S44 (2017).

32

Tricuspid Atresia

Introduction

Tricuspid valve atresia is the third most common cyanotic heart lesion, with an estimated prevalence of 0.5–1.2 per 10,000 live births. There is no difference in the incidence based on gender.

Anatomy

In tricuspid atresia (TA), there is agenesis of the tricuspid valve and no communication between the right atrium and the hypoplastic right ventricle (Figure 32.1). The tricuspid valve is embryologically part of the right ventricle. Anatomic classification is based on the presence or absence of transposition of the great arteries (TGA), the extent of pulmonary stenosis or atresia, and the size of the ventricular septal defect (VSD) (Figure 32.2). This classification and the frequency of the different lesion types are summarized in Table 32.1. Approximately 70% of patients with TA are type 1 and 30% are type 2. Type 3 lesions are very rare. The most common lesion is type 1B (50%).

Physiology

Tricuspid atresia is single-ventricle physiology lesion, with patients staged to a Fontan procedure. TA is a complex shunt with complete obstruction to right ventricular inflow and variable obstruction to right ventricular outflow. There is a communication (atrial septal defect [ASD] or patent foramen ovale [PFO]) which results in an obligatory right-to-left (R-L) shunt at the atrial level, with complete mixing of systemic and pulmonary venous blood in the left atrium. When the ASD or foramen ovale is restrictive, there will be a large right atrial to left atrial pressure gradient. This will result in poor decompression of the right atrium and systemic venous congestion.

The quantities of pulmonary blood flow associated with each type of TA are summarized in Table 32.1.

Pulmonary blood flow can be provided by a downstream shunt from one or both of the following sources.

- *Intracardiac*: the pathways are described in Table 32.1. This downstream shunt may be simple (VSD without pulmonary stenosis), complex (VSD with pulmonary stenosis), or complex with complete obstruction (pulmonary atresia with or without a VSD).
- *Extracardiac*: this is generally a patent ductus arteriosus (PDA) but in older patients, major aortopulmonary collateral arteries (MAPCAs) may have developed. When pulmonary atresia exists (types 1A and 2A), these simple shunts are the sole source of pulmonary blood flow.

In single-ventricle lesions, the degree of cyanosis will be determined largely by $Q_P:Q_S$. Therefore, patients with a Qp:Qs <1 due to stenotic or atretic pulmonary outflow tracts, restrictive VSDs, or both, will be more

The Pediatric Cardiac Anesthesia Handbook, Second Edition. Viviane G. Nasr and James A. DiNardo.
© 2025 John Wiley & Sons Ltd. Published 2025 by John Wiley & Sons Ltd.

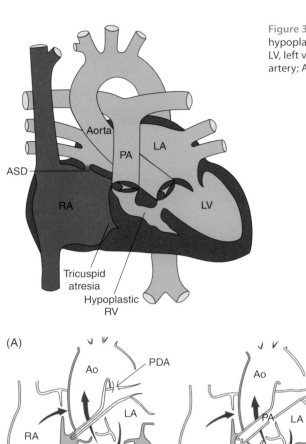

Figure 32.1 Tricuspid atresia, atrial septal defect, and hypoplastic right ventricle. RA, right atria; LA, left atria; LV, left ventricle; RV, right ventricle; PA, pulmonary artery; ASD, atrial septal defect.

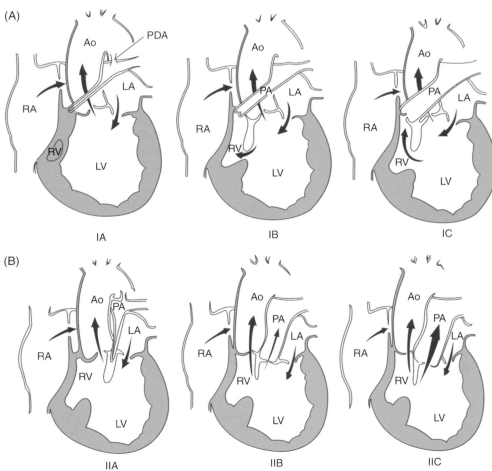

Figure 32.2 Classification of tricuspid atresia. (A) Type 1: tricuspid atresia without transposition of the great vessels. (B) Tricuspid atresia with dextro-transposition of the great vessels. RA, right atria; LA, left atria; PDA, patent ductus arteriosus; LV, left ventricle; RV, right ventricle; Ao, aorta; PA, pulmonary artery.

Table 32.1 Classification of tricuspid atresia and sources of aortic and pulmonary blood flows.

Type of tricuspid atresia	Frequency (%)	Pulmonary blood flow (amount)	Aortic blood flow pathway	Pulmonary blood flow pathway
Type 1	**70**			
1A: TA, NRGA, PA	10	Decreased	LV	PDA, MAPCAs
1B: TA, NRGA, restrictive VSD, PS	50	Decreased	LV	LV through VSD to RV
1C: TA, NRGA, nonrestrictive VSD, no PS	10	No change or increased	LV	LV through VSD to RV
Type 2	**30**			
2A: TA, D-TGA, nonrestrictive VSD, PA	2	Decreased	LV through VSD to RV	PDA, MAPCAs
2B: TA, D-TGA, nonrestrictive VSD, PS	8	No change or decreased	LV through VSD to RV	LV
2C: TA, D-TGA, restrictive VSD, no PS	20	Increased	LV through VSD to RV	LV
Type 3	**<1**			
3A: TA, D-loop ventricles, L-TGA, subpulmonic stenosis		Decreased	LV	LV through VSD to RV
3B: TA, L-loop ventricles, L-MGA, subaortic stenosis		Increased	LV through VSD to RV	LV

TA, tricuspid atresia; NRGA, normally related great arteries; PA, pulmonary atresia; LV, left ventricle; PDA, patent ductus arteriosus; MAPCAs, major aortopulmonary collaterals; VSD, ventricular septal defect; RV, right ventricle; PS, pulmonary stenosis; TGA, transposition of the great arteries; MGA, malposition of the great arteries.

cyanotic than their counterparts with normal or increased pulmonary blood flow. TA imposes a volume load on the left ventricle, and increased pulmonary blood flow produces an even larger left ventricular volume load (Figure 32.3). Therefore, patients with TA and increased pulmonary blood flow are likely to present with congestive heart failure (CHF). Furthermore, patients with increased pulmonary blood flow are at risk of developing pulmonary artery hypertension (PAH).

Surgical Therapy

More than 70% of neonates with TA have ductal-dependent pulmonary blood flow and require a modified Blalock–Thomas–Taussig shunt (mBTTS) in association with PDA ligation. This can often be done off cardiopulmonary bypass (CPB) through a median sternotomy. In the small subset of patients with increased pulmonary blood flow, the initial procedure will be placement of a pulmonary artery band to control pulmonary blood flow. In either instance, following initial repair, TA patients proceed to a superior cavopulmonary connection or bidirectional Glenn at the age of 3–6 months, and then to the Fontan procedure at 2–3 years of age.

Anesthetic Management

Goals

These patients are initially managed according to the principles of single-ventricle physiology, preinitial repair (see Chapter 28).

$$\frac{(98)\ (0.85)+(65)\ (1)}{1.85}=80$$

$Q_p:Q_s = 0.85:1$

$Q_p:Q_s = 0.85:1$

$Q_{peff} = 1.5\,l.min^{-1}.m^{-2}$

$Q_{L \to R} = 1.3\,l.min^{-1}.m^{-2}$

$Q_p = 2.8\,l.min^{-1}.m^{-2}$

$Q_{seff} = 1.5\,l.min^{-1}.m^{-2}$

$Q_{R \to L} = 1.8\,l.min^{-1}.m^{-2}$

$Q_s = 3.3\,l.min^{-1}.m^{-2}$

Figure 32.3 Depiction of saturations and blood flows in tricuspid atresia type 1B with a mildly restrictive VSD and mild pulmonary stenosis. Effective flows are shown as solid lines and shunted flows are shown as dotted lines.

Subsequent management is similar to the management of the superior cavopulmonary shunt and Fontan procedure.

References and Further Reading

Matitiau, A., Geva, T., Colan, S. *et al.* Bulboventricular foramen size in infants with double-inlet left ventricle or tricuspid atresia with transposed great arteries: influence on initial palliative operation and rate of growth. *J Am Coll Cardiol* **19**, 142–148 (1992).

Sumal, A.S., Kyriacou, H. & Mostafa, A.M.H.A.M. Tricuspid atresia: where are we now? *J Cardiac Surg* **35**, 1609–1617 (2020).

33

Heart Transplantation

The natural history of end-stage cardiac dysfunction is not well delineated in infants and children, in part because of the heterogeneity of the various congenital lesions. In addition, end-stage cardiac dysfunction may be difficult to define with clinical criteria. Growth failure secondary to severe cardiac dysfunction is useful in identifying end-stage disease. Nonetheless, heart failure (HF) is classified in children as summarized in Table 33.1.

Cardiomyopathy (CM) and complex congenital heart disease (CHD) represent the two major indications for orthotopic heart transplantation (OHT) in pediatric patients. CM is subclassified as dilated cardiomyopathy (DCM), restrictive cardiomyopathy (RCM), and hypertrophic cardiomyopathy (HCM). Specific indications for OHT are summarized in Table 33.2.

Contraindications to OHT are listed in Table 33.3.

Among patients aged less than one year, 53% of transplants are performed in children with CHD, with the vast majority (80%) of those procedures performed in children with single-ventricle anatomy. In patients aged between one and five years, the indications for heart transplantation are almost divided equally between CHD (42%) and CM (53%). Most children requiring transplantation for congenital lesions in this age group have had at least one previous cardiac surgical procedure. In patients aged between six and 10 years, the indications for OHT are more likely due to CM (56%) than to CHD (36%). In patients aged between 11 and 17 years, the primary indication (66%) for OHT is CM.

The Donor

The following guidelines are used to select donors after the diagnosis of irreversible brain death has been made. Echocardiographic assessment of donor ventricular and valvular function is routine. The final decision of whether to accept a donor heart is made by the harvesting surgeon following visual inspection of the heart and an overall assessment of donor suitability and hemodynamic stability. Important points include the following.

- No active infection or malignancy with the possibility of metastases.
- ABO compatibility and human lymphocyte antigen (HLA) screening. The donor and recipient must be ABO blood type compatible. HLA typing for cardiac transplantation is not routine. The recipient's blood is tested against a standard panel of blood cells containing a diverse human lymphocyte sample. This screen is called the panel reactive antibody (PRA) screen. If the PRA has 5–15% reactivity, most centers will proceed with transplantation based on ABO compatibility. If the PRA is greater than 15%, then a lymphocyte cross-match between donor

The Pediatric Cardiac Anesthesia Handbook, Second Edition. Viviane G. Nasr and James A. DiNardo.
© 2025 John Wiley & Sons Ltd. Published 2025 by John Wiley & Sons Ltd.

Table 33.1 Heart failure in children.

Stage	Interpretation
A	Patients with increased risk of developing HF, but who have normal cardiac function and no evidence of cardiac chamber volume overload. Examples: previous exposure to cardiotoxic agents, family history of heritable cardiomyopathy, univentricular heart, congenitally corrected transposition of the great arteries
B	Patients with abnormal cardiac morphology or cardiac function, with no symptoms of HF, past or present. Examples: aortic insufficiency with left ventricular enlargement, history of anthracycline with decreased left ventricular systolic function
C	Patients with underlying structural or functional heart disease, and past or current symptoms of HF
D	Patients with end-stage HF requiring continuous infusion of intropic agents, mechanical circulatory support, cardiac transplantation or hospice care

HF, heart failure.

Table 33.2 Indications for orthotopic heart transplantation.

Class I

- Stage D heart failure associated with systemic ventricular dysfunction in pediatric patients with cardiomyopathies or previously repaired/palliated CHD.
- Stage C heart failure associated with severe limitation of exercise and activity. If measurable, such patients would have a peak maximum oxygen consumption <50% predicted for age and sex.
- Stage C heart failure associated with systemic ventricular dysfunction in patients with cardiomyopathies or previously repaired/palliated CHD when heart failure is associated with significant growth failure attributable to the heart disease.
- Stage C heart failure in pediatric heart disease with associated near sudden death and/or life-threatening arrhythmias untreatable with medications or an implantable defibrillator.
- Stage C heart failure in pediatric restrictive cardiomyopathy disease associated with reactive pulmonary hypertension.

Class IIA

- Stage C heart failure in pediatric heart disease associated with reactive pulmonary hypertension and a potential risk of developing fixed, irreversible elevation of pulmonary vascular resistance that could preclude orthotopic heart transplantation in the future.
- Certain anatomic and physiologic conditions likely to worsen the natural history of CHD in infant patients with a functional single ventricle, which can lead to use of heart transplantation as primary therapy, including: (i) severe stenosis (stenoses) or atresia in proximal coronary arteries; (ii) moderate to severe stenosis and/or insufficiency of the atrioventricular valve and/or systemic semilunar valve(s); and (iii) severe ventricular dysfunction.
- Several anatomic and physiologic conditions likely to worsen the natural history of previously repaired or palliated CHD in pediatric patients with stage C heart failure that may lead to consideration for heart transplantation without severe systemic ventricular dysfunction, including: (i) pulmonary hypertension and a potential risk of developing fixed, irreversible elevation of pulmonary vascular resistance that could preclude orthotopic heart transplantation in the future; (ii) severe aortic or systemic atrioventricular valve insufficiency that is not considered amenable to surgical correction; (iii) severe arterial oxygen desaturation (cyanosis) that is not considered amenable to surgical correction; and (iv) persistent protein-losing enteropathy despite optimal medical/surgical therapy.

CHD, congenital heart disease; AV, atrioventricular.

Table 33.3 Contraindications to recipient selection for heart transplantation.

Absolute contraindications
- History of emotional instability, medical noncompliance, or active substance abuse.
- Fixed pulmonary hypertension >5 Wood units m^{-2} (for cardiac transplantation, not for lung or heart–lung transplantation).
- Significant cerebral vascular disease.
- Active malignancy or life-limiting coexistent disease.

Relative contraindications
- Significant peripheral vascular disease.
- Active peptic ulcer or diverticular disease.
- Severe bronchitis or chronic obstructive pulmonary disease (for cardiac transplantation, not for lung or heart–lung transplantation).
- Disease likely to recur in allograft (cardiac amyloidosis or sarcoidosis).
- Irreversible hepatic or renal disease (may be considered for combined cardiac and renal or hepatic transplantation).
- Immunological sensitization to donor antigens.
- Severe osteoporosis.
- Morbid obesity.
- Active infection.
- Diabetes mellitus with end organ dysfunction.

Table 33.4 ABO matching for ABO incompatible OHT.

ABO of heart recipient	ABO of donor heart	ABO of transfused blood products		
		Plasma	Red cells	Platelets
O	AB	AB	O	AB
O	B	AB or B	O	AB or B
O	A	AB or A	O	AB or A
B	AB	AB	O or B	AB
B	A	AB	O or B	AB
A	AB	AB	O or A	AB
A	B	AB	O or A	AB

and recipient blood can be performed. This is a time-consuming process, as donor blood must be transported to the transplant center. Pre- and post-transplant therapy with intravenous IgG or plasmapheresis may be indicated. Recently, some success with ABO-incompatible transplants has been achieved in infants due to the immaturity of infant ABO isohemagglutinins (Table 33.4).

Recipient donor size match. For older children, the donor's body weight should be within 60–150% of the recipient's weight, whereas for infants and small children the donor's weight should be between 80% and 160% of the recipient's body weight. Hearts transplanted into infants and children demonstrate normal cardiac chamber dimensional growth. Most centers prefer donors at the upper limits of size for their patients with pulmonary hypertension, although data to support this practice are lacking.

Anesthetic Management of the Recipient

Preoperative Evaluation

Cardiac transplant patients typically undergo extensive medical evaluation. A summary of this evaluation is readily available to the anesthesiologist through the transplant coordinator. The use of an antifibrinolytic should be considered for patients at risk for perioperative bleeding. Additional considerations include ventricular arrhythmias, thromboembolic phenomena, preoperative mechanical ventricular support and the artificial heart, and previous cardiac surgical procedures. All patients who have undergone previous cardiac surgical procedures are likely to have prolonged dissection times and are at risk for bleeding. Adequate intravenous access is a necessity.

At present, the limiting factor in the number of patients who can be offered a heart transplant is the availability of donor hearts. In the United States, approximately 20% of suitable pediatric transplant candidates die before a donor heart can be found. As a result, mechanical assist devices are increasingly used as a bridge to cardiac transplantation until suitable donor hearts are found.

Physical Examination

A physical examination should include an evaluation of the limitations to vascular access and monitoring sites imposed by previous surgery and catheterizations. A child who has undergone a palliative shunt procedure may have a diminished pulse or an unobtainable blood pressure in the arm in which the subclavian artery has been incorporated into the shunt. Children who have undergone multiple palliative procedures may have poor peripheral venous access, and previous surgical cut-down sites may exist. Children having multiple cardiac catheterizations may have absent or compromised femoral arterial and venous access. Such findings have obvious implications regarding arterial and venous catheter placement, noninvasive blood pressure monitoring, the use of pulse oximetry, and the mode of induction.

Premedication

Most patients will have been called into the hospital at short notice and many will have eaten solid food in the previous 6–8 hours. Premedication with midazolam 0.03–0.05 mg kg^{-1} in divided doses works well to reduce anxiety. In older children with previous multiple opioid and benzodiazepine exposures, intravenous ketamine in doses of 0.5–1.0 mg kg^{-1} may also be necessary. In children without intravenous access, oral premedication will probably be necessary. Supplemental oxygen should be administered, because hypoxemia will exacerbate existing pulmonary hypertension.

Preinduction

Some transplant patients will be receiving intravenous inotropic and vasodilator therapy when they arrive for surgery. These agents should be continued via a reliable intravenous route. Sterility is of the utmost importance because the patients will be immunosuppressed. All patients should have two large-bore peripheral intravenous lines. Placement of a central large-bore venous sheath for use as a reliable site of rapid fluid administration is warranted if peripheral access is poor. Electrocardiogram (ECG) monitoring should allow assessment of V5, I, II, III, aVR, aVL, and aVF. Normally, two leads (II and V5) are monitored simultaneously intraoperatively.

A radial artery catheter is placed after induction in infants and children. Patient size or the presence of complex intracardiac anatomy generally precludes the placement of a pulmonary artery catheter (PAC) in infants and children. Pulmonary artery pressures are monitored post cardiopulmonary bypass (CPB) with a surgically placed transthoracic PAC if needed. The disadvantages of PAC as they apply to cardiac transplant patients are as follows.

- Technical difficulties in advancing the catheter in patients with a dilated right ventricle and a low cardiac output.
- An increased risk of atrial and ventricular ectopy leading to hemodynamic compromise.
- An increased risk of infection.
- The catheter must be withdrawn into the sterile sheath during excision of the recipient's heart.
- The catheter must be readvanced across new suture lines into the donor heart as CPB is terminated.

Transesophageal echocardiography (TEE) is utilized to manage patients before and after CPB. After transplantation, TEE is used to assess left and right ventricular function, to measure pulmonary artery pressures (using a tricuspid regurgitation jet), and to guide the management of pulmonary artery hypertension and right ventricular dysfunction if necessary.

Induction and Maintenance

The patient's underlying physiology must be appreciated such that an appropriate anesthetic plan can be formulated. In patients with CHD, the individual chapters on each lesion will provide guidance. Patients with CM must be managed with an understanding of the physiologic constraints associated with DCM, RCM, and HCM (Table 33.5).

There is no single best approach to the induction or maintenance of anesthesia. It is important to keep the hemodynamic goals in mind and to titrate the anesthetic agents accordingly. The circulation time will be slow given the low cardiac output state in many of these patients. These patients require an induction that will blunt the hemodynamic response to laryngoscopy and tracheal intubation without undue myocardial depression, vasodilation, and hypotension. Careful titration of etomidate $0.1–0.3$ mg kg^{-1} in combination with $5–10$ µg kg^{-1} of fentanyl is useful for induction. A full 0.3 mg kg^{-1} dose of etomidate is rarely necessary to induce hypnosis and loss of consciousness. This drug combination has minimal direct effect on heart rate, myocardial contractility, peripheral vascular resistance, or venous capacitance. An overall diminution in central sympathetic tone will also contribute to circulatory depression. Rocuronium 1.0 mg kg^{-1} or succinylcholine $1–2$ mg kg^{-1} can be used to perform a modified rapid sequence induction (cricoid pressure during positive pressure ventilation) in the patient with questionable nil-by-mouth (NPO) status.

Anesthesia can be maintained with additional doses of opioid in conjunction with a benzodiazepine (usually midazolam in increments of 0.01 to 0.03 mg kg^{-1}), or a low inhaled concentration ($0.5–0.75$ MAC) of isoflurane or sevoflurane. N$_2$O is not a good choice as an adjuvant agent; it has a weak myocardial depressant effect that normally is counteracted by the sympathetic outflow it produces. In patients with DCM, where elevated catecholamine levels, downregulated beta-receptors, and reduced myocardial norepinephrine stores are present, the myocardial depressant effects will predominate.

In the instance of a child without intravenous access, a careful inhalation induction with 100% O$_2$ and no more than 4% sevoflurane following a heavy oral medication (ketamine $7–10$ mg kg^{-1} and midazolam 1 mg kg^{-1}) can be considered. Once intravenous access is obtained, anesthesia can be maintained as described above. An alternative for induction and maintenance in infants and children with intravenous access is a

Table 33.5 Pathophysiology characteristics of cardiomyopathies.

	Dilated cardiomyopathy (ischemic and nonischemic)	Hypertrophic cardiomyopathy (obstructive and nonobstructive)	Restrictive cardiomyopathy
Diastolic function and atrial transport function	• Biventricular diastolic dysfunction • Reduced biventricular compliance • Biatrial enlargement • Increased atrial pressures	• LV diastolic dysfunction • Reduced LV compliance • Left atrial enlargement • Increased left atrial pressure	• Severe biventricular diastolic dysfunction • Severely reduced biventricular compliance • Biatrial enlargement • Increased atrial pressures
Ventricular systolic function	• Decreased biventricular contractility; usually limited to LV in ischemic form • Exhausted preload reserve • Afterload mismatch	• Preserved or hyperdynamic LV contractility • Normal RV contractility	• Preserved biventricular contractility
Pulmonary vasculature	• Elevated LAP initially leads to passive elevation of PAP • Chronic elevation of LAP leads to reversible then irreversible elevation of PVR	• Elevated LAP initially leads to passive elevation of PAP • Chronic elevation of LAP leads to reversible then irreversible elevation of PVR	• Elevated LAP initially leads to passive elevation of PAP • Chronic elevation of LAP leads to reversible then irreversible elevation of PVR
Effect of preload alterations on hemodynamics	• Exhausted preload reserve; little or no ability to recruit SV with preload augmentation	• Retained preload reserve but reduced LV compliance results in elevated LAP with preload augmentation • In obstructive form reduced LV volumes will worsen obstruction	• Baseline LV and RV EDV are low • Severely reduced biventricular compliance results in markedly elevated atrial pressures with minimal preload augmentation
Effect of heart rate alterations on hemodynamics	• Avoid bradycardia; fixed SV due to exhausted preload reserve • Tachycardia unlikely to reduce LV filling but subendocardial perfusion may be compromised in ischemic form	• Avoid tachycardia; with retained preload reserve, LV filling will be compromised, subendocardial perfusion may be compromised • Bradycardia is well tolerated	• Avoid bradycardia; fixed SV due to severely reduced LV compliance • Tachycardia may reduce LV filling resulting in reduced SV
Effect of afterload alterations on hemodynamics	• Avoid increases in SVR; large reduction in SV will occur due to reduced contractility • SVR reduction is mainstay of medical management	• Avoid decreases in SVR particularly in obstructive form; reduced LVESV will worsen obstruction • Increases in SVR well tolerated	• Avoid decreases in SVR; with fixed SV, hypotension will result • Increases in SVR well tolerated

EDV, end-diastolic volume; LAP, left atrial pressure; LV, left ventricle; LVESV, left ventricular end-systolic volume; PAP, pulmonary artery pressure; PVR, pulmonary vascular resistance; SV, stroke volume; SVR, systemic vascular resistance; RV, right ventricle.

high-dose opioid technique (fentanyl 50–75 µg kg^{-1} or sufentanil 5–7.5 µg kg^{-1}) in conjunction with a benzodiazepine (usually midazolam), or a low inhaled concentration of isoflurane or sevoflurane and rocuronium. Caution must be exercised when benzodiazepines are used in conjunction with synthetic opioids, as they are synergistic in their effects on venous capacitance and systemic vascular resistance (SVR). This technique is a good choice in infants and children as postoperative ventilation for at least 24 hours is usually necessary.

Regardless of the choice of induction and maintenance agent, episodes of hemodynamic compromise must be treated promptly. Atropine should be used cautiously. Atropine administration may initiate tachycardia, and unlike beta-1-adrenergic agents, it increases the heart rate without any reduction in the duration of systole. Therefore, for equal increases in heart rate, atropine will cause a greater reduction in the duration of diastole and will compromise subendocardial perfusion to a greater degree than a beta-1-adrenergic agent. Ephedrine (a direct- and indirect-acting beta- and alpha-agonist) dosed at 0.03–0.07 mg kg^{-1} is a reliable agent to increase heart rate without compromising diastole. In addition, the augmentation in diastolic blood pressure obtained is beneficial when hypotension accompanies bradycardia.

Tachycardia is detrimental for patients with ischemic DCM and those with HCM; it should be treated to avoid subendocardial ischemia and hemodynamic compromise. The first strategy should be to terminate noxious stimuli and then increase the depth of anesthesia as necessary. The use of a short- or long-acting beta-blocker is not recommended considering the presence of severely depressed systolic function. If hypotension due to reduced SVR occurs, small doses of phenylephrine (0.5–1.5 µg kg^{-1}) and volume infusion (5 ml kg^{-1}) to increase preload to preinduction levels will usually correct the problem. Phenylephrine reliably increases the SVR. Caution must be exercised when alpha-adrenergic agonists are administered to patients with severe systolic dysfunction such as those with DCM. The goal should be to normalize SVR. An overzealous use of phenylephrine will increase afterload, induce afterload mismatch, and severely reduce stroke volume (SV). If the patient fails to respond with a prompt increase in aortic blood pressure, an inotropic agent should be started to avoid a downward spiral of ventricular dilation, increased wall stress, reduced SV, and further hypotension. Dopamine 3–5 µg kg^{-1} min^{-1} is a reasonable choice.

Operative Procedure

Three surgical techniques exist for OHT: the biatrial technique; the bicaval technique; and the total technique (Figures 33.1–33.3). These procedures are performed through a median sternotomy with hypothermic CPB, bicaval cannulation, and aortic cross-clamping.

After commencement of CPB using the biatrial technique, the recipient's heart is excised to just above the atrioventricular groove, leaving a large cuff of the left atrium containing all four pulmonary veins, a large cuff of the right atrium containing the superior vena cava (SVC) and inferior vena cava (IVC), the ascending aorta just distal to the aortic valve, and the main pulmonary artery just distal to the pulmonic valve. The donor left and right atria are anastomosed to the cuffs of the recipient left and right atria, while the donor and recipient aorta and pulmonary artery are anastomosed. This technique creates large atrial cavities with abnormal geometry. This results in a less than optimal contribution of atrial systole to ventricular filling. In addition, the distorted anatomy contributes to the development of functional mitral and tricuspid regurgitation. It is also associated with the development of atrial septal aneurysms, atrial thrombus, and sinus node injury.

(A)

(A)

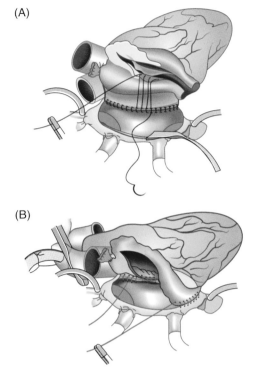

(B)

(B)

Figure 33.2 (A) The left atrial anastomosis is complete and the new intraatrial septum is being completed. (B) The right atrial anastomosis is being completed using a portion of the donor IVC. *Source:* Reproduced from DiNardo and Zvara, D.A. (2008)/with permission of John Wiley & Sons.

Figure 33.1 Operative technique for biatrial orthotopic heart transplantation. (A) The recipient heart has been excised, leaving a cuff of right atrium containing the superior vena cava (SVC) and inferior vena cava (IVC), and a cuff of left atrium containing all four pulmonary veins. The beginning of the left atrial anastomosis is depicted. The sinoatrial (SA) node of the donor heart is depicted by the dashed oval in the right atrium. The donor SVC is ligated. (B) Details of the anastomosis between the recipient and donor left atria. *Source:* Reproduced from DiNardo and Zvara, D.A. (2008)/with permission of John Wiley & Sons.

These problems have led to the application of more anatomic bicaval and total techniques. Currently, the bicaval technique is the most common technique used. These techniques result in better atrial function, a lower incidence of early and late atrial arrhythmias, and less tricuspid regurgitation. Whether they will result in long-term freedom from pacemaker implantation and better cardiac function remains to be determined.

In the bicaval technique, the recipient's atria are completely excised, leaving the SVC, the IVC, and a small cuff of left atrium containing all four pulmonary veins. In the total technique, the recipient's atria are completely excised, leaving the SVC, the IVC, and two small cuffs of the left atrium – one containing the two right pulmonary veins and the other the two left pulmonary veins. In the bicaval technique, there are five anastomoses: the donor SVC, IVC, and posterior left atrium are anastomosed to the recipient SVC, IVC, and one pulmonary vein cuff, while the donor

Figure 33.3 Details of the completed aortic and pulmonary artery anastomoses. The aortic cannula and cross-clamp are depicted. In an effort to reduce the ischemic interval, the surgeon may release the aortic cross-clamp after completion of the atrial and aortic suture lines and complete the pulmonary artery anastomosis while the heart is being reperfused. *Source:* Reproduced from DiNardo and Zvara, D.A. (2008)/with permission of John Wiley & Sons.

and recipient aorta and pulmonary artery are anastomosed. In the total technique, there are six anastomoses: the donor SVC, IVC, and posterior left atrium are anastomosed to the recipient SVC, IVC, and two pulmonary vein cuffs, while the donor and recipient aorta and pulmonary artery are anastomosed.

For children with congenital heart lesions, the technical aspects of the surgical procedure are more challenging. These patients may require extensive aortic, pulmonary artery, and caval reconstructions to create anatomically unobstructed connections to the donor heart.

Post-CPB Management

Goals

- Maintain sinus rhythm at 100–120 bpm in older children and 130–150 bpm in neonates and infants. Atrial or atrioventricular sequential pacing may be required.

- Avoid pulmonary artery hypertension by treating hypercarbia, hypoxemia, and acidosis.
- Aggressively treat pulmonary artery hypertension with vasodilator therapy to avoid right ventricular failure. If right ventricular failure does occur, inotropic support of the right ventricle and pulmonary vasodilation may be necessary.
- Maintain right and left atrial pressures to optimize SV in the setting of increased ventricular stiffness.
- Inotropic support of the left ventricle may be necessary if the ischemic interval is long.

Preparation for Termination of CPB

The following issues need to be considered when formulating a plan for the termination of CPB in a patient with a newly transplanted heart.

Impaired Systolic Function

Systolic dysfunction in the donor heart may occur for a variety of reasons.

- *Ischemia–reperfusion injury*: this is the most common cause of allograft systolic dysfunction post CPB. Preservation of the donor heart involves application of the aortic cross-clamp and delivery of cold cardioplegia to induce arrest in diastole, followed by cold storage at 4 °C. The ischemic interval – the time from when the aortic cross-clamp is applied in the donor until the aortic cross-clamp is removed after implantation of the heart in the recipient – is extremely important. The longer this ischemic interval, the more likely there is to be biventricular systolic dysfunction secondary to myocardial fibrosis. Because there is an incremental increase in mortality with ischemic times more than 3.5 hours, it is desirable to keep the interval to less than four hours. In an effort to reduce the ischemic interval, the surgeon may release the aortic cross-clamp after completion of the atrial and aortic suture lines and complete the pulmonary artery anastomosis while the heart is being reperfused. Prolonged and excessive inotropic support of the donor heart before cross-clamping also is undesirable because it contributes to post-transplant ischemic dysfunction.

- *Brain death*: abrupt increases in intracranial pressure as the source of brain death result in a greater degree of myocardial ischemia and necrosis (particularly of the right ventricle) than gradual increases in intracranial pressure. There is evidence that early survival following heart transplantation is reduced in patients receiving hearts from donors dying of gunshot wounds to the head and from donors dying from spontaneous intracranial hemorrhage. Donors who experience brain death as the result of a sudden rise in intracranial pressure exhibit a hyperdynamic cardiovascular response, massive increases in plasma epinephrine, and histologic evidence of severe myocardial ischemia and necrosis.
- *Hyperacute rejection*: this rare event is caused by ABO blood group incompatibility or cytotoxic recipient antibodies directed against donor lymphocytes. It presents as cyanosis and mottling of the allograft, in conjunction with profoundly impaired systolic function. It is impossible to separate these patients from CPB for any extended period of time. The only therapy available is excision of the allograft with placement of a total artificial heart. This type of rejection is preventable by careful donor and recipient ABO typing and PRA screening.
- *Myocardial contusion*: patients with severe myocardial contusions are excluded as donors. Patients with lesser degrees of dysfunction from blunt trauma may exhibit impaired systolic function in the post-CPB period.

Right Ventricular Afterload Mismatch

Impaired right ventricular performance is a particular risk in the presence of recipient pulmonary hypertension. Right ventricular afterload mismatch may occur as the result of severely depressed right ventricular systolic function and normal pulmonary artery pressure (PAP) and pulmonary vascular resistance (PVR) or, more commonly, as the result of less severely depressed right ventricular systolic function and elevated PAP and PVR. This may result in acute allograft right ventricular dysfunction severe enough to prevent the termination of CPB. Therapy in this setting will need to be directed towards inotropic support of the right ventricle and selective reduction of PVR. Fontan patients receiving OHT are at particular risk of right ventricular afterload mismatch because chronic pulsatile flow deprivation in the pulmonary bed leads to impaired endothelial function and NO release, reduced vascular recruitment, and impaired lung growth, all of which serve to elevate PVR. Patients late after the Fontan procedure have elevated basal PVR and exhibit a decrease in PVR with exogenous inhaled NO.

Sinus and Atrioventricular Node Dysfunction

Ischemic injury to the sinus node and atrioventricular node may produce bradycardia, nodal rhythm, or heart block. Sinoatrial node dysfunction is much more common, and approximately 10–20% of patients need permanent atrial pacing. In some instances, an appropriate sinus rate can be obtained with isoproterenol. In other instances, atrial or atrioventricular sequential pacing is necessary.

Impaired Diastolic Function

The postischemic state of the transplanted heart is characterized by increased ventricular stiffness and limited preload reserve, resulting in a fixed stroke volume. Increases in heart rate obtained with pacing will reduce diastolic filling time. This, in turn, will produce reductions in end-diastolic volume (EDV) and SV for a given end-systolic volume (ESV). The net result will be little or no change in cardiac output. Atrial or atrioventricular sequential pacing is likely to be superior to ventricular pacing due to the presence of an appropriately timed atrial systole. For a given right or left atrial pressure, atrial pacing or atrioventricular sequential pacing will provide a higher ventricular EDV than ventricular pacing.

Inotropic support is useful for patients with limited preload reserve in both sinus and paced rhythms because the SV can be augmented at a given afterload by reducing ESV. Inotropic agents allow SV to be maintained as the heart rate increases, thereby producing increases in cardiac output. This occurs because the reductions in EDV produced by reduced diastolic filling time are offset by the reductions in ESV produced by enhanced contractility. The optimal heart rate is 100–110 bpm for older children, whereas 130–150 bpm is optimal for neonates and infants. Higher heart rates result in progressive reductions in SV such that cardiac output remains constant, or falls.

Termination of CPB

Particular attention must be paid to de-airing the heart. Severe ventricular dysfunction may follow the ejection of air down the coronary arteries. The right ventricle is particularly at risk because of the anterior location of the right coronary ostia. TEE is valuable in guiding the de-airing process.

A dose of methylprednisolone (usually 10 mg kg^{-1}) will be given after aortic cross-clamp removal. In some institutions, the dose will be given after termination of CPB.

The need for additional inotropic support can be determined with either TEE or a PAC. TEE will reveal ventricular dilation and global hypokinesis. The advantage of the PAC is that it allows the measurement of PAP and calculation of PVR and SVR. PAP can be estimated with TEE using a tricuspid regurgitation jet and the central venous pressure (CVP) measurement.

Epinephrine 0.05–0.3 µg kg^{-1} min^{-1} (children) or dopamine 5–10 µg kg^{-1} min^{-1} are used as inotropic support if needed.

When right ventricular afterload mismatch exists with preserved left ventricular systolic function, there will be a low cardiac output, low systemic blood pressure, elevated CVP, elevated PAP, and low pulmonary artery occlusion pressure (PAOP). TEE will reveal a dilated right atrium and ventricle with an underfilled, hyperkinetic left ventricle. Tricuspid regurgitation will be likely.

Therapy for right ventricular failure involves inotropic support and pulmonary vasodilation. Pulmonary vasodilation with intravenous agents is problematic because a simultaneous reduction of SVR occurs. The use of the inhaled selective pulmonary vasodilator nitric oxide (NO) has revolutionized treatment of pulmonary hypertension and associated right ventricular afterload mismatch. Aerosolized, inhaled prostacyclin (PGI$_2$) has a similar profile to that of inhaled NO. These agents are selective for the pulmonary circulation as no substantial concentrations are delivered to the systemic circulation following inhalation. NO delivered at 20 ppm selectively reduces PVR in all heart transplant recipients. Evidence suggests that the peak effect in reducing PVR with NO occurs at 20–40 ppm. Continuous aerosolized PGI$_2$ is delivered at 5–50 ng kg^{-1} min^{-1}.

In addition to pharmacologic methods, efforts to reduce PVR with ventilatory interventions are essential. A combination of a high inspired FiO$_2$, an arterial PaO2 >60 mmHg, an arterial PaCO$_2$ of 30–35 mmHg, a pH of 7.50–7.60, and low inspiratory pressures without high levels of positive end-expiratory pressure (PEEP) will produce reliable reductions in PVR.

Finally, it is important to rule out two mechanical causes of increased impedance to right ventricular ejection.

- When right ventricular dysfunction exists in the presence of low pulmonary artery pressures, mechanical obstruction of the pulmonary artery anastomosis due to kinking must be ruled out. Kinking may be observed directly by the surgeon or it may be detected using TEE. It also is diagnosed readily by the direct measurement of a pressure gradient between the right ventricle and pulmonary artery.

- Mechanical obstruction of one or more of the pulmonary vein anastomoses can produce pulmonary hypertension which will be unresponsive to pulmonary vasodilator therapy. Echocardiography – either transesophageal or epicardial – is the best modality to rule out this possibility.

When univentricular or biventricular failure is severe and refractory to inotropic and vasodilator agents, a ventricular assist or circulatory assist device may be necessary to support circulation until the ventricles can recover.

Noncardiac Surgery in the Postcardiac Transplant Patient

The success of heart transplantation makes it likely that anesthesiologists will encounter patients with transplanted hearts for a variety of noncardiac surgical procedures.

Physiology of the Transplanted Heart

Autonomic Nervous System

Regardless of the surgical technique used, the orthotopically transplanted heart is devoid of sympathetic and parasympathetic innervation. The most important consequence of this is an altered baroreceptor response.

In the transplanted heart, no direct sympathetic stimulation of the heart is possible. Response to activation of baroreceptors in the patient with a transplanted heart is dependent on the generation of circulating catecholamines for inotropic and chronotropic response. It normally takes several minutes to generate appropriate levels of circulating catecholamines. Although systemic catecholamine generation in response to arterial hypotension is enhanced, reflex systemic catecholamine release in response to reduced atrial and ventricular volumes is impaired due to atrial and ventricular vagal deafferentation. As a result, abrupt decreases in blood pressure will not be compensated for quickly.

The response of baroreceptors to endogenous and exogenous vasopressors in heart transplant patients is normal, but feedback to the donor heart is absent. Therefore, increases in blood pressure will be accompanied by a reflex decrease in recipient atrial rate, but not in donor atrial rate. As a result, there will be no reflex decrease in the transplanted heart rate in response to phenylephrine- or norepinephrine-induced hypertension. Likewise, Valsalva or other vagal maneuvers will not elicit a heart rate response.

Early in exercise, increases in cardiac output are acquired by increases in SV, with EDV increasing and ESV unchanged. As exercise progresses, cardiac output increases as the result of systemic catecholamine-induced increases in heart rate with maintenance of SV. Cardiac denervation produces presynaptic supersensitivity due to denervation-associated loss of neuronal catecholamine uptake. As a result, there is an increased sensitivity to catecholamines that are taken up by adrenergic nerve terminals (epinephrine, norepinephrine) with no increase in sensitivity to catecholamines that are not taken up (isoproterenol).

Some degree of reinnervation of the left ventricle with efferent sympathetic fibers is present in 80% of transplant patients three years after transplantation. Reinnervation seems to be progressive but is likely not complete until 15 years after transplantation. Patients with reinnervation have improved heart rate and contractile response to exercise, and better exercise tolerance than patients without reinnervation. The ability of some transplant patients to experience angina is consistent with reinnervation with sympathetic afferents. Reinnervation of cardiac vagal afferents is unlikely, however. There is some evidence that over time the recipient (old) atrioventricular node may affect the donor (new) atrioventricular node via conduction over the suture line. In summary, sympathetic efferent and afferent reinnervation may occur in some patients during the years after cardiac transplantation. When reinnervation occurs, it has physiologic importance.

Heart Rate

The resting atrial rate of the transplanted human heart is approximately 90–110 bpm. This is significantly greater than the resting atrial rate of the innervated human heart, and demonstrates that the predominant effect on sinus rate in humans is a slowing effect of the parasympathetic system. The heart rate increase with exercise in heart transplant patients is achieved through the stimulation of cardiac beta-2-receptors by circulating catecholamines. The increase in heart rate does not occur until after several minutes of exercise, and it parallels the increase in serum catecholamines. Despite this, the heart rate response with exercise in transplanted hearts is attenuated relative to that seen in normal hearts due to the lack of efferent innervation of the sinoatrial node.

Left Ventricular Systolic Function

The left ventricle of the transplanted heart exhibits normal contractile function. The left ventricular EDV (LVEDV) and left ventricular ESV (LVESV) are reduced, whereas the SV and ejection fraction remain normal or low normal due to the parallel reductions in EDV and ESV. The left ventricular mass is increased due to concentric hypertrophy as the result of the arterial hypertension, which can accompany calcineurin inhibitor immunosuppression.

Right Ventricular Systolic Function

The right ventricle exhibits normal systolic function. The right ventricular EDV (RVEDV) and right ventricular ESV (RVESV)

are larger than normal, and right ventricular wall thickness is increased. This will be exacerbated in the presence of persistent tricuspid regurgitation. In patients with preoperative pulmonary hypertension, the persistence of right ventricular dilation and tricuspid regurgitation is the result of remodeling of the donor right ventricle in response to recipient pulmonary circulation. The dilation and tricuspid regurgitation may persist despite the resolution of pulmonary hypertension.

Atrial Function

Following the biatrial technique, both right and left atrial areas are larger than normal. These patients have reduced right and left atrial emptying compared with normal subjects; the portion of total atrial emptying contributed by the recipient atrium is much less than that contributed by the donor atrium. In addition, the asynchronous contraction of donor and recipient atria results in wide variations in diastolic flow. Following the bicaval technique, patients have right atrial emptying comparable to that of normal subjects. Left atrial emptying, although reduced compared with normal subjects, is superior to that seen in biatrial technique patients. In addition, the left and right dimensions are smaller in patients with the bicaval or total technique as compared with the biatrial technique.

Diastolic Function

Left ventricular diastolic dysfunction occurs immediately after orthotopic cardiac replacement, and is related to the postischemic state. This dysfunction is characterized by a restrictive ventricular filling pattern that improves during the first several months after transplantation. This restrictive pattern may manifest clinically as a reduced preload reserve in response to exercise and afterload increases. The etiology of this continued dysfunction is unclear. It may be inherent to the small allograft LVEDV. Whether patients who receive hearts from donors smaller than themselves may be at particular risk for reduced preload reserve is debatable. Rejection episodes are known to impair diastolic function, but it is unclear whether recurring rejection episodes produce progressive left ventricular and right ventricular diastolic dysfunction in the form of a restrictive/constrictive pattern.

There is also a deficient acceleration of left ventricular relaxation during exercise which, along with restrictive inflow, contributes to the elevations in LVEDP and left atrial pressure seen during exercise. This impairment of relaxation may be caused by a loss of adrenergic tone due to denervation, ischemic injury at the time of harvest, or immunosuppression-induced arterial hypertension.

Issues Unique to Heart Transplant Patients

Cardiac transplant patients have a unique set of management issues, in addition to those associated with the denervated heart. These are outlined as follows.

Cardiac Allograft Vasculopathy (CAV)

This is currently the late survival-limiting factor after heart transplantation. In children, it accounts for 40% of the deaths between three and five years after transplantation. The incidence of CAV in pediatric cardiac transplant patients is approximately 10% per year post transplant, with an incidence of approximately 50% at five years.

The pathogenesis of cardiac allograft vasculopathy is complex, multifactorial, and incompletely understood. It is believed that immunologic mechanisms (number of HLA mismatches and the number and duration of rejection episodes), in conjunction with nonimmunologic risk factors (cytomegalovirus [CMV] seropositivity, hyperlipidemia, hypertension, older age at transplantation, diabetes) produce endothelial injury with subsequent myointimal hyperplasia. Unlike atherosclerotic coronary artery disease (CAD), CAV is associated with concentric, diffuse lesions that do not disrupt the elastic lamina and that progress rapidly. Focal, traditional atherosclerotic plaques also are seen in cardiac allografts.

Surveillance for CAV is difficult. Patients with heart transplants may not experience angina or typical ECG changes with myocardial ischemia and infarction due to afferent sympathetic denervation. Noninvasive testing has poor sensitivity and specificity. Intravascular ultrasound (IVUS) is the "gold standard" for the detection of CAV but it is technically demanding, expensive, and limited by the size of the catheter to investigation of vessels of 1 mm in diameter or more. Considering these limitations, transplant centers currently use yearly coronary angiography as a screen for CAV. More frequent angiograms may be indicated to monitor progression in individual patients.

Therapeutic options are limited. More invasive approaches involve angioplasty and coronary stent placement. With this approach, short-term morbidity and success are similar to those seen in atherosclerotic disease, but the restenosis rate is high and long-term prognosis remains poor. Drug-eluting stents may prove to be more effective in the long term. Finally, in the most severe cases, coronary artery bypass surgery and retransplantation have been used. The diffuse nature of the coronary lesions makes bypass surgery an option only in selected cases. The survival rates for retransplantation are significantly less than for initial transplantation, and the incidence of malignancy is twice that of first transplants.

Hypertension

Arterial hypertension is present in 75% of transplant patients at long-term follow-up. This is not related to the conventional risk factors associated with hypertension, but rather to immunosuppression-mediated increases in SVR and the denervation of cardiac volume receptors. Immunosuppression with calcineurin inhibitors (particularly cyclosporine versus tacrolimus) and corticosteroids is implicated. Therapy is necessary to prevent severe left ventricular hypertrophy and impaired ventricular function. This usually requires treatment with multiple classes of antihypertensive agents. Calcium entry blockers, angiotensin-converting enzyme (ACE) inhibitors, or angiotensin II receptor blockers (ARB) often are used as first-line therapeutic agents.

Atrial and Ventricular Arrhythmias

The incidence of atrial and ventricular arrhythmias during initial hospitalization after transplantation is 55% and 79%, respectively. At late follow-up, the incidence of atrial and ventricular arrhythmias is 40%. In general, atrial arrhythmias during the initial hospitalization are benign, except for atrial fibrillation. The development of atrial fibrillation is associated with a threefold increase in the risk of death. The risk of death is particularly high in patients who develop atrial fibrillation more than two weeks after transplantation.

Permanent atrial pacing is required in approximately 10–20% of pediatric recipients with both symptomatic and asymptomatic bradycardia. The development of bradycardia seems to be related to a longer ischemic interval for the donor heart.

Subacute Bacterial Endocarditis (SBE) Prophylaxis

Bacterial endocarditis is a rare complication in heart transplant patients. Nonetheless, because of the extent of the suture lines and the immunosuppressed status of the patient, SBE prophylaxis is recommended by the American Heart Association (AHA).

Rejection

Most patients have at least one acute rejection episode, despite adequate immunosuppression. These episodes usually occur within the first three months after transplantation, with decreasing incidence thereafter. Surveillance during the first year is accomplished with endomyocardial biopsies of the right ventricle via the right internal jugular vein every week for the first 4–8 weeks. Some centers do not perform biopsies in children aged less than six months or less than 5 kg in weight, unless it is to confirm suspected rejection. Biopsies are graded from 0 to 4 based on histologic criteria. No rejection is 0 R, mild rejection is 1 R, moderate rejection is 2 R, severe rejection is 3 R, and very severe rejection is 4 R. After the first year, an annual biopsy is performed in most institutions in conjunction with coronary angiography to evaluate CAV. If clinical evidence of rejection exists, more frequent biopsies may be indicated to document rejection and assess regression of histologic changes with treatment.

Mild rejection frequently resolves spontaneously and is not treated. Mild rejection by biopsy usually is not associated with clinical evidence of allograft dysfunction such as hypotension, elevated jugular venous pressure, rales, sinus rate >110, atrial fibrillation, bradycardia, or systolic dysfunction by echocardiography. Moderate or more severe rejection is accompanied by evidence of allograft dysfunction, and is treated. Although normal allografts have maintained a coronary vasodilator reserve, moderate allograft rejection is associated with an impaired reserve. Normal reserve returns after treatment of rejection. Rejection also is accompanied by an attenuated coronary vasodilatory response to nitroglycerin.

First-line therapy for moderate rejection is oral or intravenous pulsed steroids. In the approximately 10% of cases in which mild rejection by biopsy is associated with allograft dysfunction, pulsed steroid therapy is necessary. Severe rejection is usually treated with steroids and a lympholytic agent such as polyclonal antithymocyte globulin (ATG) or murine monoclonal antibody (OKT3). Immunosuppressive agents are listed in Table 33.6 and their complications that may require operative intervention are listed in Table 33.7.

Table 33.6 Immunosuppressive agents.

Agent	Classification	Mechanism of action	Clinical use
Prednisone Methylprednisolone	Corticosteroid	Nonspecific blockade of T-cell cytokine and cytokine receptor production	Maintenance therapy Treatment of rejection
Cyclosporine	Calcineurin inhibitor	NFAT (nuclear factor)-mediated inhibition of IL-2 promoter gene	Maintenance therapy
Tacrolimus (FK506)	Calcineurin inhibitor	NFAT (nuclear factor)-mediated inhibition of IL-2 promoter gene	Maintenance therapy
Azathioprine	Antimetabolite, 6-mercatopurine derivative	Inhibitor of T-cell proliferation	Adjuvant therapy
Mycophenolate mofentil (MMF)	Inhibitor of *de novo* purine synthesis	Inhibitor of T-cell proliferation	Adjuvant therapy in lieu of azathioprine
Sirolimus	Antiproliferative agent (rapamycin inhibitor)	Blocks G1 to S phase of the cell cycle; inhibitor of T-cell proliferation	Adjuvant therapy in lieu of azathioprine or MMF
Everolimus	Antiproliferative agent (rapamycin inhibitor)	Blocks G1 to S phase of the cell cycle; inhibitor of T-cell proliferation	Adjuvant therapy in lieu of azathioprine or MMF
OKT3	Monoclonal antibody	Antibody to T-cell receptor complex (native and activated T cells)	Induction therapy
Basiliximab	Monoclonal antibody	Antibody to IL-2 receptor (activated T cells)	Induction therapy
Daclizumab	Monoclonal antibody	Antibody to IL-2 receptor (activated T cells)	Induction therapy
Rabbit antithymocyte gamma-globulin (RATG)	Polyclonal antibody	Antibody to T cells (native and activated T cells)	Induction therapy

Table 33.7 Complications of immunosuppression that may require operative intervention.

- Gingival hyperplasia – cyclosporine
- Pancreatitis – azathioprine, corticosteroids
- Cholelithiasis and cholecystitis – cyclosporine
- Malignancies
- Complications of corticosteroid use: cataracts, retinal detachment, aseptic bone necrosis, perforated viscus, and gastrointestinal hemorrhage
- Complications of infection

Response to Drugs

The response to various drugs is altered in heart transplant patients secondary to the denervated state of the allograft.

- *Digoxin*: digoxin prolongs AV node conduction in a biphasic manner. The initial effect is mediated vagally and is absent in the transplanted heart. The chronic effect is mediated directly and is present in the transplanted heart. The inotropic properties also are directly mediated and present.
- *Muscarinic antagonists*: atropine, glycopyrrolate, and scopolamine produce competitive inhibition of acetylcholine at the muscarinic receptors of postganglionic cholinergic nerves such as the vagus. As a result, these drugs will not increase heart rate in the denervated transplanted heart. The effects of these drugs on other organs with muscarinic cholinergic innervation will remain.

- *Acetylcholinesterase inhibitors*: the contention that agents such as neostigmine and edrophonium have no cardiac effects while they continue to have systemic muscarinic effects has been challenged recently. Bradycardia after administration of neostigmine, which is reversed with atropine, has been demonstrated in heart transplant patients. In addition, sinus arrest after the administration of neostigmine and glycopyrrolate for reversal of neuromuscular blockade reversal has been reported in heart transplant patients. Neostigmine produces direct stimulation of cholinergic receptors on cardiac ganglion cells with subsequent release of acetylcholine. In addition, there is allograft denervation hypersensitivity of both the postganglionic neurons and the muscarinic myocardial receptors. Parasympathetic reinnervation of the donor heart may also play a role. These factors, combined with intrinsic allograft sinoatrial (SA) node dysfunction, may produce severe SA node dysfunction or sinus arrest after acetylcholinesterase inhibitor administration in heart transplant patients. This discussion has become largely academic given the ready availability of sugammadex to reverse neuromuscular blockade from steroidal nondepolarizing neuromuscular blocking drugs rocuronium and vecuronium.
- *Beta-adrenergic agonists*: there is increased sensitivity to catecholamines that are taken up by adrenergic nerve terminals (epinephrine, norepinephrine) with no increase in sensitivity to catecholamines that are not taken up (isoproterenol). Improvements in systolic function with beta-adrenergic agents are obtainable during acute rejection episodes.
- *Beta-adrenergic antagonists*: these agents retain their usual activity. The sinus rate of both the donor and recipient slow equally, demonstrating that the predominant effect is caused by the blockade of circulating catecholamines. There also will be a normal increase in the refractoriness of the AV node.
- *Calcium-entry blockers*: these agents directly suppress the sinus and AV nodes and thus should have normal activity. Nonetheless, the negative chronotropic and dromotropic effects of verapamil have been demonstrated to be more pronounced in the transplanted heart. There will be no reflex tachycardia from agents with strong vasodilator properties such as nifedipine.
- *Vagolytic and vagotonic agents*: drugs with vagolytic activity (pancuronium, pethidine) will not increase heart rate, whereas drugs with vagotonic activity (fentanyl, sufentanil) will not decrease heart rate.
- *Adenosine*: the magnitude and duration of adenosine's negative chronotropic and dromotropic effects is three- to fivefold greater in the transplanted heart.
- *Ephedrine*: cardiac drugs that are both direct-acting and indirect-acting will have a diminished effect because only the direct effect will be present.

Anesthetic Considerations for Noncardiac Surgery in Patients Post Heart Transplantation

A variety of regional and general anesthetic techniques have been used safely and successfully in the anesthetic management of patients with heart transplants. In patients without evidence of allograft dysfunction, the following principles are useful.

- Aseptic technique is essential.
- Appreciate that compensation for acute alterations in preload, afterload, and contractility is incomplete and delayed; postural effects are magnified.
- Heart rate and blood pressure increases due to inadequate anesthesia will be delayed until circulating catecholamine levels increase.
- Bradycardia will compromise cardiac output. Baseline stroke volume is reduced and any reflex increase in stroke volume in response to bradycardia is delayed. Atropine will not increase heart rate. Isoproterenol and ephedrine will increase heart rate.

- Acetylcholinesterase inhibitors (neostigmine, edrophonium) for reversal of neuromuscular blockade may have cardiac effects. Anticholinergic agents (atropine, glycopyrrolate) must be given to block the peripheral muscarinic effects.
- The right internal jugular vein is typically used for access to perform endomyocardial biopsies. This should be taken in consideration when there is an indication for central venous pressure monitoring
- Reflex bradycardia will not accompany administration of vasopressor agents (phenylephrine), nor will directly induced bradycardia accompany administration of agents with vagotonic activity.
- Reflex tachycardia will not accompany administration of vasodilator agents (sodium nitroprusside, nifedipine, hydralazine), nor will directly induced tachycardia accompany administration of agents with vagolytic activity.
- Stress-dose steroid coverage should be considered for patients receiving steroids as part of their immunosuppression.

References and Further Reading

DiNardo, J.A. & Zvara, D.A. *Anesthesia for Cardiac Surgery*, 3rd edn. Blackwell, Massachusetts (2008).

Velleca, A., Shullo, M., Dhital, K. *et al*. The International Society for Heart and Lung Transplantation (ISHLT) guidelines for the care of heart transplant recipients. *J Heart Lung Transplant* **42**, e1–e141 (2023).

34

Heart–Lung and Lung Transplantation

Introduction

Heart–lung transplantation (HLT) can be considered for patients with end-stage cardiopulmonary disease that is unresponsive to maximal medical therapy and for which no surgical options exist except combined heart–lung replacement. Increasingly, in an effort to make maximum use of donated organs, double-lung transplantation (DLT) and single-lung transplantation (SLT) are being used for patients with pulmonary disease without secondary severe cardiac dysfunction. According to the Registry of International Heart and Lung Society data, the number of pediatric heart–lung transplants peaked in 1989 (at approximately 60) and has continued to decline to approximately 10 per year worldwide as the result of the increased use of DLT and SLT.

There were a total of 2323 pediatric (recipients aged <18 years) lung transplants (LTX) worldwide reported to the Registry of the International Heart and Lung Transplant Society from 1992 to 2018. During the most recent era from January 2010 to June 2018, 907 pediatric LTX procedures were recorded worldwide. The indications for LTX are age dependent. Historically, the majority (approx. 70%) of LTX were performed in older children aged 11–17 years for cystic fibrosis (CF). The frequency of LTX for CF has dramatically diminished since the introduction of novel cystic fibrosis transmembrane conductance

regulator (CFTR) modulator drugs that improve the production, intracellular processing, and function of the defective CFTR protein that causes CF. In fact, the last year to record over 30 pediatric CF-related LTX worldwide was 2013. In the age group of 1–5 years, idiopathic pulmonary arterial hypertension (IPAH) is the leading diagnosis. In infants, surfactant B deficiency, congenital heart disease, and IPAH remain the three most frequent indications. In 2020, IPAH surpassed CF as the main indication for pediatric lung transplantation in the United States. In children with CHD, the primary indication for LTX is Eisenmenger-associated severe PH. Typically these patients undergo combined concurrent intracardiac repair of CHD in association with LTX.

Contraindications for heart–lung transplant are listed in Chapter 33.

Single-lung Transplantation

Single-lung transplantation (SLT) can be considered for patients with end-stage lung disease without significant cardiac dysfunction. Generally, patients with a left ventricular ejection fraction (LVEF) >35% and a right ventricular ejection fraction (RVEF) >25% are considered candidates. SLT is used much less frequently in children than in adults, and is used for patients with Eisenmenger syndrome in conjunction with the repair of intracardiac lesions.

The Pediatric Cardiac Anesthesia Handbook, Second Edition. Viviane G. Nasr and James A. DiNardo.

Double-lung Transplantation

Double-lung transplantation (DLT) is also considered for patients with end-stage pulmonary disease without significant cardiac dysfunction. Two approaches to DLT exist, namely bilateral sequential single-lung transplantation (BSSLT) and *en bloc* DLT. Patients with LVEF >35% and RVEF >25% are suitable candidates. The trend has been to reserve DLT for patients in whom SLT is not an option.

Living Donor Lobar Lung Transplant

In the subset of patients deemed too ill to survive long enough to receive a cadaveric SLT or BSSLT, this somewhat controversial procedure can be considered. It requires two donors: one donor provides the right lower lobe and the other donor the left lower lobe. The recipient's native lungs are excised. The majority of these transplants (85%) are in patients with CF. In these patients, their small stature allows two lobes from ordinary-size donors to provide adequate lung tissue.

Absolute contraindications to lung transplant include severe scoliosis or thoracic cage deformity; irreversible, significant respiratory muscle dysfunction; numerous transpleural systemic to pulmonary artery collateral vessels; severe tracheomegaly or tracheomalacia; and *Burkholderia cepecia* genovar-3 lower respiratory tract infection in CF patients.

The Donor

Only 5–20% of all solid organ donors are suitable lung donors. Potential lungs are rejected because of blunt thoracic trauma, the potential of aspiration during resuscitation, overaggressive fluid resuscitation, and neurogenic pulmonary edema. The guidelines used to select donors for lung transplantation are summarized below.

- Age younger than 65 years.
- Adequate gas exchange. The donor should have a PaO_2 >250 mmHg on $FiO_2 = 1.0$ and PEEP = 5 cmH_2O, or PaO_2 >100 mmHg on $FiO_2 = 0.4$ and PEEP = 5 cmH_2O. Pulmonary compliance should be normal, with static pressure <20 mmHg and peak pressure <30 mmHg at a tidal volume of 15 ml kg^{-1}.
- Normal bronchoscopic examination.
- Normal serial chest radiographs.
- No history of pulmonary disease. A smoking history is acceptable at some centers.
- Donor recipient size match. Some programs compare donor and recipient lung size using chest radiography measurements. A growing practice is to compare the donor and recipient total lung capacity from nomograms based on age, height, and sex. In patients with obstructive lung disease, an allograft with a 15–20% greater volume than that predicted for the recipient can be used, as these patients have huge pleural cavities.
- No active severe infection or malignancy with the possibility of metastases.
- Negative serologies for human immunodeficiency virus (HIV) or hepatitis B or C.
- ABO compatibility and human lymphocyte antigen (HLA) screen.

The guidelines used to select donors for HLT are a combination of those for heart transplantation and those for lung transplantation.

Harvest of the lungs usually is accomplished in conjunction with harvest of the heart. The vena cavae are transected, an incision is made in the left atrial appendage, and the aorta is cross-clamped and cold cardioplegia is given. At this point, the pulmonary artery is injected directly with 500 μg of PGE_1 followed by infusion of 3–4 liters of iced preservative solution which is vented out through an incision in the left atrial appendage. The lungs are partially inflated (60%) with FiO_2 of 0.4, and the trachea or bronchi are stapled and divided. The heart–lung block is then removed. When the heart and lungs are to be used for separate recipients, adequate portions of pulmonary artery and left atrial-pulmonary vein cuff must be allocated to each recipient.

The lungs are immersed in a cold crystalloid solution at 4 °C and transported. Although the maximum ischemic time is 6–8 h, the optimal ischemic time should not exceed 5–6 h because short- and intermediate-term patient survival may be affected.

Operative Procedure and Patient Positioning

Heart–lung transplantation is performed through a median sternotomy with hypothermic cardiopulmonary bypass (CPB), bicaval cannulation, and aortic cross-clamping. The recipient undergoes resection of the heart–lung block, leaving only a right atrial cuff in continuity with the inferior vena cava (IVC) and superior vena cava (SVC), the cut end of the distal trachea, and the cut end of the proximal ascending aorta. The donor heart–lung block is implanted with anastomoses of the right atrium, distal trachea, and ascending aorta.

Single-lung transplantation is performed through a standard thoracotomy with the patient in the lateral thoracotomy position. The donor lung block contains a cuff of left atrium with two pulmonary veins, the bronchus, and the branch pulmonary artery. The other donor lung and the donor heart can be used for two other recipients. One-lung ventilation (OLV) is established and a pneumonectomy is performed, followed by implantation of the donor lung with anastomoses at the left atrium, bronchus, and branch pulmonary artery. This procedure often can be performed without CPB.

Two very different surgical procedures are used for DLT. The *en bloc* procedure is performed on CPB with hypothermia, bicaval cannulation, aortic cross-clamping, and cardioplegic arrest of the recipient heart. A median sternotomy is used. The donor double-lung block consists of the two lungs, the distal trachea, the main pulmonary artery, and a large left atrial cuff with all four pulmonary veins. The donor heart can be used for another recipient. The block is implanted with anastomoses at the trachea, posterior left atrium, and main pulmonary artery after bilateral recipient pneumonectomies. This procedure is associated with poor healing of the tracheal anastomosis and reduced long-term survival compared with BSSLT, and has been largely abandoned.

Bilateral sequential single-lung transplantation is the other approach to DLT. This procedure often can be performed without CPB, which is considerably more challenging for the anesthesiologist. This procedure is performed with the patient supine, through a sternal bithoracotomy. Proper positioning is necessary to provide adequate exposure for the thoracotomy portion of the incision. One approach is to position the patient's arms suspended over the head. This is cumbersome and consumptive of the small amount of space available at the head of the table. In addition, it exposes the patient to an increased risk of brachial plexus injuries. With proper positioning of two rolls – one on either side of the patient's spine extending from the cervical to the lumbar region – the arms can remain tucked at the patient's side.

Each donor lung block contains a cuff of left atrium with two pulmonary veins, the bronchus, and the branch pulmonary artery. The donor heart can be used for another recipient. OLV is established and a pneumonectomy is performed, followed by implantation of the donor lung with anastomoses at the left atrium, bronchus, and branch pulmonary artery. The procedure is then repeated for the next donor lung.

Use of CPB

HLT and *En Bloc* DLT

Heart–lung transplantation and *en bloc* DLT both require hypothermic CPB with aortic cross-clamping, as described previously.

SLT and BSSLT

Elective CPB is used for SLT and BSSLT for the following subsets of patients.

- Infants and small children.
- Patients with pulmonary hypertension.
- Patients undergoing lung transplantation and simultaneous repair of intracardiac defects.

For all other patients with SLT and BSSLT, CPB is initiated only when hemodynamic, gas exchange, or technical difficulties are encountered during the course of the procedure. Most SLT and BSSLT patients without pulmonary hypertension can be managed without CPB. There is a higher incidence of need for CPB in patients with restrictive lung disease.

Intraoperative criteria that predict the need for use of CPB in patients with restrictive lung disease include an SaO_2 <90% with an FiO_2 of 1.0, baseline mean pulmonary artery (PA) pressure >40 mmHg, mean PA pressure >50 mmHg with the PA clamped, severe systemic hypotension, and a cardiac index <2.0 l min^{-1} m^{-2}. Avoiding CPB when possible is important, because its use contributes to postoperative graft dysfunction in the form of an increased arterial/alveolar oxygen ratio, increased severity of radiographic pulmonary injury, and prolonged postoperative intubation. It does not appear that use of CPB affects long-term outcome.

Full CPB is used for infants and small children, and for all patients undergoing simultaneous repair of an intracardiac lesion. Aortic cross-clamping and cardioplegic arrest are only necessary when intracardiac defects are repaired. Normothermic partial CPB is used for all other cases of SLT and BSSLT. Cannulation of the ascending aorta and the right atrium is used for bilateral SLT and right SLT. For patients undergoing left SLT, descending aorta and pulmonary artery cannulations have been used. Alternatively, femoral vein and artery cannulations can be used.

Anesthetic Management

Goals

- With the initiation of positive pressure ventilation, patients with obstructive lung disease may exhibit air trapping and auto-positive end-expiratory pressure (PEEP) with progressive increases in lung volumes leading to high intrathoracic pressure and hemodynamic compromise. This is particularly likely if a short expiratory time interval and/or a high respiratory rate are present. Ventilatory interventions will be necessary.
- Preexisting left ventricular or right ventricular dysfunction requires that contractility be maintained or enhanced.
- Avoid hypercarbia, hypoxemia, and acidosis, which will exacerbate pulmonary hypertension and may result in acute right ventricular decompensation.
- Avoid increases in the pulmonary vascular resistance (PVR):systemic vascular resistance (SVR) ratio in patients with Eisenmenger syndrome. This will increase right-to-left (R-L) shunting and worsen hypoxemia.

Preoperative Evaluation

Lung transplant patients typically undergo extensive medical evaluation. A summary of this evaluation is readily available to the anesthesiologist through the transplant coordinator.

Premedication

Most patients are called into the hospital at short notice, and many will have eaten solid food during the previous 6–8 h. To reduce the risk of aspiration in older children, a non-particulate antacid (30 ml) can be given in addition to intravenous metoclopramide (10 mg) and an intravenous H_2 receptor blocker such as ranitidine (50 mg). For infants and smaller children, a period of 2–3 h of NPO status is sufficient and usually transpires before induction.

Premedication for children is most safely and effectively titrated by the anesthesiologist before induction and while lines are placed and the history and physical examination are completed. Midazolam 0.03–0.05 mg kg^{-1} in divided doses works well to reduce anxiety. Supplemental oxygen should be administered because hypoxemia will exacerbate existing pulmonary hypertension.

Preinduction

Some transplant patients will be receiving intravenous inotropic and vasodilator therapy when they arrive for surgery. These agents should be continued via a reliable intravenous route. Sterility is of the utmost importance because the patients will be immunosuppressed. Patients with bronchospastic disease should receive bronchodilator therapy before induction. Likewise, patients with CF should receive nebulized acetylcysteine or rhDNase to help break up tenacious secretions.

Placement of an intravenous catheter before induction is optimal. Patients with preserved ventricular function, an appropriate NPO interval, and cardiopulmonary stability will likely tolerate an inhalation induction. Electrocardiogram monitoring should allow the assessment of V5, I, II, III, aVR, aVL, and aVF. Baseline recording of all seven leads should be obtained for comparative purposes. Normally, two leads (II and V5) are monitored simultaneously intraoperatively. If a left thoracotomy incision is used, V5 is not an option because the lead will be in the operative field.

A radial or femoral artery catheter is placed after the induction of anesthesia. Central venous pressure monitoring is placed after induction. For older children undergoing SLT or BSSLT with or without CPB, a PA catheter may be placed in some institutions. Alternatively, an appropriately sized double-lumen (DL) central venous line is placed; the right internal jugular vein is the preferred site. A transthoracic PA catheter can be placed by the surgeon directly into the PA, or advanced out to the PA via the right atrium if postoperative PAP monitoring is desired. A pediatric transesophageal echocardiography (TEE) probe can be used for children weighing less than 15–20 kg, and the adult TEE probe for children weighing more than 20–30 kg to help manage the patient before and after CPB.

Management of One-lung Ventilation

In procedures performed with full CPB, lung isolation and OLV are not necessary. These procedures can be managed with a standard single-lumen endotracheal tube. The anesthetic plan for SLT and BSSLT in adults and older children must include a method of lung isolation and OLV because these procedures are being performed increasingly without CPB or with partial CPB. When partial CPB is used, OLV to the perfused, nonoperative lung is necessary. A number of methods of lung isolation and OLV are available. The advantages and disadvantages of the various methods are summarized in Table 34.1.

Endobronchial Intubation

A standard endotracheal tube (ETT) is used, with a bronchoscope being employed to direct the ETT down the mainstem bronchus of the lung that is to be ventilated.

Single-lumen Endotracheal Tube Plus a Bronchial Blocker

This technique involves use of a Fogarty catheter or an Arndt blocker and a standard ETT. Laryngoscopy is performed and the blocker is placed in the trachea, followed by placement of the endotracheal tube. Alternatively, the blocker can be placed within the lumen of the ETT. In either case, a fiberoptic bronchoscope is then used to guide the bronchial blocking catheter down the appropriate bronchus. Fogarty catheters with balloon sizes from 0.5 to 3 ml are available. Arndt blockers are available in three sizes. When using a pediatric (3.4 mm) fiberoptic bronchoscope to position the catheter,

Table 34.1 Advantages and disadvantages of one-lung ventilation (OLV) techniques.

Type of OLV	Advantages	Disadvantages
Endobronchial intubation	• Any size patient • Use of appropriate-sized fiberoptic bronchoscope • Suctioning is possible • Use the same ETT at the end of the procedure	• Deflation of the nonventilated lung will occur passively • Suctioning of the nonventilated lung and application of CPAP to the nonventilated lung are impossible • In taller patients, a standard ETT may not be long enough to extend far enough into the mainstem bronchus to provide isolation
Bronchial blocker (Fogarty catheter or Arndt blocker)	• Applicable to any size patient with use of an appropriate-sized ETT and bronchial blocker • Suctioning of secretions via the ETT before placement of the blocker • When the procedure is completed, the ETT does not have to be replaced and the blocker can be removed	• The Fogarty catheter balloon is a high-pressure, low-volume balloon that may compromise bronchial mucosal blood flow. There is no internal lumen to allow lung decompression or suctioning • The internal lumen of the Arndt blocker is too small to allow adequate suctioning of secretions • Occlusion of the RUL bronchus by the balloon of the blocker may occur due to the high take-off of the RUL bronchus • Maintaining the position of the blocker in the mainstem bronchus during surgical manipulation may be difficult or impossible
Univent	• The blocker being an integral part of the ETT provides better stability of the blocker • The internal lumen of the blocker will allow some decompression of the nonventilated lung and will allow the application of CPAP • When the procedure is completed, the Univent tube does not have to be replaced with a standard ETT	• Due to the large external diameter, these tubes are useful only for adult patients and older children • The internal lumen of the blocker is too small to allow adequate suctioning of secretions • As with a standard bronchial blocker, occlusion of the RUL bronchus by the balloon of the blocker may occur
E-Z endobronchial blocker	• It is securely placed at the carina without the need for navigation of the cuff into either of the bronchi • Cuff inflation can be performed just before lung isolation, which minimizes the need to manipulate the catheter after placement and reduces the potential for the cuffs to become dislodged	• The bronchial blocker balloon is a high-pressure, low-volume balloon that may compromise bronchial mucosal blood flow • Only one size (7 Fr) is available
Double-lumen endotracheal tubes	• Deflation and suctioning of the nonventilated lung are easily accomplished • Application of CPAP to the nonventilated lung is easy • The endobronchial tube is not dislodged easily with surgical manipulation • Visualization of the RUL bronchus with the DL tube in place is accomplished easily with a fiberoptic bronchoscope	• Alignment of the RUL lumen of a right-sided DL tube with the patient's RUL can be difficult, particularly in the presence of thick secretions • The smallest available DL tube is appropriate for children aged 7–8 years • Suctioning tenacious secretions through the small lumens of the DL tube is more difficult than through the lumen of a standard ETT • When the procedure is completed, the DL tube must be exchanged for a standard ETT

CPAP, continuous positive airway pressure; DL, double-lumen; ETT, endotracheal tube; RUL, right upper lobe.
Credit: Reproduced from Benden and Kucheryavaya (2013)/with permission of Elsevier.

the 5 Fr catheter can be placed in a 4.5 mm ETT, the 7 Fr catheter can be placed in a 6.5 mm ETT, and the 9 Fr catheter can be placed in a 7.5 mm ETT. Ardnt blockers have a small central lumen which can be used for lung deflation and continuous positive airway pressure (CPAP) application.

Single-lumen Endotracheal Tube Plus an E-Z Bronchial Blocker

The E-Z blocker is a Y-shaped catheter with a low-pressure balloon bronchial blocker on each arm. Each arm has a small central lumen which can be used for lung deflation and CPAP application. Placement involves intubation with a 7.0 mm ETT or larger. A multiport adaptor is attached and a fiberoptic bronchoscope is used to confirm that the ETT is 4 cm above the carina to allow sufficient space for deployment of the bifurcated arms of the blocker. The E-Z blocker is then inserted through the adaptor until the bifurcated arms each enter a bronchus. The bronchoscope is used to verify the position and to confirm that the cuff of the bronchus to be blocked is inflated properly.

Univent™ Tube

This is a standard endotracheal tube with a 3 mm outer-diameter bronchial blocker, which passes through a 4 mm channel incorporated within the lumen of the ETT. The bronchial blocker has a 2 mm internal-diameter lumen. These tubes are available with internal diameters ranging from 6.0 to 9.0 mm in 0.5 mm increments, and in a 3.5 mm uncuffed and 4.5 mm cuffed version. Because of the presence of the enclosed bronchial blocker, the external diameter of these tubes is considerably larger. The external diameter of the 8 mm Univent tube is 13 mm, which is the same as the external diameter of a 39 Fr DL tube. The external diameter of the 3.5 mm Univent tube is the same as a 6 mm ETT or a 26 Fr DL tube. These tubes have a small central lumen in the blocker which can be used for lung deflation and CPAP application. Optimal placement of the bronchial blocker requires the use of a fiberoptic bronchoscope.

Double-lumen Endotracheal Tube

Double-lumen tubes are available in sizes 26, 28, 32, 35, 37, 39, 41, and 43 Fr. The outer diameter of a 26 Fr DL tube is equivalent to a 6.0 mm ETT, and thus is an appropriate size for a patient weighing approximately 30 kg or aged 8–10 years. Both right- and left-sided tubes are available. Right-sided tubes have a side lumen in the bronchial tube that must be positioned over the right upper lobe (RUL) bronchus so that the balloon of the bronchial lumen does not occlude the RUL bronchus. Fiberoptic bronchoscopy is necessary to ensure proper positioning of both right- and left-sided DL tubes.

Induction and Maintenance

Anesthetic techniques should allow for early postoperative extubation. Many patients with end-stage pulmonary disease will be unable to lie flat due to severe dyspnea. These patients are induced in the sitting position and, as they lose consciousness, they are slowly placed supine. For patients in whom there is a risk of aspiration, induction is performed with the patient in a slightly head-up position and cricoid pressure is applied until the trachea is intubated.

Difficult mask ventilation can have disastrous consequences for these patients. Careful titration of etomidate (0.1–0.3 mg kg^{-1}) in combination with fentanyl 5–10 µg kg^{-1} or sufentanil 1–2 µg kg^{-1} is useful for induction. A full dose of etomidate 0.3 mg kg^{-1} is rarely necessary to induce hypnosis and loss of consciousness in these patients. This drug combination has minimal direct effect on heart rate, myocardial contractility, peripheral vascular resistance, or venous capacitance. An overall diminution in central sympathetic tone will also contribute to circulatory depression. These drugs in combination with rocuronium (1.0 mg kg^{-1}) or succinylcholine (1–2 mg kg^{-1}) can be used to perform a modified rapid-sequence induction (cricoid pressure during positive pressure ventilation) in the patient with questionable NPO status.

Anesthesia can be maintained with additional doses of opioid in conjunction with a benzodiazepine (usually midazolam in increments of 0.01–0.03 mg kg^{-1}) or a low inhaled concentration (0.5–0.75 MAC) of isoflurane or sevoflurane. N$_2$O is not a good choice as an adjuvant agent; it has a weak myocardial depressant effect that normally is counteracted by the sympathetic outflow it produces.

For patients with obstructive lung disease (emphysema, alpha-1-antitrypsin deficiency, CF), induction and positive pressure ventilation may produce profound hypotension. The possibility that a pneumothorax is present must always be considered. This cardiovascular compromise is secondary to air trapping or auto-PEEP. This auto-PEEP reduces the stroke volume and cardiac output through the following.

- Reductions in venous return to the right ventricle resulting in a decrease in right ventricular end-diastolic volume (RVEDV).
- Increased impedance to right ventricular ejection by mechanical compression of the pulmonary arterial system, resulting in an increase in right ventricular end-systolic volume (RVESV).
- Shift of the interventricular septum into the left ventricle, which reduces left ventricular compliance and left ventricular end-diastolic volume (LVEDV).

This combination is particularly detrimental for patients with compromised right ventricular systolic function and right ventricular afterload mismatch. Treatment requires volume administration (10–15 ml kg^{-1} of a balanced salt solution) to normalize RVEDV, and inotropic support to improve right ventricular systolic function and normalize RVESV. Dopamine 5–10 μg kg^{-1} min^{-1} or epinephrine 0.05–0.3 μg kg^{-1} min^{-1} are effective for inotropic support. In addition, ventilation with a rapid initial inflation followed by an inspiratory hold or pause and a long expiratory time is necessary (low inspiration:expiration [I:E] ratio). This may require hand ventilation, although pressure-controlled ventilation with an intensive care unit ventilator works well. PEEP should not be used.

Transesophageal echocardiography is extremely valuable in assessing ventricular filling and contractile function in this setting, because filling pressures will not provide an accurate measure of ventricular volumes.

In the most severe instances, intermittent periods of apnea may be necessary. This apneic oxygenation may exacerbate preexisting pulmonary hypertension via CO$_2$ retention and hypoxemia. Evaluation of pulmonary artery pressures and cardiac output with a PA catheter, right and left ventricular functions with TEE, and arterial saturation with pulse oximetry are necessary to determine the extent of hypoventilation that can be tolerated. Marked acidosis (pH of 6.94) and hypercarbia (PaCO$_2$ of 150 mmHg) can be tolerated during lung transplantation as long as systemic blood pressure and oxygen delivery are maintained. In some instances, the initiation of CPB may be necessary.

Blood loss may be impressive during dissection for pneumonectomy in HLT, SLT, and DLT patients with dense adhesions from previous thoracic surgery, or for patients with cystic fibrosis or bronchiectasis. A rapid transfusion device may be necessary in some cases. Some centers use antifibrinolytics when CPB is used or when there are dense adhesions, regardless of whether CPB is used. In addition to red cells, component therapy with fresh frozen plasma and platelets is often necessary, particularly when CPB is used. Manipulation of the lungs in patients with CF or bronchiectasis may result in the release of endotoxins with a subsequent decrease in SVR, hyperpyrexia, and increased metabolic rate. Management of the recipient without use of CPB under these conditions is extremely difficult.

After one or both of the lungs have been implanted and perfused, most centers administer methylprednisolone (10 mg kg^{-1}). After lung implantation has been completed, PEEP of 5–10 cmH$_2$O is applied and the FiO$_2$ selected is the lowest necessary to obtain a

PaO_2 of 90–100 mmHg. This is done because the postischemic lung is vulnerable to oxygen free radical toxicity. In some institutions, inhaled nitric oxide or a prostacyclin analog is routinely used because they can reduce PVR, improve V/Q mismatch, and mitigate ischemia/reperfusion injury.

At the termination of the procedure, patients with DL tubes have the DL tube replaced with a large single-lumen ETT. A large tube size should be used to allow easy access for postoperative fiberoptic bronchoscopy.

Special Considerations for SLT and BSSLT

Management of OLV and pulmonary artery clamping for recipient pneumonectomy and allograft implantation in SLT and BSSLT patients without CPB is a challenge. The task is made easier for patients undergoing SLT if the lung with the poorest ventilation and perfusion is removed and replaced. For patients undergoing BSSLT, the lung with the poorest ventilation and perfusion should be removed first and replaced.

Maintenance of body temperature is difficult when CPB is not used. A warming blanket under the patient, an actively humidified breathing circuit, a fluid/blood warmer, and a forced warming air blanket over the patient are necessary.

One-lung Ventilation

Collapse of the operative lung and OLV is likely to exacerbate air trapping and the subsequent hemodynamic compromise and CO_2 retention. Treatment with volume administration, inotropes, and ventilatory interventions is warranted, as described previously. Marked hypercarbia with acidosis is likely and is generally well tolerated. Aggressive suctioning may be necessary to facilitate collapse of the operative lung. PaO_2 also is likely to decrease, due to intrapulmonary shunting, until the ipsilateral pulmonary artery is clamped. Administration of CPAP to the nonventilated lung, insufflation of O_2 to the nonventilated lung, or high-frequency jet ventilation (HFJV) of the nonventilated lung may improve oxygenation.

Clamping of the PA

Recipient pneumonectomy requires clamping of the ipsilateral PA. Before clamping, the PA catheter is withdrawn into the main PA. Palpation by the surgeon will confirm its position proximal to the proposed cross-clamp site. After the ipsilateral PA has been clamped, the catheter is advanced into the contralateral PA. Clamping of the PA may compromise right ventricular function due to afterload mismatch. This is most likely in patients with mild to moderate preexisting pulmonary hypertension, and in those with impaired right ventricular function. This is the primary reason why patients with severe pulmonary hypertension require elective CPB. If there is any doubt regarding the ability of the patient to tolerate PA clamping, a trial of clamping is recommended. TEE is used to assess right ventricular function. In addition, increased PAP and central venous pressure (CVP), falling cardiac index, and S_VO_2 may occur.

Allograft Implantation

Immediately after allograft implantation and washout of the preservative solution and prostaglandin, there may be profound, transient systemic hypotension. Treatment requires fluid administration and alpha-adrenergic support. After implantation of the donor lung, there usually is an immediate reduction in PA pressures and an improvement in pulmonary compliance and gas exchange. This period may be followed by allograft dysfunction characterized by deteriorating gas exchange, decreasing pulmonary compliance, and elevated PA pressures. This is the result of noncardiogenic, reperfusion pulmonary edema. Two factors predispose to this process: (i) preexisting pulmonary hypertension which results in overperfusion of the donor lung; and (ii) a long ischemic interval, which enhances capillary permeability.

Positive end-expiratory pressure (5–15 cmH_2O) usually is necessary to maintain adequate gas exchange when allograft dysfunction occurs. Increased capillary permeability and the lack of pulmonary lymphatic drainage in the allograft dictate judicious crystalloid administration. Excessively large tidal volumes should be avoided because overinflation of the allograft will contribute to elevated PA pressures through mechanical compression of the pulmonary vasculature.

If allograft dysfunction is severe, implantation of the second lung in BSSLT patients may require CPB. If CPB is not used, implantation of the second lung is managed as described for the first lung.

Indications for CPB

The decision to use CPB is individualized for each patient. The use of CPB may become necessary at any time during the procedure. The combination of a cardiac index <2 l min^{-1} m^{-2}, S_VO_2 $<60\%$, mean arterial pressure (MAP) <50–60 mmHg, SaO_2 <85–90%, and pH <7.00, despite aggressive ventilatory and pharmacologic intervention, is an indication for use of CPB. The latter process is not necessary for increased PA pressures unless there is evidence of deteriorating right ventricular function. TEE assessment of right ventricular function is supplemented by use of CVP determinations. Increasing CVP, right ventricular distension, worsening global hypokinesis, and new or worsening tricuspid regurgitation, despite inotropic support with epinephrine, norepinephrine, or dopamine in combination with inhaled NO (20–40 ppm) or intravenous pulmonary vasodilation (milrinone 0.5–1.0 µg kg^{-1} min^{-1}, nitroglycerin 0.5–5 µg kg^{-1} min^{-1}, PGE$_1$ 0.05–0.2 µg kg^{-1} min^{-1}, or PGI$_2$ 5–20 ng kg^{-1} min^{-1}), are indications for use of CPB. Norepinephrine (0.01–0.1 µg kg^{-1} min^{-1}) is the most effective agent for maintaining coronary perfusion pressure in patients with right ventricular hypertension, but its use must be tempered with the knowledge that it may also increase PVR.

Transesophageal echocardiography assessment of left ventricular function is supplemented by use of pulmonary artery occlusion pressure (PAOP) determinations.

Hypoxemia, hypercarbia, and reduced systemic blood pressure can all contribute to left ventricular dysfunction. Progressive deterioration in left ventricular function (new wall motion abnormalities, left ventricular distension, new or worsening mitral regurgitation) despite aggressive pharmacologic and ventilatory interventions is an indication for CPB.

A metabolic acidosis is difficult to treat because sodium bicarbonate administration will produce CO_2, which must be eliminated by increased alveolar ventilation. Obviously, increasing alveolar ventilation often is not possible in these patients.

Post-CPB Management

Particular attention must be paid to de-airing the heart. Severe ventricular dysfunction may follow the ejection of air through the coronary arteries. The right ventricle is particularly at risk due to the anterior location of the right coronary ostia. TEE is valuable in guiding the de-airing process.

Patients undergoing HLT have a denervated heart and are managed during the post-CPB period in the same manner as that described for heart transplant patients.

Right ventricular function usually improves dramatically after lung implantation due to the immediate reduction in PA pressures. Despite this, patients with *en bloc* DLT, BSSLT, or SLT may require inotropic support. Patients requiring aortic cross-clamping and cardioplegic arrest are at particular risk for post-CPB right and left ventricular dysfunction. In addition, the presence of lung allograft dysfunction may contribute to post-CPB right ventricular dysfunction as the result of elevated PA pressures.

Postoperative Care

In rare instances, extracorporeal membrane oxygenation (ECMO) and independent lung ventilation may be necessary after SLT in patients with pulmonary hypertension secondary to reperfusion pulmonary edema. Postoperative independent lung ventilation with a DL tube has been used for patients with SLT to minimize preferential ventilation and air trapping in the native lung in patients with obstructive lung disease. For these patients, the native lung has high compliance, and air trapping can result in hyperinflation with subsequent displacement of the mediastinum and compression of the donor lung.

Differential ventilation with hypoventilation of the native lung has been used successfully to avoid this problem. Preferential perfusion of the donor lung occurs after SLT, especially for patients with pulmonary hypertension. In cases of severe V/Q mismatch, selective hypoventilation of the native lung, combined with positioning the patient in the lateral position with the donor lung in the nondependent position, may be necessary during the postoperative period. This will minimize overventilation of the native lung and overperfusion of the donor lung. In patients with SLT with a fibrotic native lung, positioning the patient with the donor lung dependent may help equalize ventilation to the both lungs.

Noncardiac Surgery in Lung Transplant Patients

As with heart transplant patients, lung transplant and HLT patients may require other surgical procedures. Some are purely elective, whereas others are likely to be urgent or emergent. Most surgical procedures are the direct result of complications of immunosuppressive therapy. (Such complications and immunosuppressive agents are listed in Tables 33.6 and 33.7.) The incidence of complications requiring general surgical consultation and intervention in lung transplant patients is 16%. In addition, lung transplant patients suffer airway and vascular anastomotic complications that require operative intervention. The incidence of airway complications in SLT and BSSLT is

12–17% per anastomosis, with an associated mortality rate of 2–3%. Some 9% of nonlethal airway complications require operative intervention. Similar statistics exist in pediatric patients, where the most common intervention required is for the treatment of bronchial stenosis. This usually involves flexible and rigid bronchoscopy for laser excision of granulation tissue, stent placement, or balloon dilatation.

Lung transplant and HLT patients present a unique set of management issues.

- *Loss of cough reflex due to transection of vagal fibers.* This makes the patient with a transplanted lung prone to retention of secretions and at risk for pulmonary infections. The risk of aspiration should not be significantly increased, as the innervation of the larynx, epiglottis, and proximal trachea remains normal. However, laryngeal nerve injury during dissection can result in loss of protective airway reflexes.
- *Reduction in lung volumes.* Mild proportional reductions in all lung volumes are seen long term in patients after HLT, DLT, and SLT. These reductions are not due to reduced elastic properties of the transplanted lung, but are secondary to the volume constraints of the recipient chest cavity and to the strength and efficiency of the thoracic musculature. In fact, the improvement in elastic recoil and the reduced chest wall distension that follow SLT for emphysema substantially reduce the work of breathing and dyspnea.
- *Ventilatory response to CO_2.* HLT and DLT patients have total vagal denervation, whereas SLT patients retain vagal innervation to the native lung. HLT, BSSLT, and SLT patients all increase minute ventilation in response to CO_2 rebreathing-induced hypercapnia. However, while SLT patients increase both tidal volume and respiratory rate, HLT and BSSLT patients exhibit an increase in tidal volume with little or no respiratory rate response.
- *Ventilatory response to hypoxia.* Lung transplant patients have an increase in

tidal volume and respiratory rate comparable to that in normal patients in response to hypoxia.

- *Rejection.* Acute rejection of the transplanted lungs can be diagnosed both clinically and with transbronchial biopsies via a flexible bronchoscope. In the absence of clinical evidence of rejection (dyspnea, fever, diffuse perihilar infiltrate on chest radiography), biopsies are performed at regular intervals postoperatively. Obviously, if clinical evidence of rejection exists, more frequent biopsies may be indicated to document rejection and assess regression of histologic changes with treatment. Biopsies are graded from 0 to 4 based on histologic criteria. Acute rejection of the lungs is very common; approximately 50% of patients experience an acute rejection episode in the first 3–6 months post transplantation. Rejection of the heart in HLT patients, on the other hand, is uncommon. Because rejection of the heart and lungs is not synchronous, heart biopsies are performed in HLT patients only if there is clinical evidence of heart rejection. Rejection is treated with oral or intravenous pulsed steroids. Persistent rejection unresponsive to steroids usually is treated with a lympholytic agent such as polyclonal antithymocyte globulin (ATG) or murine monoclonal antibody (OKT3).
- *Bronchiolitis obliterans syndrome (BOS) and bronchiolitis obliterans (BO).* BOS is a clinical entity characterized by declining FEV_1, FEF_{25-75}, and FEF_{50}/FVC. BOS is graded based on the reduction in FEV_1 compared with the best baseline value (grade 0: FEV_1 >90% and FEF_{25-75} >75%; grade 1: FEV_1 66–80%; grade 2: FEV_1 51–65%; grade 3: FEV_1 <50%). BO is a pathologic diagnosis based on histologic evidence of fibrous scarring of membraneous and respiratory bronchioles with partial or complete obliteration of the lumen. BOS and BO are the main sources of morbidity and mortality after lung transplantation. The prevalence of BOS

and BO for HLT, SLT, and BSSLT patients is 25% at one year, 50–60% at three years, 60% at five years, and 80% at 10 years in large series. The survival rate for lung transplant patients is 76% at one year, 60% at three years, 49% at five years, and 24% at 10 years. Once established, BOS and BO follow a progressively worsening course. Patients with BOS and BO ultimately develop severe obstructive pulmonary disease and progressive hypoxemia. Augmented immunosuppression may attenuate this downhill course and improve survival. In severe progressive cases, retransplantation is the only option. However, the results are not encouraging, with a five-year survival of 45%, as BOS and BO usually recur within a short time. The etiology is multifactorial, with rejection and cytomegalovirus infection both implicated. It is believed that an alloimmune injury occurs with subsequent release of immunologic mediators and the production of growth factors that lead to luminal obliteration and scarring of the small airway. Monitoring for BO is accomplished with transbronchial biopsies or open-lung biopsy when transbronchial biopsy specimens are equivocal.
- *Response to drugs.* HLT patients have a denervated heart and have drug responses identical to those described for heart transplant patients.
- *HLT patients.* These patients will have all of the cardiac problems outlined previously for heart transplant patients.

Anesthetic Considerations for Noncardiac Surgery in Patients Post Lung Transplantation

Sterile technique is essential.

- Patients with stenotic airways and those with BOS and BO may exhibit air trapping and auto-PEEP.
- Diminished cough reflex makes clearing of secretions difficult. Laryngeal damage will predispose to aspiration.

- Lymphatic interruption necessitates careful fluid administration to avoid interstitial pulmonary fluid accumulation.
- Placement of an ETT must take into account the position of the tracheal or bronchial anastomoses.
- Patients with preoperative CO_2 retention may exhibit CO_2 retention for 2–3 weeks postoperatively as the central chemoreceptors reset.
- HLT patients will present the same cardiac challenges as heart transplant patients.

- Stress-dose steroid coverage should be considered for patients receiving steroids as part of immunosuppression.

References and Further Reading

Avdimiretz, N. & Benden, C. The changing landscape of pediatric lung transplantation. *Clin Transplant* **36**, e14634 (2022).

35

Anomalous Origin of the Left Coronary Artery from the Pulmonary Artery and Anomalous Aortic Origin of a Coronary Artery

Anomalous Origin of the Left Coronary Artery (ALCAPA)

Introduction

Anomalous origin of the left coronary artery or Bland–White–Garland syndrome is a rare anomaly occurring in 1 in 300,000 live births. Although it commonly occurs in isolation, it has been reported with other cardiac lesions.

Anatomy

The most common origin of the left main coronary artery (LMCA) in ALCAPA is the leftward posterior sinus of the pulmonary artery, followed by the rightward and posterior sinus, the posterior wall of the main pulmonary artery, and the posterior aspect of the origin of the right pulmonary artery.

Physiology

Dramatic changes occur in the coronary circulation in infants with ALCAPA within the first weeks of life. While the fetus remains *in utero*, the heart will develop quite normally. Initially after birth, the relatively high pulmonary vascular resistance (PVR) and pulmonary artery pressure (PAP) allow the myocardium supplied by the anomalous artery to remain well perfused. In the few days after birth, as the PVR decreases, the pressure in the pulmonary trunk decreases.

This will result in coronary steal and subsequent compromise of the left ventricular subendocardial perfusion. In addition, all antegrade left coronary artery flow is deoxygenated mixed venous blood. Severe left ventricular dysfunction and associated mitral insufficiency generally develop rapidly. Left untreated, 90% of infants will not survive the first year of life. A small subset of patients survives beyond infancy due to the rapid development of collaterals from the right coronary artery to the territory of the LMCA (Figure 35.1).

Echocardiography can be used to delineate the origin of the coronary arteries following presentation. However, cardiac catheterization and angiography remain the "gold standard." Increasingly, computed tomography angiography is also being utilized. Once the diagnosis of ALCAPA is made, urgent surgery is indicated.

Surgical Treatment

Surgical treatment can be classified into one-coronary and two-coronary system repairs. The one-coronary approach involves ligating the anomalous LMCA at its origin with the pulmonary artery to eliminate the steal phenomenon. This approach has been largely abandoned due to poor outcomes associated with inadequate coronary blood flow to the LMCA system via the collateral network from the right coronary. The two-coronary system approach involves one of the following.

The Pediatric Cardiac Anesthesia Handbook, Second Edition. Viviane G. Nasr and James A. DiNardo.
© 2025 John Wiley & Sons Ltd. Published 2025 by John Wiley & Sons Ltd.

(A)   (B)   (C)

Figure 35.1 Varying functional states in anomalous origin of the left coronary artery from the pulmonary trunk. (A) During fetal life the aortic (A) and pulmonary arterial (P) pressures are essentially equal. Flow in the anomalous artery is from the pulmonary trunk into the myocardium. (B) In early postnatal life, the pulmonary artery pressure has fallen below levels that pertain during fetal life. Rich intercoronary collateral channels have not yet developed. In this phase, flow through the anomalous coronary artery is probably at a low level. The anomalous vessel may be perfused either from the pulmonary trunk or from the right coronary artery through developing collateral systems. (C) In the final phase, a rich collateral system has developed between the two coronary arteries. Characteristics of an arteriovenous fistula now pertain, with the major contribution to fistulous flow coming from the right coronary artery. Mediastinal arteries, which make communication with the coronary arterial system, may also contribute to such flow. *Source:* Reproduced from Lopez and Geva (2016)/with permission of John Wiley & Sons.

- Reimplantation of the LMCA into the aorta using a coronary button technique. This is the preferred technique.
- Creation of an intrapulmonary artery baffle to establish continuity between the LMCA orifice and the aorta (Takeuchi procedure).
- Ligation of the anomalous LMCA at its origin with the pulmonary artery and placement of a coronary artery bypass graft(s) to the left coronary artery territory (coronary artery bypass grafting; CABG).

Mitral valve repair is generally not undertaken as the origin of mitral regurgitation, including severe mitral regurgitation, is ischemic and not mechanical in origin.

Anesthetic Management

These patients are managed in a manner similar to any patient with a severe dilated cardiomyopathy. The additional management

issue in these patients is PVR. The patients generally have systemic or near-systemic PAPs due to passive elevation from a very high left atrial pressure and reactive pulmonary vasoconstriction. In theory, a reduction in PVR will worsen the coronary steal phenomenon by reducing PAP.

Following surgical repair, a comprehensive TEE or epicardial echo exam (see Chapter 8 and and Figure 35.3) should be performed to examine regional wall motion in all myocardial segments, with attention paid to the coronary artery supplying any segment with impaired wall motion. Regional wall motion abnormalities should be assumed to be the result of a technically imperfect coronary artery repair unless proven otherwise (Figure 35.2). Left ventricular assist device (LVAD) support may be necessary following repair if an immediate improvement in left ventricular function following revascularization does not occur.

RCA
LAD
CX
RCA or CX
LAD or CX
RCA or LAD

Figure 35.2 Regional wall motion abnormalities should be assumed to be the result of a technically imperfect coronary artery repair unless proven otherwise. *Credit:* Reproduced from Lang (2015)/with permission of Oxford University Press.

Anomalous Aortic Origin of a Coronary Artery (AAOCA)

Introduction

Anomalous aortic origin of a coronary artery from the inappropriate sinus of Valsalva is a rare congenital cardiac anomaly with an estimated prevalence of 0.01–2%. These lesions may be associated with myocardial ischemia and sudden cardiac death (SCD) and are increasingly recognized by cardiac imaging. Because invasive angiography and echocardiography provide limited visualization of these lesions, coronary computed tomography angiography (CTA), magnetic resonance angiography (MRA), and intravascular ultrasound (IVUS) are the diagnostic tools of choice.

Anatomy

Anomalous aortic origin of a coronary artery arising at or above the inappropriate

sinus of Valsalva is characterized by its course subtype: interarterial and/or intramural, subpulmonic, prepulmonic, retroaortic, and retrocardiac. Figure 35.3 summarizes the most common variations of AAOCA.

Physiology

The major concerns with AAOCA lesions are limitation of coronary reserve leading to myocardial ischemia and/or lethal ventricular arrhythmias and sudden cardiac death (SCD). While the precise mechanism involved is unknown, it is clear that an intramural or interarterial (aortic wall) coronary course, particularly a long one, where compression of the anomalous coronary artery is likely a risk factor, is a possibility.

The management of AAOCA lesions, once indentified, must include assessment of the risk of an ischemic event using a provocative test for ischemia. This approach is summarized in Figures 35.4 and 35.5.

Surgical View

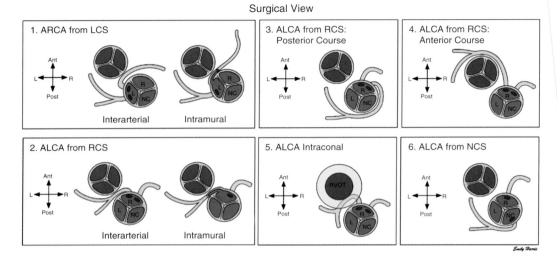

Figure 35.3 Surgical view of the most common variations of AAOCA. ARCA, anomalous right coronary artery; LCS, left coronary sinus; ALCA, anomalous left coronary artery; RCS, right coronary sinus.

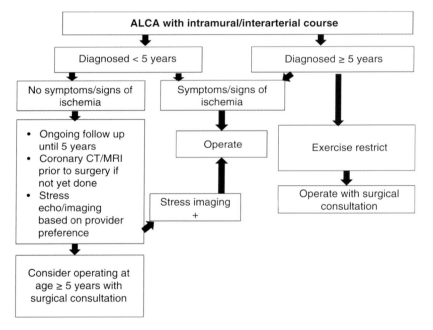

Figure 35.4 Management of anomalous left coronary artery (ALCA) with an intramural/interarterial wall course. CT/MRI, computed tomography/magnetic resonance imaging.

Surgical Treatment

Unroofing is the procedure of choice for interarterial, intramural AAOCA in the young patient. This is accomplished via an anterior aortotomy and consists of incising the common wall between the aorta and intramural segment of the anomalous coronary artery. This procedure relocates the functional orifice to the appropriate sinus,

Figure 35.5 Management of anomalous right coronary artery (ARCA) with an intramural/interarterial wall course. CT/MRI, computed tomography/magnetic resonance imaging; QoL, quality of life; IM, intramural.

enlarges the orifice, eliminates the intramural component of the artery, and decompresses the portion of the vessel that lies between the great arteries. For patients with a very short or minimal intramural course and two separate ostia, reimplantation is undertaken. The anomalous vessel is mobilized over its proximal course. A few millimeters of aortic wall containing the ostium of the anomalous coronary are excised from their abnormal location, and then reimplanted in the correct sinus of Valsalva.

An alternative to reimplantation is osteoplasty wherein a neo-ostium is created for the anomalous vessel in the sinus from which it would normally have exited. An incision is created in the aortic sinus with a matching incision in the coronary artery away from the aortic wall. A neo-ostium is created when the incisions are joined and the opened areas augmented with an autologous pericardium patch. Coronary bypass grafting is performed in the presence of atherosclerotic narrowing or if a previous AAOCA reconstruction procedure has failed.

Anesthetic Management

The anesthetic management of these patients should focus on avoiding any stimulus or change in hemodynamics that migh lead to myocardial ischemia. If a provocative test for ischemia was performed, the results of that test should be carefully reviewed to determine the hemodynamic thesholds at which ischemia was induced.

Following surgical repair, a comprehensive TEE or epicardial echo exam (see Chapter 8) should be performed to examine regional wall motion in all myocardial segments with attention paid to the coronary artery supplying any segment with impaired wall motion.

References and Further Reading

Lopez, L. & Geva, T. Double outlet ventricle. In: Lai, W.W., Mertens, L.L., Cohen, M.S. & Geva, T. (eds) *Echocardiography in Pediatric and Congenital Heart Disease: From Fetus to Adult*, 2nd edn. John Wiley & Sons, Chichester (2016).

Wesselhoeft, H., Fawcett, J.S. & Johnson, A.L. Anomalous origin of the left coronary artery from the pulmonary trunk. Its clinical spectrum, pathology, and pathophysiology, based on a review of 140 cases with seven further cases. *Circulation* **38**, 403–425 (1968).

36

Heterotaxy

Introduction

Heterotaxy is present in 3% of all congenital heart disease cases, with an incidence of 1 in 10,000.

Anatomy

Heterotaxy is said to exist when the thoraco-abdominal viscera are abnormally arranged across the right–left axis of the body. Patients with situs solitus (normal arrangement across right–left axis) and with situs inversus (mirror-image arrangement across right–left axis) are not included in this characterization. Heterotaxy is synonymous with "visceral heterotaxy" and "heterotaxy syndrome."

Defining the anatomy in heterotaxy requires a dedicated segmental approach.

Position of the Heart in the Chest

The position of the heart in the chest can be determined using chest radiography. The position does not reliably predict segmental anatomy or associated cardiac lesions. Dextrocardia is defined as a right-sided ventricular mass, where the heart is predominantly in the right hemithorax and typically the apex points to the patient's right (dextroversion) (Figure 36.1). Levocardia is defined as a left-sided ventricular mass, where the heart is predominantly in the left hemithorax and typically the apex points to the patient's left (levoversion). Mesocardia is defined as a central/midline ventricular mass, where the heart is predominantly midline and typically the apex points to the patient's midline.

Atrial Anatomy

The current level of echocardiographic expertise combined with high-resolution ultrasound systems generally allows the delineation of atrial appendage anatomy, which is a key feature in any description of the anatomy. Heterotaxy patients have either bilateral left atrial anatomy (left atrial isomerism [LAI]) or bilateral right atrial anatomy (right atrial isomerism [RAI]) (Figure 36.2). The right atrial appendage is characterized by a broad junction to the right atrium, a short and blunt shape (Snoopy's nose), and separation from the smooth walls of the atrium by pectinate muscles.

The left atrial appendage is characterized by a narrow junction to the left atrium, a long, narrow shape (Snoopy's ear), and the presence of pectinate muscles within the appendage itself.

Venoatrial Connections

A wide variety of venoatrial connections exist in heterotaxy. These connections do not define atrial situs; that is defined by appendage anatomy. Several important points deserve discussion.

The Pediatric Cardiac Anesthesia Handbook, Second Edition. Viviane G. Nasr and James A. DiNardo.

(A)   (B)

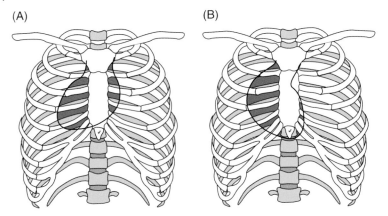

Figure 36.1 (A) Dextrocardia. (B) Dextroposition. *Source:* Reproduced from Lytrivi and Lai (2016)/with permission of John Wiley & Sons.

- *SVC* – may be unilateral (right or left) or bilateral with or without a connecting vein.
- *IVC* – LAI is associated with an absence of the suprarenal (between the renal vein and liver) segment of the IVC. In this setting, the hepatic veins drain directly into the floor of the atrium and the abdominal inferior vena cava (IVC) drains via the azygos system to either a right or left superior vena cava (SVC).
- *Coronary sinus* – RAI is associated with an absence of the coronary sinus septum such that no discrete coronary sinus is seen.
- *Pulmonary veins* – totally and partially anomalous pulmonary venous connections are seen. Purists would say that with RAI, the pulmonary venous connection is always abnormal even if all four veins connect directly to a left-sided atrium because the morphologic connection (to a right atrium) is abnormal.

Ventricular Anatomy

A chamber is considered a ventricle if it receives more than 50% of the ventricular inlet or fibrous ring of an atrioventricular (AV) valve. The AV valve need not be patent for the chamber to be considered a ventricle, as is the case with tricuspid or mitral atresia. Likewise, the chamber does not need to be large to be considered a ventricle, as is the case with

hypoplastic left heart syndrome. The right and left ventricles have different morphologies.

- Right ventricle.
  - Tricuspid valve (three leaflets) with one of the leaflets having chordal attachments to the septum; there are three papillary muscles that are located apically.
  - The septal leaflet of the tricuspid valve inserts slightly lower on the intraventricular septum than the anterior leaflet of the mitral valve.
  - Triangular shape and a trabeculated endocardial surface.
  - Has the moderator band, a band of tissue that stretches from the lower intraventricular septum to the anterior right ventricle wall.
- Left ventricle.
  - Mitral valve (two leaflets) with no chordal attachment to the septum; there are two papillary muscles that are located at the junction of the apical and middle two-thirds of the chamber.
  - Ellipsoid shape and a smooth endocardial surface.

The right ventricle wraps around the left ventricle in either a D-loop or L-loop configuration. With D-loop ventricles, when an observer's right palm is placed on the patient's chest, the thumb will be positioned in the right ventricle inlet (tricuspid valve)

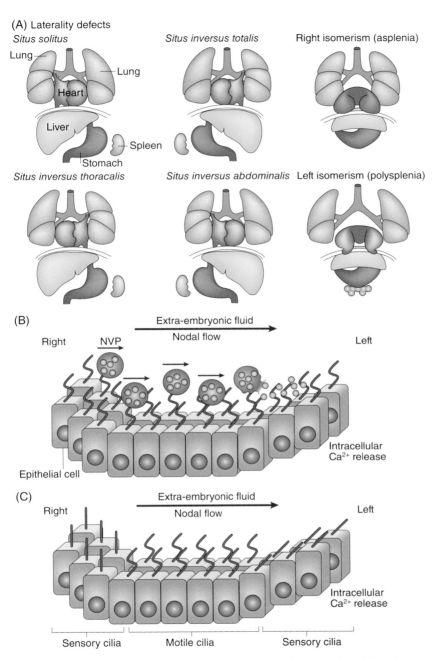

Figure 36.2 Human laterality disorders and current models for establishing left–right asymmetry. (A) Schematic illustration of normal left–right body asymmetry (situs solitus) and five laterality defects that affect the lungs, heart, liver, stomach, and spleen. By their vigorous circular movements, motile monocilia at the embryonic node generate a leftward flow of extraembryonic fluid (nodal flow). (B) The nodal vesicular parcel (NVP) model predicts that vesicles filled with morphogens (such as sonic hedgehog and retinoic acid) are secreted from the right side of the embryonic node and transported to the left side by nodal flow, where they are smashed open by force. The released contents probably bind to specific transmembrane receptors in the axonemal membrane of cilia on the left side. The consequent initiation of left-sided intracellular Ca^{2+} release induces downstream signaling events that break bilaterality. In this model, the flow of extraembryonic fluid is not detected by cilia-based mechanosensation. (C) In the two-cilia model, nonsensing motile cilia in the center of the node create a leftward nodal flow that is mechanically sensed through passive bending of nonmotile sensory cilia at the periphery of the node. Bending of the cilia on the left side leads to a left-sided release of Ca^{2+} that initiates the establishment of body asymmetry. Source: Reproduced from Fliegauf et al. (2007)/with permission of Springer Nature.

and the other four fingers will represent the right ventricular outflow tract (RVOT). With L-loop ventricles, when an observer's left palm is placed on the patient's chest, the thumb will be positioned in the right ventricle inlet (tricuspid valve) and the other four fingers will represent the RVOT.

Atrioventricular Junction

The manner in which the atria and ventricles are connected must be described. This connection can be either univentricular (double inlet right ventricle or left ventricle, mitral or tricuspid atresia), or biventricular (common or separate mitral and tricuspid valve orifices).

Ventriculoarterial Connections

Normally, the great vessels are oriented at 45° to each other when they leave the heart with the pulmonary artery (PA) anterior to the aorta. Echocardiographically, when one vessel is observed in the short axis to be circular, the other will have an oblong shape in the same plane. When the great vessels are malposed, they are oriented parallel to each other when they leave the heart. Echocardiographically, both vessels will appear circular in the short axis and tubular in the long axis. The rule of thumb when viewing malposed vessels in the short axis is that the anterior vessel is invariably the aorta. When the vessels are aligned side to side, the determination is more difficult and usually requires finding the arch of the aorta, the coronary arteries, or the branch pulmonary arteries to make the determination.

After the great vessel orientation is determined, the relationship of the vessels to the ventricles must be delineated. When the left ventricle is in continuity with the aorta and the right ventricle is in continuity with the PA, the ventriculoarterial relationship is concordant. When the left ventricle is in continuity with the PA and the right ventricle is in continuity with the aorta, the ventriculoarterial relationship is discordant. Isomerism of the right atrial appendages is more frequently associated with discordant or double-outlet ventriculoarterial connections and with severe pulmonary stenosis or atresia. Isomerism of the left atrial appendages is more frequently associated with concordant ventriculoarterial connections and with subaortic obstruction and coarctation.

Tracheobronchial Anatomy

The normal relationship of the bronchi to the pulmonary arteries differs between the right and left lungs. The right bronchus is said to be eparterial as the right pulmonary artery courses anterior to the right mainstem bronchus. The left bronchus is said to be hyparterial as the left pulmonary artery courses over and behind the left mainstem bronchus prior to the take-off of the left upper lobe bronchus.

General Characterizations

Wide variability in cardiac anatomy is the hallmark of heterotaxy, and while no "typical" heterotaxy patient exists, the following very general characterizations are helpful.

- RAI (asplenia syndrome or Ivemark syndrome).
  - Bilateral right-sidedness (two right lungs with eparterial bronchi and two right atria).
  - Absence of spleen.
  - Midline liver.
  - Bilateral SVC.
  - Bilateral sinoatrial nodes
  - Twin atrioventricular (AV) nodes, creating a substrate for a macroreentrant tachycardia.
  - Double-outlet right ventricle.
  - Complete atrioventricular canal (CAVC) defect, often unbalanced with right ventricular dominance.
  - Pulmonary stenosis or atresia.
  - Total anomalous pulmonary venous return (TAPVR).
- LAI (polysplenia syndrome).
  - Bilateral left-sidedness (two left lungs with hyparterial bronchi, two left atria).
  - Multiple spleens.

- Midline liver.
- Interrupted IVC with azygos continuation to SVC.
- Hypoplastic or absent SA node and sinus node dysfunction; prone to complete heart block.
- CAVC defect.

Extracardiac anomalies include respiratory abnormalities, gastrointestinal abnormalities, hepatic dysfunction, splenic dysfunction, and associated midline defects. Heterotaxy is associated with ciliary dysfunction. The absence of coordinated cilia-generated waves to clear mucus results in recurrent respiratory tract, sinus, and ear infections. Respiratory complications resulting from ciliary dysfunction can significantly impact postoperative recovery.

Surgical Therapy

Single-ventricle palliation of patients with heterotaxy is challenging due to the constellation of cardiac abnormalities that accompany the syndrome. A subset of patients may be amenable to biventricular repair. This is a particularly challenging pathway given the constellation of lesions and abnormal venous connections that must be corrected. An example of a typical complicated repair is illustrated in Figure 36.3a, b.

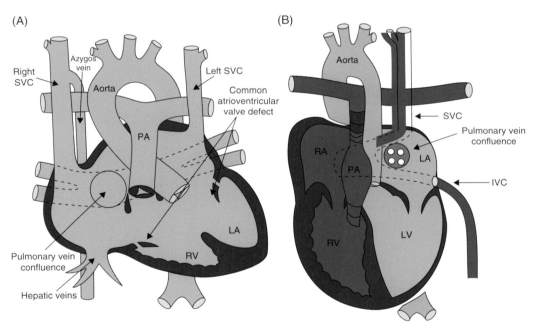

Figure 36.3 Examples of heterotaxy anatomy and repair. (A) Example of complex heterotaxy anatomy. Depicted here is levocardia, normally related great vessels, left atrial isomerism (polysplenia syndrome or bilateral left sidedness), bilateral SVCs without a connecting (innominate) vein, complete atrioventricular canal (CAVC) defect with almost complete absence of the intraatrial septum and a very large ventricular septal defect, anomalous pulmonary venous connection to the right side of the atrium, interrupted IVC with hepatic venous drainage directly to the floor of the right side of the atrium and drainage of the infrahepatic portion of the IVC via the azygos vein to the right SVC. (B) Complete repair in a patient with CAVC, double-outlet right ventricle (DORV), pulmonary stenosis (PS), total anomalous pulmonary venous return (TAPVR) to the SVC, and drainage of the SVC and IVC to the morphologic left atrium (LA). Repair consists of CAVC repair, ventricular septal defect closure to baffle the left ventricle (LV) to the aorta, placement of a right ventricle (RV) to pulmonary artery (PA) conduit, anastomosis of the pulmonary venous confluence to the posterior wall of the LA, and a Mustard procedure to baffle caval blood across the tricuspid valve to the RV and pulmonary venous blood across the mitral valve to the LV. Also seen are stents placed in the SVC baffle and in the PA postoperatively in the cardiac catheterization laboratory. IVC, inferior vena cava; SVC, superior vena cava.

References and Further Reading

Fliegauf, M., Benzing, T. & Omran, H. When cilia go bad: cilia defects and ciliopathies. *Nat Rev Mol Cell Biol* **8**, 880–893 (2007).

Lytrivi, I.D. & Lai, W.W. Cardiac malpositions and heterotaxy syndrome. In: Lai, W.W., Mertens, L.L., Cohen, M.S. & Geva, T. (eds) *Echocardiography in Pediatric and Congenital Heart Disease: From Fetus to Adult*, 2nd edn. John Wiley & Sons, Chichester (2016).

Williams, G.D. & Feng, A. Heterotaxy syndrome: implications for anesthesia management. *J Cardiothorac Vasc Anesth* **24**, 834–844 (2010).

Yim, D., Nagata, H., Lam, C. *et al.* Disharmonious patterns of heterotaxy and isomerism: how often are the classic patterns breached? *Circ Cardiovasc Imaging* **11**, e006917 (2018).

37

Ebstein Anomaly

Introduction

Ebstein anomaly is an uncommon disorder occurring in about 3–5 babies in 100,000 live births, and accounts for 0.38–0.50% of all congenital heart diseases. The incidence of Ebstein anomaly in the fetus is higher due to the fact that the fetal form is generally very severe and easily detected, whereas milder forms may not be detected until late childhood or adolescence.

Anatomy

Ebstein anomaly is characterized by downward displacement of the septal and posterior leaflet hingepoints of the tricuspid valve (TV) from the atrioventricular junction into the right ventricular cavity (Figures 37.1 and 37.2). This is the result of adhesion of the leaflets to the underlying ventricular wall, with underdevelopment of the chordae and papillary muscles. The septal leaflet is commonly small and also dysplastic. The anterior leaflet is not adherent and the hingepoint is located at the true TV annulus. The anterior leaflet, however, is elongated ("sail-like"), malformed, may have multiple fenestrated orifices, and has abnormal chordal attachments.

As a consequence of these changes, the true TV annulus is dilated and there is atrialization of the right ventricular cavity. At the severe end of the spectrum, the right ventricle consists of only the trabecular and outflow portions. Anatomic pulmonary stenosis or atresia may also be present which must be distinguished from functional pulmonary atresia. The TV orifice(s) is typically directed toward the right ventricular outflow tract (RVOT). The TV is usually regurgitant. There is a patent foramen ovale (PFO) or secundum atrial septal defect (ASD). Left ventricular geometry can be altered by leftward bowing of the ventricular septum. A Wolff–Parkinson–White type of accessory pathway is present in 10–20% cases. These pathways are usually located around the orifice of the TV.

Physiology

There is a broad spectrum of physiology present in patients with Ebstein anomaly. In the mildest form, mild tricuspid regurgitation (TR), diminished right ventricular function, and/or atrial and reentrant arrhythmias lead to disease detection in late childhood or adolescence. As the TR progresses and right ventricular function diminishes, there will be cyanosis due to right-to-left (R-L) physiologic shunting at the PFO or ASD secondary to elevated right atrial pressures. In the severest form, the presence of severe TR and a small, poorly contractile functional right ventricle combined with the physiologic elevation in the PVR after birth and ductus blood flow will result in little or no antegrade pulmonary

The Pediatric Cardiac Anesthesia Handbook, Second Edition. Viviane G. Nasr and James A. DiNardo.
© 2025 John Wiley & Sons Ltd. Published 2025 by John Wiley & Sons Ltd.

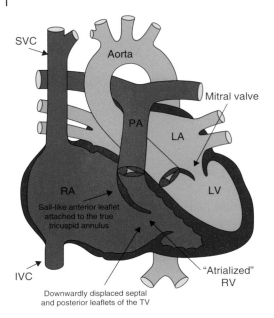

Figure 37.1 Ebstein anomaly of the tricuspid valve. RA, right atria; LA, left atria; LV, left ventricle; RV, right ventricle; PA, pulmonary artery; Ao, aorta, TV, tricuspid valve.

blood flow (PBF), leading to functional pulmonary atresia (PA). These patients present *in utero* or immediately after birth with cardiomegaly, hydrops, and arrhythmia, with mortality rates as high as 48%. Many of these patients have a massive right atrium and atrialized right ventricular enlargement with the size of these two structures equal to or greater than the size of the other three cardiac chambers (left atrium, left ventricle, true right ventricle) combined.

The Great Ormond Street Echocardiogram (GOSE) score utilizes the Celermajer index to stratify the risk of death in the neonate. The Celermajer index is derived from a four-chamber view at end-diastole obtained echocardiographically. It is the calculated ratio of the sum of the right atrium and atrialized RV areas to the sum of the remaining chambers (RV + LV + LA) as follows:

- Ratio < 0.5 Grade 1
- Ratio 0.5–0.99 Grade 2
- Ratio 1–1.4 Grade 3
- Ratio ≥1.5 Grade 4.

The relationship between the Celermajer ratio and the GOSE score and mortality is summarized as shown in Table 37.1.

The heart can occupy the majority of the thoracic cavity, resulting in lung hypoplasia. Pulmonary blood flow will be supplied by L-R physiologic shunting across the ductus arteriosus and whatever antegrade flow across the RVOT is present; the patients will be prostaglandin E_1 (PGE_1) dependent. There will be obligatory R-L physiologic shunting at the atria due to a very high right atrial pressure. These patients are cyanotic because the systemic cardiac output will be dependent on blood delivered to the left atrium and left ventricle across the atrial septum from the right atrium (deoxygenated) and from the pulmonary veins (oxygenated). Furthermore, paradoxical motion of the intraventricular septum and rightward shift of the septum of the ventricular septum into the LV will further impair systemic blood flow by impairing LV filling.

Approximately 30% of patients presenting as neonates will have pulmonary regurgitation (PR). The latter develops as a consequence of severe TR, a lack of antegrade pulmonary valve flow, retrograde ductal flow, low right ventricular pressure, and the high pulmonary vascular resistance (PVR) of the newborn. The presence of PR, TR, and a ductus arteriosus creates circular shunt physiology whereby the path of blood flow is aorta to ductus to pulmonary artery to right ventricle to right atrium to left atrium to left ventricle to aorta. This results in a compromised systemic oxygen delivery and further volume overloading of the right atrium and atrialized right ventricle. This shunt physiology is associated with very high fetal and neonatal mortality.

Medical Management

Neonates who are reasonably stable are treated with supplemental oxygen and PGE_1 to maintain ductal patency and are closely observed for the adequacy of the cardiac output and oxygen saturations.

Figure 37.2 Anatomic specimen (A), apical four-chamber echocardiographic image (B), and cardiac computed tomography image (C) in severe Ebstein anomaly all demonstrate severe displacement of the tricuspid valve leaflets into the apex of the right ventricle with severe enlargement of the right atrium and atrialized portion of the right ventricle. The left ventricle is compressed due to the massive right-sided volume overload. The anterior TV leaflet has multiple muscular tethering points along its length. The septal leaflet is not delaminated in all three images. aRV, atrialized right ventricle; LA, left atrium; LV, left ventricle; RA, right atrium. *Source:* Reproduced from Cetta F et.al. 2015/with permission of John Wiley & Sons.

Table 37.1 Relationship between Celemajer ratio, GOSE score, and mortality.

GOSE score	Celermajer ratio	Mortality
1–2	< 1.0 (Grade 1 and 2)	8%
3 (acyanotic)	1.1–1.4 (Grade 3)	10% early, 45% late
3 (cyanotic)	1.1–1.4 (Grade 3)	100%
4	> 1.5 (Grade 4)	100%

Treatment of unstable patients involves intubation, deep sedation, and muscle relaxation to reduce systemic oxygen consumption and facilitate mechanical ventilation. Large tidal volumes (10–12 ml kg^{-1}) are utilized to offset the effects of gross cardiomegaly on lung expansion, and ventilation is further adjusted to decrease PVR. In addition to the initiation of PGE_1, inhaled nitric oxide (iNO) is utilized to reduce PVR and promote antegrade pulmonary blood flow.

If the patient remains physiologically stable without cyanosis and there is echocardiographic and physiologic evidence that antegrade PBF is present, a trial of discontinuing PGE$_1$ is undertaken to initiate ductal closure to determine the next steps (Antegrade PBF pathway in Figure 37.3). If there is functional PA, it should be determined over the course of 1–2 days if antegrade PBF has developed as PVR drops. Here again, a trial off PGE$_1$ is undertaken to initiate ductal closure to determine the next steps (Functional PA, Stable pathway in Figure 37.3). The critically unstable neonate with functional PA is likely to have a circular shunt due to the presence of PR (Functional PA, Critically unstable pathway in Figure 37.3).

Surgical Treatment

Surgical therapy for children and adolescents involves the cone procedure, so named because the shape of the TV following the repair resembles a cone. In this procedure, the septal, anterior, and posterior tricuspid valve leaflets are delaminated from their attachments in the right ventricle, and the chordal attachments to the apical portion of the right ventricle are left. After the three leaflets are sutured together to form a cone-shaped structure that is tethered only by apical and some infundibular chords, they are reattached at the native atrioventricular (AV) valve annulus. TV inflow will then be directed toward the right ventricular apex rather than the outflow tract. Plication of the thin inferior free wall of the right ventricle (atrialized portion) is also done. A TV

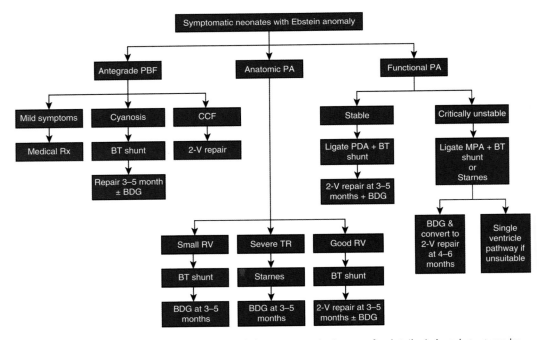

Figure 37.3 Management algorithm for neonatal Ebstein anomaly. See text for details. A ductal stent can be utilized as an alternative to a BT shunt in any circumstance where a BT shunt is the only proposed surgical procedure. An alternative to the modified Starnes procedure is the Sano right ventricular exclusion procedure. PBF, pulmonary blood flow; PA, pulmonary atresia; CCF, congestive cardiac failure; BT, Blalock–Thomas–Taussig; BDG, bidirectional Glenn; RV, right ventricle; TR, tricuspid regurgitation; PDA, patent ductus arteriosus; MPA, main pulmonary artery. *Source:* Reproduced from Knott-Craig and Boston (2021)/with permission of Elsevier.

annuloplasty ring may also be placed. The PFO or ASD may be left with a 4 mm fenestration if there is concern that a small R-L physiologic shunt will be necessary to augment cardiac output in the presence of right ventricular dysfunction.

In instances where TV repair is adequate but right ventricle function or size is insufficient to support adequate cardiac output, a 1.5 ventricle repair as employed in PA/IVS patients (see Chapter 23) should be considered. This consists of a bidirectional Glenn (BDG) in conjunction with a cone procedure and a fenestrated ASD (R-L "pop off") or ASD closure. This repair allows all or most IVC blood to cross the tricuspid valve and be ejected by the right ventricle antegrade into the pulmonary bed, while SVC blood is delivered directly to the pulmonary arteries.

The surgical management of neonates is challenging, and there is no clear consensus on optimal management strategy. An example of a comprehensive decision tree which considers PGE$_1$ dependency to maintain pulmonary blood, the presence of anatomic or functional pulmonary atresia, RV size, and the presence of tricuspid regurgitation is illustrated in Figure 37.3.

The modified Starnes right ventricular exclusion procedure involves:

- ligation of the main pulmonary artery if the valve is incompetent, and ligation of the PDA
- patch closure of the TV with a Gore-Tex® or pericardial patch; the patch has a 4 mm fenestration to allow for RV decompression. Patch placement allows the coronary sinus to drain to the right atrium
- creation of an unrestricted atrial septum
- creation of Blalock–Thomas–Taussig shunt
- atrioplasty to reduce the size of the right atrium to allow for growth of the lungs.

A further modification of the modified Starnes procedure is the Sano right ventricular exclusion procedure. In addition to all the components of the modified Starnes procedure, it includes excision of the redundant thinned-out right ventricular free wall and repair of the resultant defect. This results in the volume reduction of a dilated RV and prevention of late leftward diastolic movement of the ventricular septum and compression of the LV.

Anesthetic Management in Ebstein Anomaly

For children presenting for an elective cone procedure, the primary management issues are TR, reduced right ventricular function, potential for R-L physiologic shunting at the atrial level and, in some patients, dysfunction from an abnormal left ventricular geometry.

Goals

- Maintain sinus rhythm when possible.
- Maintain heart rate at a faster rate, better than slower rate.
- Decrease right ventricular afterload; increases are poorly tolerated. Decreasing the afterload will improve cardiac output by decreasing regurgitation, but the preload must be maintained.
- Maintain contractility; there may be significant right ventricular dysfunction.
- When pulmonary vascular resistance is high, or when right ventricular systolic dysfunction exists, the right ventricular afterload reduction will improve the right ventricular and subsequently the left ventricular output. The concurrent systemic vasodilation also will directly reduce regurgitation.
- Avoid hypercarbia, hypoxemia and acidemia, which tend to cause pulmonary hypertension and may result in acute right ventricular decompensation.
- Cardiac output can be maintained at the expense of cyanosis in the presence of poor antegrade pulmonary blood flow (right ventricular dysfunction or high PVR) if there is significant R-L physiologic shunting at the atrial level.

Neonates with Ebstein anomaly presenting for surgery are critically ill. In the absence of antegrade pulmonary blood flow, they have ductal-dependent, single-ventricle physiology that is complicated by the presence of massively dilated, mechanically ineffective right heart structures (right atrium and atrialized right ventricle). They are dependent on mechanical ventilation managed to minimize mean airway pressure so as not to mechanically impede any antegrade pulmonary blood flow. The presence of lung hypoplasia can make the achievement of adequate alveolar ventilation at a low mean airway pressure difficult.

These neonates are usually sedated and paralyzed to facilitate mechanical ventilation and to reduce systemic oxygen consumption in the setting of marginal systemic oxygen delivery. Neonates with ductal-dependent pulmonary blood flow must have ductal patency maintained with PGE_1. Those with antegrade pulmonary blood flow may be able to be weaned off PGE_1 to allow ductal closure or reduction in ductal size. In all likelihood, they will be receiving iNO to reduce PVR and promote antegrade flow.

Post-CPB Management

Repaired tricuspid valves may exhibit some residual mild TR and tricuspid stenosis (TS). Transesophageal echocardiography (TEE) or epicardial echocardiography is essential in evaluating valvular repairs. In the absence of significant residual TR or TS, the management of patients having undergone the cone procedure will be dictated by the size and pressure-generating capacity of the true right ventricle. It is necessary to maintain right ventricular contractile function and to reduce the PVR. Inotropic support may be necessary. Dopamine 5–10 µg kg^{-1} min^{-1} or epinephrine 0.05–0.1 µg kg^{-1} min^{-1} are reasonable choices. Milrinone 0.5–1.0 µg kg^{-1} min^{-1} may also be employed to reduce PVR. However, milrinone's weak inotropic properties and its potent effects on systemic vascular resistance (SVR) limit the effectiveness of this drug. A better alternative would be inhaled nitric oxide. Mechanical ventilation should be managed to avoid hypercarbia and to minimize mean airway pressure so as not to mechanically impede antegrade pulmonary blood flow.

Neonates undergoing aortopulmonary shunt insertion (modified Blalock–Thomas–Taussig shunt) and ductus arteriosus ligation are managed according to the principles outlined in Chapter 28.

References and Further Reading

Dearani, J.A. Ebstein repair: How I do it. *JTCVS Tech* **3**, 269–276 (2020).

Lang, R.M., Badano, L., Mor-Avi, V. *et al.* Recommendations for cardiac chamber quantification by echocardiography in adults: an update from the American Society of Echocardiography and the European Association of Cardiovascular Imaging. *J Am Soc Echocardiogr* **28**, 1–39. e14 (2015).

Sainathan, S., da Silva, L.F. & da Silva, J.P. Ebstein's anomaly: contemporary management strategies. *J Thorac Dis* **12**, 1161–1173 (2020).

Index

Note: Page numbers with figures in *italic* and and tables in **bold**.

22q11.2 deletion syndrome 24–25. *See also* DiGeorge syndrome
22q11.2 microdeletion 235

a
ABO compatibility, heart transplantation 289, 291, **291**
acetylcholine 6, 7, 304, 305
acetylcholinesterase inhibitors 305–306
acetylcysteine 311
acid–base management 70, 71–72, 265
acid–base status 36, 38, 65
acidemia 135, 201, 202, 205, 337
acidosis 4, 72, 241, 314, 315
  intracellular 71
  lactic 237
  marked hypercarbia with 315
  metabolic 131, 156, 185, 189, 216, 236
activated clotting time (ACT) 73–74
  monitoring of UFH anticoagulation **112**
  prolongation 74, 75
activated form of PC (APC) 44, 45

activated partial thromboplastin time (aPTT) 41, 73, 74, 113
acute kidney injury (AKI) 141
acute normovolemic hemodilution (ANH) 46, 68
adenosine **29**, 305
"adult" coarctation 153
adult structure correspondences, embryologic structures 3, **4**, **6**
adverse events (AEs) 103
afterload mismatch 7, 147, 295
  left ventricular 202, 279
  left ventricular decompensation 239
  right ventricular 168, 170, 175, 186, 189, 220, 298, 299, 314
air entrainment 63
air-trap filters in IV lines 28
airway equipment 28
airway management 38, 165
akinetic areas 52–53
albumin 141, 220
alcohol abuse, environmental factors causing CHD 3
alkalosis 19, 72, 237
allergies 23

allograft implantation 315
allograft replacement 198
alpha-2-antiplasmin 46
alpha-2-macroglobulin 46
alpha-stat management 71–72
alpha-stat regulation 70–71
alveolar ventilation 4, 7, 110, 111, 230, 316, 338
American Heart Association (AHA) 303
amiodarone **29**, 223
Amplatzer™ 146
anaerobic metabolism 8, 251
analgesics 66, 127. *See also* pain management
anastomosis 297
  atriopulmonary 258
  BDG 211
  cavopulmonary 258, *258*, *259*, 273
  distal 220
  DKS 181, *257*, 271, 278
  end-to-end *156*, *157*, 185, 217, 282
  nonrestrictive surgical 190
  pulmonary artery *297*, 298, 299
  of pulmonary venous 189
  right atrial *296*
  stenotic 260
  tracheal 309

The Pediatric Cardiac Anesthesia Handbook, Second Edition. Viviane G. Nasr and James A. DiNardo.
© 2025 John Wiley & Sons Ltd. Published 2025 by John Wiley & Sons Ltd.

anatomic coronary artery
lesions   22
anatomic coronary
lesions   54–55
anatomic repair. *See* arterial
switch operation (ASO)
anatomic shunts   10, 15
anatomic R-L shunt   14
complex shunts   17–18
orifice size and total outflow
resistance   *17*
simple shunts   15, **16**
anatomy:
anomalous aortic origin
of coronary
artery   323
anomalous left coronary
artery from pulmonary
artery   321
aortopulmonary
window   149
atrial septal defects   161
atrioventricular canal
defects   171–173, *172*
coarctation of aorta
153, *155*, *156*
congenitally corrected
transposition of great
vessels   *243*, 243–244
coronary anatomy
53–54, *54*
of double cavopulmonary
anastomosis   *258*
double outlet right
ventricle   177–179
Ebstein anomaly   333
heterotaxy   327
hypoplastic left heart
syndrome   269
interrupted aortic arch
275, **278**
left ventricular outflow tract
193–195
mitral valve regurgitation
203
mitral valve stenosis
199–200, *200*
patent ductus arteriosus
145

pulmonary atresia with
intact ventricular
septum   207, *208*
pulmonary vascular
anatomy   58–60
segmental anatomy   **97**
Tetralogy of Fallot
213, *214*
Tetralogy of Fallot with
absent pulmonary
valve   229
Tetralogy of Fallot with
pulmonary atresia
225, *226*
total anomalous pulmonary
venous return
187–188
transposition of great
arteries   233–234
tricuspid atresia   285
truncus arteriosus   183
vascular rings   281
ventricular septal
defects   167
anemia   23, 24, 66
anesthesia   18, 293, 314
deployment of PDA
occlusion devices   146
hypercarbia   18
hypoxemia   18
"Tet spells" under   216
anesthesiologist(s)
challenges   9, 27, 216, 220,
300, 309
preoperative
evaluation   292
anesthetic agents   21
anesthetic induction
27, 120, 150,
293–295, 313–315.
See also ventricular assist
device (VAD)
intramuscular
induction   39
intravenous induction
39–40, 169, 175, 221, 253
anesthetic maintenance
39–40, 120, 150, 221,
293–295, 313–315

anesthetic management   292
AAOCA   325
ALCAPA   322
DORV   181
in Ebstein Anomaly
337–338
goals   310
heart–lung transplantation
310
hypoplastic left heart
syndrome   271–272
interrupted aortic
arch   278–279
left ventricular outflow
tract   196–198
management of one-lung
ventilation   311–313
mitral valve regurgitation
204–205
mitral valve stenosis
201–202
pathophysiology
characteristics of
cardiomyopathies
294
physical examination   292
pre-bypass   120
pre-Fontan   264–265
preinduction
292–293, 311
preinitial repair   251–253
premedication
292, 310–311
preoperative evaluation
292, 310
presuperior cavopulmonary
shunt   259
pulmonary atresia/intact
ventricular septum   211
regional wall motion
abnormalities   323
risk factors for adverse
cardiac events in
children   **197**
special considerations for
SLT and BSSLT
315–316
Tetralogy of Fallot
220–221

Tetralogy of Fallot with
absent pulmonary
valve   230
Tetralogy of Fallot with
pulmonary atresia   227
total anomalous pulmonary
venous return   189–190
tricuspid atresia   287–288
truncus arteriosus
185–186
vascular rings   283–284
aneurysms   157, 167, 229, 295
angina   300, 302
angiographic data   26
angiography   49
angiotensin-converting
enzyme (ACE) inhibitors
30, 159, 174, 303
angiotensin II receptor
blockers (ARB)
30, 303
annuloplasty   122, 203,
204, 337
anomalous aortic origin of
coronary artery
(AAOCA)   101,
323–325, *324*
anomalous left coronary
artery from pulmonary
artery (ALCAPA)
22, 101, 321–322, *322*
anomalous origin of right
coronary artery from
pulmonary artery
(ARCAPA)   101
anomalous right coronary
artery (ARCA)   *325*
antegrade cerebral perfusion
(ACP)   72–73
anterior leaflets   98, 164, 199,
203, 328, 333
anterolateral
commissures   199
antibodies   76, 298
anticholinergic agents   306
anticoagulation   73–74, 77,
112, **112**, 200. *See also*
activated clotting time
(ACT); heparin

antidysrhythmics   **29**
antifibrinolytics   83, 120, 314
antihypertensive drugs   **30**
antithrombin III (ATIII)
44, 74
antithymocyte globulin (ATG)
303, 318
anxiety   27, 28, 30, 292, 311
aortic cross-clamping   158
aortic diastolic pressure
21–22
aortic pressure waveform   51
aortic regurgitation (AR)   51,
61, 196, 204
aortic saturation   12, 15
aortic valve stenosis
153, *194*, 195
aortography   51
aortopulmonary collaterals
(APCs)   72
aortopulmonary shunts,
patency of   101
aortopulmonary window
(AP)   149–151, *150*
aortotomy   198, 324
apnea   130, 237, 314
Ardnt blockers   303
argatroban   112
arrhythmias   165, 175, 200
atrial   263, 296, 303, 333
ventricular   219, 223, 292,
303, 323
arterial blood, fetal circulation
4–5, *5*
arterial hypertension
302–303
arterial line catheter sizes   **34**
arterial line filter (ALF)   64
arterial saturation (SaO$_2$)   12,
15, 40, 155, 214, 236, 241,
250, *257*, 314
arterial switch operation (ASO)
237–239, *238*
artery:
axillary   33, 50, 219
brachial   33, 50, 73
carotid   110, 219
femoral   33, 50, 65, 146,
219, 311

radial   33, 73, 311
subclavian   23, 33,
145, 153, 157, 219,
275–279, 281,
282, 292
artificial heart   292
ascites   23, 141, 264
asphyxia   10
aspiration risks   313
asplenia syndrome   330
associated congenital
abnormalities, CHD
24–27
atelectasis   19, 120, 220, 253
atrial anatomy   327
atrial and ventricular
arrhythmias   303
atrial fibrillation   303
atrial function   296, 301
atrial hypertension   59–60,
91, 155, 156, 190, 211,
236, 242–243, 267,
272, 279
atrial identity and
location   98
atrial kick   49
atrial reentrant
tachycardia   223
atrial septal aneurysms   295
atrial septal defects (ASDs)
39, 50, 100, 156, 161, 171,
188, 207, 233, 269, 285,
333. *See also* ventricular
septal defects (VSDs)
anatomy   161
anesthetic management
164–165
catheterization laboratory
intervention   164
device closure   *164*
induction and
maintenance   165
noncardiac surgery   165
ostium primum   *162*
ostium secundum   *163*
physiology   163–164
post-CPB management   165
surgical therapy   164
types   *162*

atrial septectomy   250, 260,
   271
atrial situs   327
atrial switch-Rastelli
      procedures   244–246
atrial thrombus   295
atriopulmonary
      anastomosis   258
atrioventricular (AV)
   canal-type VSDs   177
   groove   53, 295
   junction   330
   nodal branch   53
   relationship   99
   valve   167, 171, 244,
      328, 336
atrioventricular canal (AVCs)
      defects   171
   anatomy   171–173, *172*
   anesthetic management
      174, 174–175
   induction and maintenance
      174–175
   noncardiac surgery   175
   physiology   173–174
   post-CPB management
      175
   surgical therapy   174
atropine   **29**, 295,
      304–306
autonomic innervations   8
autonomic nervous system
      300–301
A wave   49
axial continuous flow devices
      115–118
axial pump
      technology   116–118
axillary artery   33, 50, 219
azathioprine   **304**
azygous veins   187, 256

b

bacterial endocarditis   303
baffle obstruction   100
baffle pressure   265, 267
balloon angioplasty   26, **105**
balloon atrial septostomy
      (BAS)   236, 250

balloon septostomy   26
balloon valvuloplasty   26
basiliximab   **304**
BDG anastomosis   211
benzodiazepine   129, 202,
      253, 293
Berlin Heart EXCOR®
      VAD   113, *114*
beta-adrenergic
      agonists   217, 305
beta-adrenergic
      antagonists   305
beta-adrenergic
      catecholamines   7
beta-blockers   **30**, 159
biatrial heart transplant
      technique   295, 301
bicarbonate   216
bicaval heart transplant
      technique   296
bidirectional Glenn shunt
      (BDG)   210, 247,
      254–264, 337
bidirectional shunting   15,
      185, 236
bilateral sequential single-lung
      transplantation
      (BSSLT)   308–310,
      315–316
BiVAD insertion   123
bivalirudin   74, *75*, 112
biventricular conversion   273
biventricular repair   272–273
bladder   71
Blalock–Taussig shunt   24
Blalock–Thomas–Taussig
      shunt (BTTS)
      33, 73, 217
Bland–White–Garland
      syndrome   321
blood bank   120
blood gas
      management   69–71
blood pressure   33–34
blood pressure cuffs   33, 34
blood urea nitrogen
      (BUN)   120
blood volumes   66, 68, 69, 71,
      73, 74

B-natriuretic peptide
      (BNP)   120
body surface area (BSA)
      56, 60, 65
"borderline" left heart   272
brachial arteries
      33, 50, 73
brachiocephalic trunk
      277, 281
bradycardia   204, 305
bradykinin   7, 77
brain cooling   72
brain death, donors   298
brain emboli   38
bridge-to-bridge
      transplantation   113
bridge to decision   113
bridge to recovery   113
bridge to transplantation   113
bronchial blockers
      311, **312**, 313
bronchial vein blood   63
bronchiolitis obliterans
      (BO)   318
bronchiolitis obliterans
      syndrome (BOS)   318
bronchoscope/bronchoscopy
      283–284, 313
   fiberoptic   311, 313, 315
   rigid   284, 317
bulboventricular foramen
      (BVF)   98
bulbus cordis   **4**
Burkholderia cepecia   308

c

calcineurin inhibitors   303
calcium   7, 20
calcium entry blockers   303,
      305
calcium gluconate   **29**
canal-type VSDs   167, 177
cannulas   63
   aortic   63, 69, 73
   arterial   65, 73, 74
carbohydrates   8
cardiac allograft vasculopathy
      (CAV)   302
cardiac catheterization   209

cardiac catheterization data
  interpretation   49
  angiographic data   26
  assessment of pulmonary
    vascular anatomy   58–60
  assessment of valve lesions
    60–61
  cardiac output determination
    55–56
  cardiac shunts evaluation
    56–58
  coronary angiography
    53–55
  functional status   26
  left ventriculography
    51–53
  left-heart catheterization
    50–51
  pressure data   26
  prior surgical
    interventions   26
  pulmonary arterial
    hypertension   59
  pulmonary vascular
    anatomy assessments
    58–60
  resistances   58
  right-heart catheterization
    49–50
  saturations   56, 58
  valve lesions'
    assessments   60–61
cardiac index (CI)   58, 60,
  131, 202, 310, 316
cardiac MRI scans   27
cardiac output (CO)   55–56, 58
cardiac shunts evaluation
  56–58
cardiac surgery   103–105
cardinal venous system   187
cardiomyopathy (CM)
  109, 289
cardiopulmonary bypass
  (CPB)   19, 28, 33, 63, *64*,
  145, 149, 157, 165, 169,
  197, 217, 241, 248, 277,
  287, 309
  ACP   72–73
  adult and pediatric   **65**

anesthesia during   66
anticoagulation   73–74
blood gas management
  69–71
circuit size and component
  selection   65–66
configurations   *67*
DHCA   71–72
differences between adult
  and pediatric   65–69
flow rates   65, **66**
indications for   316
monitoring during   66
post-CPB hemostasis
  77–83
protamine reversal of
  heparin   74–77
rate relative to patient
  temperature   **66**
use of   309–310
cardiopulmonary bypass
  (CPB)   293
cardiotomy suction   64
cardiovascular
  development   3
cardiovascular
  physiology   3–7
  embryology   3, **4**
  myocardial performance in
    neonate   **7**, 7–8
carotid artery   110, 219
catheter-based therapy
  209–211
catheterization   103. *See also*
  cardiac catheterization
  data interpretation
  laboratory intervention
  146, 150, 157, 164, 169,
  185, 196, 200, 204, 219,
  278, 283
  left-heart   50–51
  right-heart   49–50
Catheterization Risk Score for
  Pediatrics (CRISP)   103
cavopulmonary anastomosis
  258, *258*, *259*, 273
cavopulmonary shunts,
  patency of   101
Celermajer index   334

central shunt   217
central venous pressure
  (CVP)   34–35, **35**, 58,
  66, 221, 299, 315
centrifugal continuous flow
  devices   118–119
centrifugal pump
  technology   118–119
CentriMag™   118
cerebral metabolic rate for
  oxygen (CMRO$_2$)   71
cerebral microemboli   38
cerebral oximetry   36
cerebral oxygenation   72
cerebral spinal fluid (CSF)   157
chest:
  heart position in   327
  radiograph   25
Chiari network   4
Children's Hospital
  Boston   *75*, 145
ciliary dysfunction   331
cineangiograms   26, 52, 54
cis-atracurium   39
classic cascade   41, *42*
clot formation   43
coagulation, inhibition of
  44–45
coarctation of aorta   153
  anatomy   153, *155*, *156*
  anesthetic management
    157–159
  appearance of   *154*
  catheterization laboratory
    intervention   157
  echocardiography of
    coarction   *154*
  induction and
    maintenance   158
  management after
    cross-clamp removal
    158–159
  noncardiac surgery   159
  physiology   153–156
  surgical therapy   157
coils   146
Collett and Edwards
  classifications, truncus
  arteriosus (TA)   5

color flow (CF) Doppler
91, 99
COMFORT-B scale   131
complete atrioventricular canal
defect (CAVC defect)
330, *331*
complete AVC (CAVC)
171–173, *172, 173*
complex congenital
heart disease
(CHD)   289
complex shunts   17–18
comprehensive
echocardiographic exam
goals   96
atrial identity and
location   98
atrioventricular
relationship   99
great vessel orientation and
identity   99
intracardiac shunts and
obstructive lesions
99–100
segmental anatomy   **97**
surgical repair
evaluation   100–101
ventricular size and
identity   98–99
ventriculoarterial
relationship   99
computed tomography
angiography (CTA)
321, 323
conal morphology
177, *179*
conduction defects   170
cone procedure
336–338
Congenital Cardiac
Catheterization Project
on Outcomes
(C3PO)   103
Congenital Cardiac
Interventional Study
Consortium
(CCISC)   103
congenital diaphragmatic
hernia   109

congenital heart disease
(CHD)   3, 9, 24, 33, 153,
171, 187
anatomic shunts   15–18
common syndromes and
associated   **25**
control of pulmonary
vascular resistance
19–21
intercirculatory mixing
13–15
myocardial ischemia
21–22
pathophysiology   9
pulmonary vascular
pathophysiology   18–19
shunting   9–10
single-ventricle physiology
10–12
Congenital Heart Surgery
Nomenclature and
Database Project   177
congenitally corrected
transposition of great
vessels (C-TGV)
243–246, *243*
congestive heart failure
(CHF)   169, 174, 185,
216, 238, 287
conoventricular defects   167
conoventricular septal
defect   214, 275
conoventricular septum
169, 277
continuous-wave (CW)
Doppler   91, 99, 101
continuous positive airway
pressure (CPAP)   313
contractile capacity,
reduced   7
conventional ultrafiltration
(CUF)   69
cooling and rewarming
35, 40
Cornell Assessment of
Pediatric Delirium
(CAPD)   131
coronary anatomy   53–54,
235, 237

coronary angiography   53–55
coronary artery:
anatomy in C-TGV   244
in D-TGA   233
supply   **55**
coronary artery bypass
grafting (CABG)   322
coronary artery disease
(CAD)   302
coronary bypass grafting   325
coronary collaterals   55
coronary ostia   22, 53,
209, 237, 242–243,
299, 316
coronary perfusion pressure
(CPP)   21, 36,
145, 253
coronary sinus (CS)   328
coronary sinus (CS)
defects   161, 163
coronary stenotic lesions   54
coronary vascular reserve
(CVR)   22
corticosteroids   303
cor triatriatum   18, 59,
199, 200
cough reflexes   317, 318
creatinine   120
cross-clamp removal,
management after
158–159
crux cordis   53
crystalloid prime   66, 67
custom tubing packs   65
C wave   49
cyanosis   18, 23–24, 46,
185, 333
differential   276
reverse differential   236
in single-ventricle
lesions   285
cyclic adenosine
monophosphate
(cAMP)   20
cyclic guanosine
monophosphate
(cGMP)   20
cyclosporine   303, **304**
cystic fibrosis (CF)   307

cystic fibrosis transmembrane conductance regulator (CFTR) 307
cytomegalovirus (CMV) 302, 318

d
daclizumab **304**
Dacron® patch aortoplasty 157
Damus–Kaye–Stansel anastomosis (DKS anastomosis) 181, 249, *257*, 271, 278
de-airing needs, heart transplants 299
decannulation 111
deep hypothermic circulatory arrest (DHCA) 28, 254
  background 71–72
  definition 35
definitive repair for TOF 218, 221
dehydration 28
delirium 131
deoxyhemoglobin 23, 36
dependent shunts 15
desflurane 21
desmopressin (DDAVP) 81–81
destination therapy 113
dexmedetomidine 21, 127, 130–131
dextro (D) 99
dextrocardia 327
dextrose 28
diabetes. *See also* obesity
  environmental factors causing CHD 3
  heart transplant contraindications 289
diagnosis:
  congenital heart disease 23–30
  cyanosis 23, 155, 276
  respiratory tract infections 23
diaphoresis 149

diastolic function impairments, heart transplants 301–302
diastolic pressure 7–8, 21–22, 49, 51, 120, 122, 195, 263–264
DiGeorge syndrome 24, 213
digoxin 30, 304
dilated cardiomyopathy (DCM) 289, 322
dilution effects on blood volume **65**
direct thrombin inhibitor (DTI) 74, 112
direct vasodilators 170
distal anastomosis 220
distal aortic blood flow 269
distal conus 177
distal limb ischemia 33
diuretics 30, 141
diverticular disease **291**
dobutamine 21, 203, 221, 248
donor 308–309
  brain death 298
  double-lung block 309
  double-lung transplantation 307, 308
  heart–lung transplants 307
  heart transplants 302, 305
  living donor lobar lung transplants 308
  single-lung transplants 309
dopamine 8, **29**, 132, 190, 202, 203, 248, 265, 279, 295, 299
  in hypotension 198
  LVOT 198
  Tetralogy of Fallot 221
Doppler echocardiography 60
Doppler probes 36
dorsalis pedis arteries 33
doses, medications 8, 20–21, 28, 30, 39–40, 66, 73–74, 77, 79, 81, 113, 129–130, 135, 141, 159, 169, 175, 186, 198, 202–203, 216, 253, 295, 314

double-lumen endotracheal tube 313
double-lung transplantation (DLT) 307, 308
  anesthetic management 310–316
  definition 308
  donors 308–309
  noncardiac surgery 317–318
  operative procedure 309–310
  patient positioning 309–310
  post-CPB management 316
  postoperative care 316–317
  preoperative evaluation 310
  statistics 317
double-inlet left ventricle (DILV) 13
double-lung block 309
double outlet right ventricle (DORV) 99, 177
  anatomy 177–179
  anesthetic management 181
  conal morphology *179*
  distance from tricuspid valve to pulmonary valve *179*
  physiology 179–180
  post-CPB management 181
  surgical therapy 180–181
  variants of *178*
double switch procedure 244–246, *245*
drainage 18–19, 38, 63, 65, 110, 141, 162, 165, 187, 254, 256
drugs, environmental factors causing CHD 3
d-transposition of great arteries (D-TGA) 99, 233, 234, **236**
Duchenne muscular dystrophy **25**

ductal closure   154–155
ductal-dependent
    circulation   11
ductus arteriosus (DA)
    4, 154
    background   4–6, 154, 189,
        208, 275, 334, 338
    closure   5–6
ductus venosus   6
dyspnea   23
dysrhythmias   25, 131, 165,
    170, 240

e
early tracheal extubation
    138–139
Ebstein anomaly   333
    anatomy   333
    anesthetic management in
        337–338
    apical four-chamber
        echocardiographic
        image in   *335*
    medical management
        334–336
    physiology   333–334
    post-CPB management
        338
    relationship between
        Celemajer ratio, GOSE
        score, and mortality
        335
    surgical treatment
        336–337
    of tricuspid valve   334
ecarin clotting time
    (ECT)   74
echocardiography   27, 85,
    149, 248, 272, 300, 321
    goals of comprehensive
        echocardiographic
        exam   96–101
    TEE   85–96
    TTE   85
edema   18–19, 23, 38, 59,
    123, 140, 147, 155, 189,
    190, 200, 242, 254,
    272, 279
edrophonium   305, 306

effective arterial elastance
    (Ea)   132
effective blood flow   10, 236
effective pulmonary blood
    flow   10, 14, 236, 256
effective systemic blood
    flow   10, 14–15, 58,
    188, 236
Ehlers–Danlos syndrome   **25**
Eisenmenger syndrome   307
ejection fraction (EF)   51, 53,
    263
elastin gene
    microdeletion   193
electrocardiogram (ECG)   25,
    33–34, 292, 311
electrochemical
    neutrality   69–70
electrolytes   25
Ellis–van Creveld
    syndrome   **25**
emboli   38, 242
embryologic structures   3
embryology   3
en bloc DLT   309
end-diastolic volume
    (EDV)   22, 51, 169,
    204, 219, 251, 264,
    298, 314
endobronchial
    intubation   311
endocardial cushion defects.
    See atrioventricular canal
    defects (AVCs)
endocardial fibroelastosis
    (EFE)   272
endocarditis prophylaxis   165
endomyocardial
    biopsies   303, 306
end-organ dysfunction
    113, 119
endothelial NO synthase
    (eNOS)   20
endothelial protein C receptor
    (EPCR)   44
endotracheal tubes (ETT)
    311, 313
end-stage cardiac dysfunction,
    heart transplants   289

end-systolic volume
    (ESV)   219, 298
end-tidal carbon dioxide
    (ETCO$_2$)   34, 216, 253
enhanced recovery after
    surgery (ERAS)
    138–139
environmental factors causing
    CHD   3
ephedrine   **29**, 295, 305
epicardial A-V sequential
    pacing   170, 175
epicardial echocardiography
    (e-Echo)   95–96, 338
epinephrine   6, **29**, 132,
    135, 202, 203, 248,
    279, 299
epoprostenol   20
epsilon-aminocaproic acid
    (Amicar®)   45, 83
EQUANOX 7600 NIRS   36
erythrocytosis   46
esmolol   197–198, 217
esophageal compression   281
esophageal temperatures   35
esophagus, vascular
    rings   281
estimated blood volume
    (EBV)   68
etomidate   21, 39, 165, 197,
    205, 293, 313
Eustachian valve   4, 98
everolimus   **304**
expanded
    polytetrafluoroethylene
    (ePTFE)   217
extended CICU care
    139–141
extracardiac pulmonary
    blood flow   285
extracorporeal
    cardiopulmonary
    resuscitation
    (E–CPR)   109
extracorporeal life support
    (ECLS). *See*
    extracorporeal
    membrane oxygenation
    (ECMO)

extracorporeal membrane oxygenation (ECMO) 109, 237, 316
circuit in venoarterial support mode *110*
common terminology 111
device and patient complications 110–111
indications 109
intraoperative considerations for patients 111–113
modes of ECMO support 109
multitest monitoring of UFH anticoagulation during ECMO **112**
relative contraindications 109
E-Z blocker 313

f

Faces, Legs, Activity, Cry, and Consolability (FLACC) 131
facial dysmorphia 24
factor eight-inhibitor bypass activator (FEIBA™) 81
Fallot, Etienne 213
fasting periods 267–268
femoral arteries 33, 50, 65, 146, 216, 219, 279, 311
femoral vein 40, 49, 118, 146, 219, 271, 310
fenestrated Fontan 210, 264
fenoldopam mesylate 141
fentanyl 39–40, 66, 127–129, 146–147, 158, 165, 169, 175, 186, 190, 197–198, 202, 221, 241, 279, 293, 295, 305, 313
ferric iron gluconate 24
ferumoxytol 24
fetal alcohol syndrome **25**
fetal channels, closure 4
fetal circulation 3
ductus arteriosus 5–6
ductus venosus 6
fetal structures and structure in adults **6**

foramen ovale 6
in late gestation *5*
pulmonary vascular changes 6–7
fetal IVC blood 3
fetal shunts 4
fetus 6
fiberoptic bronchoscope 311, 313, 315
fibrin-bound plasminogen 45
fibrin degradation products (FDP) 45
fibrinogen repletion 79
fibrinolysis *45*, 45–46
Fick determination 55–56
Fick method for cardiac output determination 56
FIII. *See* tissue factor (TF)
FIO₂, 12, 20–21, 36, 57, 111, 174, 186, 227, 250, 252–253, 258–259, 265, 299, 308, 310, 314
FIX deficiency (hemophilia B) 41
flolan 20
fluid-filled catheter 49–50
fluid retention 141, 237
fluid therapy, preoperative evaluations 28
Fogarty catheter 311
Fontan baffle evaluation 100
Fontan physiology 12
Fontan procedure 260–264, *263*
anesthetic management, pre-Fontan 264–265
fenestrated Fontan 264
fenestrated Fontan procedure *267*
hydraulic schematic of Fontan circulation *261*
normal and Fontan circulation *262*
physiology 260–264, **266**
post-CPB management, post-Fontan procedure 265–267

foramen ovale (FO) 4, 6, 233, 270, 285
Fore-Sight instrument 36
fossa ovalis **6**, 98, 161
four-factor prothrombin complex concentrates (4FPCCs) 79
Frank–Starling mechanism 7
fresh frozen plasma (FFP) 68
Friedreich ataxia **25**
functional closure 5
functional residual capacity (FRC) 253
functional status, interpretation of catheterization data 26
FVIII deficiency (hemophilia A) 41
FXI deficiency 41
FXII 41

g

gamma-aminobutyric acid (GABA) 83
gastric tube (G-tube) 30
genetic predisposition to CHD 3
gingival hyperplasia **304**
glomerular filtration rate (GFR) 120
glucose 28
glycoprotein (GP) 41
glycopyrrolate 30, 39, 306
Gore-Tex. *See* expanded polytetrafluoroethylene (ePTFE)
gravity drainage, cardiopulmonary bypass (CPB) 63
Great Ormond Street Echocardiogram (GOSE) 334
great vessel orientation and identity 99
Gross, Dr Robert 145
group B streptococcal sepsis 109

h

haematocrit 24, 28, 67–68
haemoglobin 12, 20, 36
halothane 39
head circumferences, congestive heart failure 23
heart blocks 165, 170, 175, 244, 298, 331
heart failure (HF) 289
heart–lung block 308–309
heart–lung transplantation (HLT) 307
  anesthetic management 310–316
  donor 308–309
  double-lung transplantation 308
  living donor lobar lung transplant 308
  noncardiac surgery in lung transplant patients 317–319
  operative procedure 309–310
  patient positioning 309–310
  post-CPB management 316
  postoperative care 316–317
  single-lung transplantation 307
HeartMate II™ 116, *117*
HeartMate 3™ 118, 122
heart murmurs **26**
heart rate 22, 301
  heart transplants 302
  myocardial ischemia 21–22
heart transplantation:
  ABO compatibility 289, 291, **291**
  anesthetic considerations for noncardiac surgery 305–306
  anesthetic management of recipient 292–295

arrhythmias 223
atrial function 296, 301
atrial hypertension 236
autonomic nervous system 300–301
body weight factors 291
cardiac allograft vasculopathy 302
cardiopulmonary bypass 63–83
catheterization 49
completed aortic and pulmonary artery anastomoses *297*
contraindications to recipient selection for **291**
de-airing needs 299
diastolic function impairments 301–302
donor 289–292
drug responses 318
end-stage cardiac dysfunction identification 289
heart failure in children **290**
heart rates 299
human lymphocyte antigen 289
IgG therapy 291
indications for orthotopic **290**
left atrial anastomosis *296*
left ventricular systolic function 299
lung transplant 308
monitoring 292
noncardiac surgery in postcardiac transplant patient 300–305
operative procedure 295
operative technique for biatrial orthotopic heart transplantation *296*
panel reactive antibody screen 289
physical examination 292

physiology of the transplanted heart 300–302
post-CPB management 297–300
postoperative periods 27
premedications 310–311
preoperative evaluation 292
reinnervation 300
right ventricular afterload mismatch 314
right ventricular systolic function 314
sinus and atrioventricular node dysfunction 298
statistics 317
suture lines 303
systolic dysfunction in donor heart 242
termination of CPB 279
heat-exchanger units 64
hematoma **35**
hemi-Fontan procedure 258
hemodilution 66, 77
hemodynamics:
  background 7, 27–28, 74, 129, 138
  donors 289–292
hemolysis 111, 115
hemostasis 41
  amplification 44
  classic waterfall model of coagulation *42*
  cyanosis 46
  fibrinolysis 45–46
  hemostatic factor concentrations and activities between neonates and adults **46**
  inhibition of coagulation 44–45
  initiation 44
  primary platelet plug and secondary *43*
  propagation 44
  special considerations in neonates and infants 46
  stabilization 44

heparin:
   background   74
   protamine reversal   74–77
heparin-induced
   thrombocytopenia
   (HIT)   74
heparin-induced
   thrombocytopenia with
   thrombosis (HITT)   74
heparin dose–response test
   (HDR)   73
hepatic dysfunction
   119–120, 156, 331
hepatic veins   3, 12, 98
hepatomegaly   23
Hepcon® heparin management
   system (HMS)   73
heterotaxy syndrome   12, 327
  anatomy   327
  atrial anatomy   327–328
  examples of heterotaxy
    anatomy and
    repair   *331*
  general characterizations
    330–331
  human laterality disorders
    and current models   *329*
  surgical therapy   331
  tracheobronchial
    anatomy   330
  venoatrial connections
    327–328
  ventricular anatomy
    328–330
  ventriculoarterial
    connections   330
high-frequency jet ventilation
   (HFJV)   315
high-intensity transient signals
   (HITS)   38
high molecular weight
   kininogen (HMK)   41
high Q_P:Q_S 60
histamine   7
Holt–Oram syndrome   **25**
homograft   180, 185
HQ curves   117, *118, 118*
human immunodeficiency
   virus (HIV)   308

human lymphocyte antigen
   (HLA)
   heart transplants   289
   lung transplants   308
humidification   28
Hunter, John   207
hydralazine   306
hydrogen   69
hydroxyl   69
hyperacute rejection, heart
   transplants   298
hypercapnia   317
hypercarbia   4, 18–19, 21,
   186, 201–202, 236, 241,
   252–253, 260, 267, 297,
   310, 314
hypercyanotic episodes. *See*
   hypoxic episodes
hyperglycemia   28
hyperinflation   19
hyperlipidemia   302
hyperpnea   216
hypertension   302–303
hyperthermia   136
hypertrophic cardiomyopathy
   (HCM)   289
hyperventilation   19, 260
hypocalcemia   25
hypocarbia   19, 260
hypogastric artery   5
hypoglycaemia   25
hypoglycemia   28
hypokinesis   52, 122, 228,
   299, 316
hyponatremia   **26**
hypoplastic left heart
   syndrome (HLHS)
   11, 22, 72, 250, 269
  anatomy   269
  anesthetic management
    271–272
  apical four-chamber view
    of   *270*
  biventricular repair
    272–273
  noncardiac surgery   273
  physiology   269–271
  post-CPB management   272
  surgical therapy   271

hypoplastic ventricles   10–11
hypotension   21, 30, 120,
   129–130, 134–135, 139,
   147, 158, 190, 198, 202,
   205, 221, 223, 248, 254
hypothermia   4, 20, 65,
   70–71, 222, 278, 309
hypoxemia   18
hypoxia   4, 8, 19, 216, 268,
   317–318
hypoxic episodes   216–217
hypoxic pulmonary
   vasoconstriction
   6, 21, 253

i
iatrogenic withdrawal
   syndrome (IWS)   131
idiopathic pulmonary arterial
   hypertension
   (IPAH)   307
IgG therapy, heart
   transplants   291
IIase   44
iliac artery occlusion   33
iloprost   20
imidazole buffering
   system   69
immature myocardial
   metabolism, neonatal/
   adult comparisons in
   myocardial
   performance   8
immunodeficiency   24
immunoglobulin E (IgE)   76
immunoglobulin G (IgG)   76
immunosuppression
   302, **304**
immunosuppressive
   agents   303, **304**
impaired diastolic
   function   298–299
impaired systolic
   function   297
Impella® 2.5/5.0/CP/RP
   115–116
Improving Pediatric and Adult
   Congenital Treatment
   (IMPACT)   103

incomplete autonomic innervations, neonatal/adult comparisons 8
increased intraventricular dependence, neonatal/adult comparisons 7–8
indexed pulmonary flow 56
indexed systemic flow 56
indomethacin 6
"infantile" coarctation 153
infants:
  with aortic stenosis 195
  special considerations in 46
infections 23, 25, 169, 317, 331
inferior and superior sinus venosus defects 161
inferior vena cava (IVC) 3, 56, 63, 162, 187, 211, 295, 309, 328
infracardiac drainage 187
infundibular stenosis 17, 213
inhalation agents 253
inhaled nitric oxide (iNO) 335
inhaled pulmonary vasodilators 260, 265
inlet defects 167
innominate artery 72–73, 213, 217, 219, 271
innominate vein 187
inodilators 21
inodilators therapy 132
inotropes 111, 120, 122, 315
inotropic agents 8
inspiratory:expiratory (I:E) ratio 20, 221, 314
intact ventricular septum (IVS) 207, 233
intensive care unit (ICU) 33, 259
intercirculatory mixing 13–15, *14*
intermediate AVC 171
interobserver variability 54
interrupted aortic arch (IAA) 183, 275
  anatomy 275, **278**

anesthetic management 278–279
catheterization laboratory intervention 278
oxygen saturation **278**
physiology 275–276
post-CPB management 279
surgical management 276
interventricular septum (IVS) 161, 171
intraarterial catheter 66
intraatrial physiologic repair 239
intraatrial septum (IAS) 161
intracardiac baffles 181
intracardiac drainage 187
intracardiac pulmonary blood flow 285
intracardiac shunts 99–100
intracellular acidosis 71
intramuscular induction 39
intraoperative
  management 33
  airway management 38
  anesthesia induction and maintenance 39–40
  central and arterial line catheter sizes **34**
  central venous pressure 34–35
  ECG and blood pressure 33–34
  end-tidal carbon dioxide 34
intraoperative monitoring 33–38
intraoperative NIRS data *37*
NIRS 36
systemic oxygen saturation 34
TCD 36–38
TEE 38
temperature 35
intraoperative TEE 91
intravascular ultrasound (IVUS) 55, 302, 323
intravenous (IV)
  catheters 28, 169, 311

intravenous (IV) line 30, 241, 292
intravenous induction 39–40, 169, 175, 221, 253
intravenous pulmonary vasodilation 316
intraventricular dependence 7–8
intraventricular haemorrhage (IVH) 145
intraventricular septum (IVS) 213
intrinsic Xase 44
in vitro coagulation 41
INVOS 5100 NIRS 36
iron deficiency anemia 24
irritability symptoms, congestive heart failure 25
ischemia 21, 33, 71, 139, 157, 195, 204, 221
ischemia–reperfusion injury 297–298
isoflurane 21, 39
isolated aortic valve stenosis 195
isolated ostium primum ASDs 161
isoproterenol **29**, 203, 300, 305
Ivalon plug 146
Ivemark syndrome 330

j

Jervell and Lange Nielsen long QT syndrome **25**
jitteriness symptoms, congestive heart failure 25
jugular vein 40, 49, 110, 303
junctional ectopic tachycardia (JET) 221

k

ketamine 21, 30, 127, 131, 221
Konno procedure 196

l

labetalol **30**

laboratory data, preoperative evaluations 24–27

lactate 8, 120

laparoscopic gastrostomy 273

laryngeal nerve injury 147, 317

laryngoscopies 120, 253, 293, 311

Lecompte procedure 180, 240

left anterior descending artery (LAD) 55

left anterior oblique (LAO) projection 52

left aortic arch *243, 282*

left atrial hypertension 59

left atrial isomerism (LAI) 327

left atrial pressure (LAP) waveform *50,* 51, 94, 202, 221

left atrium (LA) 4, 9

left common carotid artery 183, 275

left coronary anatomy 53–54, *54*

left-heart catheterization 50–51

left heart rehabilitation 272

left lung 5, 146, 158

left main coronary artery (LMCA) 321

left posterolateral thoracotomy 281

left pulmonary artery (LPA) 145, 330

left subclavian artery (LSCA) 145, 153

left superior vena cava (LSVC) 163

left thoracotomy 145

left-to-right (L-R) shunt 9, 56, 63, 145, 149, 156, 162, 168, 174

left ventricle (LV) 98–99, 153, 157, 161, 163, 175, 177, 195, 198, 216, 220

left ventricular assist device (LVAD) 322

left ventricular diastolic filling 7

left ventricular ejection fraction (LVEF) 307

left ventricular end-diastolic pressure (LVEDP) 51, 195

left ventricular end-diastolic volume (LVEDV) 51, 204, 301, 314

left ventricular end-systolic volume (LVESV) 51, 301

left ventricular hypertrophy (LVH) 8, 303

left ventricular outflow tract (LVOT) 153, 179, 193, 233

  anatomy 193–195

  anesthetic management 196–198

  catheterization laboratory intervention 196

  long-axis view of left ventricle *194*

  physiology 195

  post-CPB management 198

  supravalvar and subvalvar aortic stenosis *194*

  surgical therapy 195–196

left ventricular outflow tract obstruction (LVOTO) 275

left ventricular pressure (LVP) waveform 51, *52*

left ventricular segments *53*

left ventricular systolic function, heart transplants 301

left ventricular volume overload 186

left ventriculography 51–53

Leopard syndrome **25**

lethargy 120

leukocytes 120

leukotrienes 7

levo (L) 99

levocardia 327

lidocaine **29**

ligamentum arteriosum 6

ligamentum teres **6**

ligamentum venosum 6

limited preload reserve, neonatal/adult comparisons in myocardial performance 7

lipophilicity 20

liver 3, 261

living donor lobar lung transplants (LDLLTs) 308

long QT syndromes **25**

low cardiac output syndrome (LCOS) 131

  detection and treatment of 131–136

  key pain, agitation, neuromuscular blockade, and delirium scales *133*

  left ventricular pressure–volume loops *134–135*

low heparin sensitivity (LHS) 74

lumen 6

lungs 4, 38, 85, 111, 230, 261, 308, 317, 330

lung transplants (LTX) 307, 308

lung volumes, variation in 19

  heart–lung transplants (HLTs) 317

  pulmonary vascular resistance (PVR) 19

lymphocytes 298

lympholytic agent 318

lysine analog antifibrinolytics 45, 83, 120

m

magnesium **29**

magnetic resonance angiography (MRA) 225, 323

magnetic resonance cardiac imaging   60
magnetic resonance imaging (MRI)   225, 272
major aortopulmonary collateral arteries (MAPCAS)   223, 249, 285
malnutrition   **26**
Marfan syndrome   **25**
Masimo O3 NIRS   36
mask induction   39
masks   23, 28
mean arterial blood pressure (MAP)   58, 123, 316
mean pulmonary artery pressure (mPAP)   18, 58
mechanical circulatory support (MCS)   109
  extracorporeal membrane oxygenation   109–113
  VAD   113–123
mechanical ventilation   136–138
meconium aspiration syndrome   109
medial umbilical ligaments   **6**
medical management   334–336, *336*
medications   23, 28, 113, 128
  doses   8, 20–21, 28, 30, 39–40, 66, 73–74, 77, 79, 81, 113, 129–130, 135, 141, 159, 169, 175, 186, 198, 202–203, 216, 253, 295, 314
  preoperative evaluation   310
  respiratory depression problems   30
Melody™ valve   200
membrane oxygenators   64
membranes, extracorporeal membrane oxygenation (ECMO)   109–113
membranous defects   167
mesocardia   327
methemoglobin   20
methylprednisolone   299

methylprednisolone   **304**
metoclopramide   310
midazolam   30, 129, 311
middle cerebral artery (MCA)   36
mild pulmonary stenosis   249
milrinone   21, 134, 203, 221, 248, 265, 279
mitochondria   7
mitral annulus   199
mitral regurgitation (MR)   161
mitral valve:
  hypoplasia   199
  regurgitation   203–205
  stenosis   199–203, *200, 201*
mixed drainage   187
M-mode capabilities   91
modified Blalock–Thomas–Taussig shunt (mBTTS)   209, 217, 226, 247, 271, 287
modified Norwood stage 1   271
modified Starnes right ventricular exclusion procedure   337
modified ultrafiltration (MUF)   69
monitoring:
  blood pressure cuffs   34
  cardiopulmonary bypass   63–83
  central venous pressure   34–35
  extracorporeal membrane oxygenation   109–113
  heart transplants   302
  intraoperative management   33–38
  near-infra-red spectroscopy   36
  non-invasive blood pressure   158
  temperature   35
  transcranial Doppler   36–38
  transesophageal echocardiography   38

urine output   66
ventricular assist devices   109
morphine   129
mortality rates   103, 334
mucopolysaccharidosis   **25**
multiplane imaging   100
multiple aortopulmonary collateral arteries (MAPCA)   11, 225, 226
murine monoclonal antibody (OKT3)   303, **304**, 318
muscarinic antagonists   304
muscular defects   167
Mustard procedures   *239*, 239–240
mycophenolate mofentil (MMF)   **304**
myocardial contusion   298
myocardial depression   211
myocardial hypertrophy   159
myocardial ischemia   21–22
myocardial oxygen consumption:
  in mitral regurgitation   204
  Williams–Beurin and nonsyndromic SVAS   195
myocardial performance in neonate   7–8
myocardial rhabdomyoma   **25**
myocarditis   109, 113

n

nasopharyngeal temperatures, monitoring   35
near-infra-red spectroscopy (NIRS)   36, 66, 158, 279
neonatal platelets   46
neonates:
  with ductal-dependent pulmonary blood flow   338
  myocardial performance in   7, 7–8
  special considerations in   46
  surgical management of   337

neo-ostium   325
neostigmine   305, 306
neuromuscular blocking
    agents (NMBA)   127
nicardipine   198
nifedipine   306
Nikaidoh procedure
    101, 240–241
nil-by-mouth status (NPO
    status)   293
nil-per-os (NPO) orders   28
nitric oxide (NO)   20, 60,
    203, 209, 227, 299
nitroglycerin   20, **30**, 202,
    242, 303, 316
nitroprusside   20, **30**,
    134–135, 139, 141,
    158–159, 170, 198,
    254, 306
nitrosylhemoglobin   20
nodal vesicular parcel (NVP)
    model   *329*
nomogram   70
noncardiac procedures
    106–107
noncardiac surgery:
    anesthetic considerations
        305–306, 318–319
    hypoplastic left heart
        syndrome   273
    issues unique to heart
        transplant patients   302
    in lung transplant
        patients   317
    physiology of transplanted
        heart   300–302
    in postcardiac transplant
        patient   300
    single-ventricle
        lesions   267–268
    Tetralogy of Fallot   223
    transposition of the great
        arteries   243
noncommitted VSD
    physiology   179–180
non invasive blood pressure
    (NIBP)   158, 279
nonrestrictive surgical
    anastomosis   190

nonrestrictive VSDs   168
nonsyndromic SVAS   195
Noonan syndrome   **25**
norepinephrine   6, 8, 21, **29**,
    135, 316
normally related great arteries
    (NRGAs)   13, 249, 287
normocarbia   19, 186,
    252, 260
Norwood procedure
    72–73, 269

o

obesity   **291**. *See also*
    diabetes
oblique vein of left atrium   **4**
obstructed TAPVR   189
obstructive lesions   99–100
oliguria   141
one-coronary approach   321
one-lung ventilation (OLV)
    309, 311–313, 315
opioids   21, 39–40, 129–130,
    150, 165, 190, 197, 202,
    205, 259, 265, 295
orthotopic heart
    transplantation
    (OHT)   289
osteoporosis   **291**
ostium primum defects, ASD
    161, *162*
ostium secundum defects,
    ASD   161, *163*
outflow tract obstruction
    131, 179, 195–196,
    219, 272
oxidative phosphorylation   5
oxygen   5–6, 21, 27, 39, 49,
    55, 60, 63, 70, 110, 139,
    256, 315
    debt   136
    saturations   10, 56,
        58, 109
    trials   60
oxygenators   40, 64–67, 109,
    113
oxyhemoglobin dissociation
    curve   72
Ozaki procedure   198

p

pacemaker   120, 244, 296
packed red blood cells   67, 68
$PaCO_2$ 6, 19–21, 34, 36, 38,
    70–71, 111, 158, 174, 216,
    253, 273, 299, 314
pain management   129.
    See also analgesics
palliative shunts   217, 220
pancreatitis   **304**
pancuronium   39, 305
panel reactive antibody
    (PRA)   289
PaO_2 19
parachute mitral valve   199
paraplegia   157
parasympathetic reinnervation
    of donor heart   305
paroxysmal hyperpnea   216
partial anomalous pulmonary
    venous return
    (PAPVR)   183
partial atrioventricular canal
    defects. *See* isolated
    ostium primum ASDs
partial AVC   171
partially anomalous
    pulmonary venous return
    (PAPVR)   162
partial thromboplastin time
    (PTT)   24
patch leaks   100
patent ductus arteriosus
    (PDA)   11, 51, 63,
    145–147, *146*, 149, 153,
    195, 208, 210, 219, 225,
    233, 247, 269, 285
patent foramen ovale
    (PFO)   50, 161, 188, 207,
    233, 269, 285, 333
pathophysiology:
    characteristics of
        cardiomyopathies
        294
    congenital heart disease   9
    pulmonary vascular   18
patient blood
    management   46–47
pediatric circle system   28

Pediatric Confusion
    Assessment Method for
    ICU (pCAM-ICU)   131
PediMag™   118
peptic ulcers   91
percutaneous mechanical
    circulatory assist
    devices   *116*
perfusion pressure   **65**, 145,
    250
perimembranous defects   167
perimembranous
    septum   169
perimembranous VSD   100
perioperative management
    9, 269
peripheral arterial
    catheter   34
peripherally inserted central
    catheter (PICC)   273
permanent anatomic
    closure   5
persistence of the fetal
    circulation (PFC)   4
PGI_2 (prostacyclin)   7
pH   19–20, 38, 70–72, 252,
    299, 314, 316
pH-stat regulation   70–71
phenylephrine   **29**, 216,
    295, 306
physiologic shunts   10
physiology:
    ALCAPA   321
    anomalous aortic origin of
        coronary artery   323
    aortopulmonary
        window   149
    atrioventricular canal
        defects   173–174
    C-TGV   244
    cardiovascular   3–7
    coarctation of aorta
        153–156
    congenital heart disease   9
    DORV   179–180
    Ebstein anomaly   333–334
    Fontan   12
    hypoplastic left heart
        syndrome   269–271

LVOT   195
mitral valve regurgitation
    203–204
mitral valve stenosis   200
PA/IVS   207–209
patent ductus
    arteriosus   145
single-ventricle
    lesions   247
single-ventricle
    physiology   10, 180
TAPVR   188–189
Tetralogy of Fallot
    213–216
TOF/APV   229
TOF/PA   225
of transplanted
    heart   300–302
transposition   10, 14
truncus arteriosus   185
vascular rings   281
ventricular septal
    defects   167–169
'pink Tet' patients   18, 214
placenta   3–5, 43
plasma   21, 25, 77
plasmin   45
plasminogen   45
plasminogen activator
    inhibitor 1 (PAI-1)   45
platelet repletion   77–79
platelets   41
pneumatic pulsatile flow
    devices   113–115
pneumothorax   314
point-of-care (POC)   46
polyclonal ATG   318
polyphosphate (PolyP)   44
polysplenia syndrome   330
portal venous system   3
positive-pressure ventilation
    (PPV)   136
positive end-expiratory
    pressure (PEEP)
    19, 138, 253, 299, 310
postcapillary PH   18–19, 59
post-cardiopulmonary
    bypass (CPB)
    hyperventilation   19

post-CPB hemostasis   77–83
post-CPB management   297
    DORV   181
    Ebstein anomaly   338
    goals   297
    heart–lung
        transplantation   316
    hypoplastic left heart
        syndrome   272
    interrupted aortic
        arch   279
    left ventricular outflow
        tract   198
    mitral valve
        regurgitation   205
    mitral valve stenosis
        202–203
postinitial repair   253
postsuperior
    cavopulmonary shunt
    259–260
preparation for termination
    of CPB   297–299
pulmonary atresia/intact
    ventricular septum   211
TAPVR   190
termination of CPB
    299–300
Tetralogy of Fallot
    221–223
Tetralogy of Fallot with
    absent pulmonary
    valve   230
Tetralogy of Fallot with
    pulmonary atresia
    227–228
transposition of the great
    arteries   241–243
truncus arteriosus   186
posterior leaflets   199, *200*,
    244, 333
posterior tibial arteries   33
posteromedial
    commissures   199
postligation cardiac
    syndrome   147
postoperative cardiac
    intensive care unit
    care   127

context-sensitive half-times *129*

coordinated, goal-directed postoperative management strategy *140*

detection and treatment of low cardiac output syndrome 131–136

enhanced recovery after surgery and early tracheal extubation 138–139

extended CICU care 139–141

heart lung interactions and hemodynamic changes *137*

management of sedation/analgesia 131

mechanical ventilation 136–138

sedation/analgesia medications 127–131

structured hand-off from OR to CICU team 127

postoperative care 127, 269, 316–317

postoperative junctional ectopic tachycardia (POJET) 222–223

postoperative periods 27, 138, 139, 272, 317

post-transplant therapy 291

post-VAD placement management 120–123, *121*

pre-bypass management 120

pre-transplant therapy 291

precapillary PH (PAH). *See* pulmonary arterial hypertension (PAH)

precardiopulmonary bypass (CPB) 186

prednisone **304**

pregnancy tests 27

prekallikrein (PK) 41

preload reserve 7

preoperative evaluation **26**

associated congenital abnormalities 24

clinical history 23

laboratory data 24–27

physical examination 23–24

pregnancy 27

preoperative preparation 27–30

psychological considerations 27

preoperative fluid therapy 28

preoperative medications 28–30

pressure data, interpretation of 26

pressure gradients 26, 202

pressure-limited ventilation 28

preterm neonates 6

primary hemostasis 43

priming solution 66–68

primitive atrium **4**

primitive ventricle **4**

prior surgical interventions 26

procainamide **29**, 222

Procedural Risk in Congenital Cardiac Catheterization (PREDIC3T) score 103, **105**

propofol 21, 127, 130

propranolol 217

prostacyclin 20

prostaglandins (PGEs) 5

prostaglandin D$_2$ 7

PGE$_1$ 7, 156, 189, 203, 225, 236–237, 247, 276, 334

PGE$_2$ 7

protamine reversal of heparin 74–77, *76*

protein C (PC) 44

protein kinase A 20

protein S (PS) 44

prothrombin 44

prothrombinase complex 44

prothrombin complex concentrates (PCC) 47, 79–81

prothrombin time (PT) 24

psychological considerations 27

pulmonary arterial blood flow: classification of tricuspid atresia **249**

initial procedures to optimizing 247–249

repair sequence for hypoplastic left heart syndrome *248*

pulmonary arterial hypertension (PAH) 18, 59, 185, 189, 234, 247

pulmonary arteriovenous malformations (PAVMs) 259

pulmonary artery (PA) 4, *5*, 9, 11–12, 13–14, 49, 99, *115*, 189, 207, 225, 310, 330

anastomosis *297*, 298, 299

catheters for pediatric patients 34

clamping of 315

wedge angiogram 59

pulmonary artery band (PAB) 245, 248–249

pulmonary artery catheter (PAC) 293

pulmonary artery hypertension (PAH) 149, 168, 217, 227, 287

pulmonary artery occlusion pressure (PAOP) 58, 60, 299, 316

pulmonary artery pressure (PAP) 34, 50, *51*, 94, 200, 221, 236, 248, 298, 321

pulmonary artery wedge pressure (PAWP) 18, 59

pulmonary atresia (PA) 11, 334

pulmonary atresia with intact ventricular septum (PA/IVS) 22, 207, 247

algorithm for surgical management of *210*

pulmonary atresia with intact
　　ventricular septum
　　(PA/IVS) (cont'd)
　anatomy   207, *208*
　anesthetic management
　　211
　moderately hypoplastic
　　right ventricle in   *208*
　physiology   207–209
　post-CPB management
　　211
　surgical and catheter-based
　　therapy   209–211
pulmonary blood flow (PBF)
　　210, 285, 333–334
pulmonary edema   189
pulmonary hypertension (PH)
　　18, 59, **60**
pulmonary obstructions
　　17, 243
pulmonary regurgitation (PR)
　　219, 223, 334
pulmonary stenosis (PS)   151,
　　179, 195, 213, 229, 234,
　　244, 246, 249, 285, 330
pulmonary trunk   145, 180,
　　322
pulmonary valve (PV)   207
pulmonary valvotomy   209
pulmonary vascular:
　anatomy assessment
　　58–60
　disease   59–60
　pathophysiology   18–19
　system   9, 18, 59
　changes   6–7
pulmonary vascular resistance
　　(PVR)   7, 15, 38, 58, 60,
　　122, 145, 149, 156, 168,
　　174, 185, 189, 202, 216,
　　234, 247, 270, 298, 310,
　　321, 334
　anesthetic agents   21
　control of   19
　PaCO$_2$ 19
　PaO$_2$ 19
　pH   19
　sympathetic nervous system
　　stimulation   20–21
　variation in lung
　　volumes   19
　vasoactive agents   21
　vasodilator agents   20
pulmonary vascular resistance
　　index (PVRI)   18, 58, 59
pulmonary vasculature
　　evaluation   58–59
pulmonary veins   328
pulmonary vein wedge
　　angiogram   59
pulmonary venous atrium   9
pulmonary venous blood
　　flow   249–250
pulmonary venous
　　obstruction   59
pulmonary venous
　　plexus   187
pulmonary venous
　　saturation   12
pulsatile/axial device
　　comparisons   120–121
pulsatile pump technology
　　114–115
pulsatility index (PI)   122
pulsed-wave (PW) Doppler
　　probe   36, 91, 99, 101
pulse oximetry   24, 36, 66,
　　248, 292, 314
pulse rates, congestive heart
　　failure   22
pumps:
　arterial   64
　axial flow   117
　centrifugal   118–119
pyrexia   237

q
q11.23 deletion syndrome
　　193
quantification method, shunt
　　56–58

r
rabbit antithymocyte gamma-
　　globulin (RATG)   **304**
radial artery   33, 73, 279, 311
radial artery catheter
　　292–293
radiographic contrast
　　material   49, 51, 53
rales, congestive heart
　　failure   23, 303
ranitidine   310
Rashkind–Miller balloon atrial
　　septostomy   250
Rastelli A   171
Rastelli B   171
Rastelli C   173
Rastelli procedure   180
recirculated flow   10
recirculation of pulmonary
　　venous blood   9
recombinant erythropoietin
　　(rEPO)   24
recombinant FVIIa
　　(rFVIIA)   47
rectal temperatures   35
recurrent laryngeal nerve
　　(RLN)   282
red blood cell (RBC)   68
red cell repletion   81–83, *82*
reduced contractile capacity   7
reduced ventricular
　　compliance   7
regional cerebral perfusion
　　278, 279
regional wall motion
　　abnormalities   53
regurgitant fraction   61, 204
regurgitant lesions   61
regurgitant stroke volume   61
regurgitant valves   100
reimplanted coronary
　　arteries   242
reinnervation issues, heart
　　transplants   305
rejection:
　heart transplant   303
　lung transplants   318
remifentanil   129–130
renal anomalies   24
renal arteries   *5*
renal dysfunction   120, 189
renal vein   328
reparation á l'étage
　　ventriculaire procedure
　　(REV procedure)   180

residual VSD   221

resistances   58, **58**

respiratory depression problems, medications   30

respiratory distress syndrome   109, 146, 281

respiratory failure   109, 113

respiratory rate (RR)   221

respiratory tract infections   23, 308

response to drugs   304–305

restenosis   191, 302

resting heart rates   301

restrictive cardiomyopathy (RCM)   289

restrictive simple shunts   220

reverse differential cyanosis   236

rhDNase   311

right-heart catheterization   49–50

right-to-left shunt (R-L shunt)   10, 56, 168

right anterior oblique (RAO) projection   52

right atrial anastomosis   *296*

right atrial appendage (RAA)   98

right atrial isomerism (RAI)   327

right atrial pressure (RAP)   49, 202

right atrium (RA)   4, 5, 9, 19, 49, 50, 63, 69, 74, 98, 115, *115, 162,* 310

right bundle branch block   170

right common carotid artery (RCCA)   *276–278*

right coronary anatomy   53–54, *54*

right coronary artery   53–54, 101, 219, 233, 237, 244, 321

right lung   *5,* 163, 234, 330

right pulmonary artery (RPA)   34, 73, *86,* 149, 163, 211, 217, 254, 258, *259,* 262, 321, 330

right subclavian artery   275, 277, 279

right upper lobe (RUL)   313

right ventricle-dependent coronary circulation (RVDCC)   209

right ventricle-to-pulmonary artery conduit   138, 181, 185, *240,* 240, 250, 271–273

right ventricle (RV)   4, 7, 98, 226

right ventricular afterload mismatch   298

right ventricular diastolic filling   8

right ventricular ejection fraction (RVEF)   307

right ventricular end-diastolic volume (RVEDV)   301, 314

right ventricular end-systolic volume (RVESV)   301, 314

right ventricular outflow tract (RVOT)   179, 198, 209, 213, 219, 330, 333

right ventricular pressure (RVP) waveform   49, *50*

right ventricular systolic function   301

right ventricular volume overload (RVVO)   163–164

rigid bronchoscope/ bronchoscopy   284, 317

Risk Adjustment for Congenital Heart Surgery (RACHS)   103

risk scoring systems   103

cardiac surgery   103–105

individual procedures by RACHS category   **104**

multivariate analysis of predictors   **106**

mutivariate risk stratification   **106**

noncardiac procedures   106–107

for original 20-point risk score   **104**

systematic approach to patients with congenital heart disease   *107*

rocuronium   39, 40, 165, 253, 293, 295, 305, 313

Romano–Ward syndrome   **25**

Ross/Konno procedure   278

Ross procedure   101, 198, 278

Rotaflow II   118

rotational thromboelastometry (ROTEM)   77, **78,** *80, 81*

RUPV draining   163

rVIIA   79–81

S

saline   220

Sano procedure. *See* modified Norwood stage 1

Sano shunt   269, 271

sarcoplasmic reticulum (SR)   7

saturation   26

aortic   12, 15

in atrial septal defect   *11*

data   58

interpretation of catheterization data   49

oxygen   10, 56, 253, **278**

pulmonary venous   12

systemic oxygen   34

systemic venous   12

threshold level of capillary   251

in tricuspid atresia   *14,* 15, *288*

Scimitar syndrome   163

scopolamine   304

secondary hemostasis   43

sedation/analgesia management   131

sedation/analgesia medications   127

benzodiazepines   129

dexmedetomidine   130–131

ketamine   131

opioids   129–130

propofol   130

sedatives 66, 127, 205
Senning procedures *239*,
    239–240
Senning–Rastelli
    procedure 245
sepsis 4
septal leaflets 171
septation 3, 174
seropositivity 302
severe neonatal aortic
    stenosis 11, 247
sevoflurane 21, 39
Shprintzen syndrome **25**
shunting 9–10
    anatomic 15–18
    bidirectional 57–58
    blood flows in normal cardiac
        physiology without *10*
    dynamics of 4
    location 56
    palliative 217, 220
    quantification 56–58
    types 217
sildenafil 20
simple shunts 15, **16**
single-lumen endotracheal
    tube plus bronchial
    blocker 311
single-lung transplantation
    (SLT) 307, 310
    allograft implantation
        315–316
    clamping of PA 315
    indications for CPB 316
    one-lung ventilation 315
    special considerations
        for 315
single-ventricle lesions 247
    depiction of saturations and
        blood flows in
        neonate *257*
    initial procedures to
        optimizing pulmonary
        arterial blood flow
        247–249
    initial procedures to
        optimizing pulmonary
        venous blood flow
        249–250

initial procedures to
    optimizing systemic
    blood flow 250
management of single-
    ventricle physiology
    250–251, *251*
noncardiac surgery
    267–268
physiology and initial
    procedures 247
single-ventricle pathway,
    superior cavopulmonary
    shunt or BDG
    254–264
single-ventricle pathway
    (SVP) 269
single-ventricle physiology
    10, 180
    anatomic subtypes **13**
    anesthetic management,
        preinitial repair
        251–253
    management of 250–251,
        251, **255–256**
    post-CPB management,
        postinitial repair 253
    systemic SaO_2 versus
        Qp:Qs *15*
sinoatrial node dysfunction
    (SA node
    dysfunction) 305
sinus and atrioventricular
    node dysfunction 298
sinus node injury 295
sinus of Valsalva
    194, 323
sinus venosus **4**
sinus venosus defects
    162–163
sirolimus **304**
sizes, catheter **34**
smooth part of left ventricle
    (aortic vestibule) **4**
smooth part of right atrium
    (sinus venarum) **4**
smooth part of right ventricle
    (conus arteriosus) **4**
Snoopy's ear 98, 327
Snoopy's nose 98, 327

Society of Thoracic Surgeons
    European Association for
    Thoracic Surgery
    (STAT) 103
sodium bicarbonate 216, 316
sodium nitroprusside 134,
    158–159, 170, 198, 306
somatic NIRS 73
Sophia Observation
    Scale 131
spinal cord ischemia 157
spironolactone 141
spleen *329*
$SpvO_2$ 250, 251
staged left ventricular
    recruitment 272–273
State Behavioral Scale
    (SBS) **132**
stenotic anastomosis
    100–101, 260
stenotic lesions 60
stenotic valves 100
stent placement **105**
sterile technique 318
sterility 292, 311
sternotomy 282
stomach 38
stranger anxiety 27
stress-dose steroid 306
stroke volume (SV) 51, 132,
    196, 295
subacute bacterial
    endocarditis prophylaxis
    (SBE prophylaxis) 303
subaortic stenosis 193
subclavian artery 23, 33, 145,
    153, 158, 219, 275–279,
    281, *282*, 292
subendocardial perfusion 21
subendocardial pressure 22
subpulmonary defects
    167, 169
subpulmonary VSDs 99, *168*,
    177, 179
subpulmonic stenosis 233
succinylcholine 39, 293, 313
sudden cardiac death
    (SCD) 323
sufentanil 129

Super Glenn procedure 258–259, *259*
superior cavopulmonary shunt 247, 254
  anatomy of double cavopulmonary anastomosis *258*
  anesthetic management, presuperior cavopulmonary shunt 259
  post-CPB management, postsuperior cavopulmonary shunt 259–260
superior vena cava (SVC) 4, 35, 56, 63, 162, *163*, 183, 211, 247, 295, 309, 328
superior vesicular artery **6**
suppression of CMRO$_2$ 72
supracardiac drainage 187
supracristal defects 167, 169
supravalvar stenosis 193
supravalvular aortic stenosis (SVAS) 193, 198, 199
supravalvular mitral stenosis 199
surfactant B deficiency 307
surgeon-performed epicardial imaging 95
surgical repair evaluation 100–101
surgical therapy/management:
  AAOCA 324–325
  ALCAPA 321–322
  with aneurysmal dilation of pulmonary arteries *230*
  for DORV *180*, 180–181
  double switch procedure and atrial switch-Rastelli procedures 244–246
  Ebstein anomaly 336–337
  heterotaxy 331
  hypoplastic left heart syndrome 271
  left ventricular outflow tract 195–196
  mitral valve regurgitation 204

mitral valve stenosis 200
pulmonary atresia/intact ventricular septum 209–211
surgically created systemic-to-pulmonary artery shunts *218*
TAPVR 189
Tetralogy of Fallot 217–219
Tetralogy of Fallot with absent pulmonary valve 229–230
Tetralogy of Fallot with pulmonary atresia 225–227
traditional repair for C-TGV 244
transposition of the great arteries 237–241
tricuspid atresia 287
truncus arteriosus 185
vascular rings 281–282
"sutureless" techniques 189
sweating 23
sympathetic innervation 8
sympathetic nervous system stimulation 20–21
SynCardia® TAH 114, *115*
systemic blood flow 250, 270
systemic hypotension 221
systemic hypothermia 65
systemic oxygen saturation 34
systemic vascular resistance (SVR) 15, 58, 129, 145, 150–151, 168, 174, 185, 216, 234, 270, 295, 310, 338
systemic vascular resistance index (SVRI) 58
systemic venous saturation 12
systolic dysfunction in the donor heart 297
systolic function 297
systolic pressure 21

t
tachycardia 197–198, 295
tachypnea 149
tacrolimus (FK506) **304**
Takeuchi procedure 322
TandemHeart® *116*, 118
target heparin concentration (THC) 73
"temperature-uncorrected" values 70
temperature 35
  cooling and rewarming 35, 40
  monitoring 35
tenase complex 44
Tetralogy of Fallot (TOF) 11, 17, 173, 179, 183, 213, 247
  anatomy 213, *214*
  anesthetic management 220–221
  catheterization laboratory intervention 219
  hypoxic episodes 216–217
  noncardiac surgery 223
  parasternal long-axis view *214*
  physiology 213–216
  post-CPB management 221–223
  spectrum of infundibular stenosis *215*
  surgical therapy 217–219
Tetralogy of Fallot with absent pulmonary valve (TOF/APV) 213, 229–230
Tetralogy of Fallot with pulmonary atresia (TOF/PA) 213, 225–228, *226*
tetralogy of Fallot with pulmonary stenosis (TOF/PS) 213
"Tet Spells". *See* hypoxic episodes
Thebesian vein blood 63
thermodilution cardiac output 55
thermodilution technique 55

thiopental   39
thoracotomy approach   220
Thoratec® PVAD   113–115
three-factor prothrombin
    complex concentrates
    (3FPCCs)   79, 81
thrombin-activatable
    fibrinolysis inhibitor
    (TAFI)   45
thrombin   44
thromboelastography
    (TEG)   77, *77–78*, **78**,
    80, 81
thrombomodulin (TM)   44
thromboxane   76
time-velocity integral
    (TVI)   36
tissue factor (TF)   41–42
tissue factor pathway inhibitor
    (TFPI)   41
tissue plasminogen activator
    (tPA)   45
tissue thromboplastin. *See*
    tissue factor (TF)
total anomalous pulmonary
    venous return
    (TAPVR)   187, 330
  anatomy   187–188
  anesthetic management
    189–190
  connection   *188*
  etiologies of pulmonary
    hypertension   *191*
  long-term outcomes
    191–192
  physiology   188–189
  post-CPB management
    190
  surgical therapy   189
total artificial heart
    (TAH)   109
total cavopulmonary
    connection (TCPC)
    209, 247, 260–264
totally anomalous pulmonary
    venous return
    (TAPVR)   12
total pulmonary blood flow
    (Q$_p$)   10, *11*, 12

total systemic blood
    flow (Q$_s$)   10, 12
tracheal anastomosis   309
tracheobronchial malacia
    (TBM)   281
tranexamic acid (TXA)
    45, 83, **83**
transcatheter pulmonary valve
    replacement
    (TPVR)   219
transcranial Doppler
    (TCD)   36–38, 73
transesophageal
    echocardiography (TEE)
    38, 85–96, *90*, 120, 158,
    175, 190, 198, 202, 222,
    248, 293, 311, 314, 316, 338
  conventional display and
    orientation   *91*
  views in comprehensive
    TEE exam   *92–97*
transitional AVC   171
transmembrane pressure
    gradient (TMP)   69
transposition of great arteries
    (TGA)   13, 179, 233,
    285. *See also* congenitally
    corrected transposition of
    great vessels (C-TGV)
  anatomy   233–234
  anesthetic management
    241
  arterial switch operation
    237–239, *238*
  coronary artery patterns
    in   *235*
  with intact ventricular
    septum   *234*
  Lecompte procedures
    240–241
  Mustard and Senning
    procedures   *239*,
    239–240
  Nikaidoh procedures
    240–241
  noncardiac surgery   243
  physiology   234
  post-CPB management
    241–243

Rastelli procedures   240
  surgical therapy   237–241
  transposition physiology
    10, 14
transpulmonary gradient
    (TPG)   58, 60, 260, 267
transthoracic
    echocardiography (TTE)
    85, 93, 181, 209
  apical four-chamber
    sweep   *87*
  apical long-axis view   *88*
  parasternal long-axis
    sweep   *88*
  parasternal short-axis
    sweep   *89*
  subxiphoid long-axis
    (frontal) sweep   *86*
  subxiphoid short-axis
    (sagittal) sweep   *87*
  suprasternal notch aortic
    arch view   *89*
  suprasternal view of
    pulmonary veins   *90*
  transducer locations   *86*
transthoracic intracardiac
    lines   35
transthoracic PA
    catheter   311
tricuspid atresia (TA)
    11, 285, *286*
  anatomy   285
  anesthetic management
    287–288
  classification of
    286, **287**
  depiction of saturations and
    blood flows in   *288*
  physiology   285–287
  surgical therapy   287
tricuspid regurgitation (TR)
    245, 333
tricuspid stenosis (TS)   338
tricuspid valve (TV)
    177, 333
  atresia   285
  Ebstein anomaly of   334
trisomy   13, 24, 18, and 21,
    167, 177, 207

trisomy 21 microdeletion
235
truncus arteriosus (TA)   183
  anatomy   183
  anesthetic management
    185–186
  catheterization laboratory
    intervention   185
  classification of   *184*
  parasternal short-axis
    view   *184*
  physiology   185
  post-CPB
    management   186
  subcostal coronal
    view   *184*
  surgical therapy   185
  type I TA   183
  type II TA   183
  type III TA   183
  type IV TA   183
truncus arteriosus   **4**
T tubules   7
twin atrioventricular nodes
  (AV nodes)   330
two-coronary system
  approach   321
two-dimensional
  echocardiography   237
Type A interrupted aortic
  arch   275, *276*, **278**
Type B interrupted aortic
  arch   275, *277*, **278**
Type C interrupted aortic
  arch   275, *278*, **278**

u
ultrafiltration   68–69
ultrafiltrators   68
umbilical artery   50
umbilical artery catheters   34
umbilical cord   *5*
umbilical vein   3, *5*, 6, **6**, 49
umbilical vessels   6
umbilicovitelline drainage
  system   187
umbilicus   *5*
unbalanced AVC   173
unconsciousness   130

unfractionated heparin
  (UFH)   73, 112
unifocalization   226, 227, 228
Univent™ Tube   313
univent tubes   313
unroofing procedure   324
urine output   66
urokinase plasminogen
  activator (uPA)   45
uterus   188

v
VACTERL association   24
vacuum-assisted venous
  drainage   63
vagolytic and vagotonic
  agents   305
vagus nerve   *155, 156*
valve lesions, assessment of
  60–61
valvular aortic stenosis   193
valvular mitral stenosis   199
valvular stenosis   213
valvuloplasty   **105**
Van Praagh and Van Praagh
  classifications, truncus
  arteriosus (TA)   183
vascular anomalies, types of
  281, **284**
vascular rings   281–284
vascular smooth muscle
  (VSM)   20
vasoactive agents   21
vasoactive drugs   **29**
vasoactive infusions   132
vasoconstriction   7
vasodilator   159
  agents   20
  therapy   205
vasopressin   21, **29**
vasopressor agents   306
VATER association   24
vecuronium   39, 305
venoarterial (VA)
  ECMO   110, **111**
venodilation   265
venous blood   9, 10, 111, 216
venous cannulas   63
venous filters   *67*

venous reservoirs   63–64, 69,
  71, *261*
venovenous (VV) ECMO
  109, **111**
ventricles   236, 279, 330
ventricular anatomy
  328–330
ventricular assist device
  (VAD)   109, 113
  anesthetic considerations
    for patients receiving
    VAD   119–120
  BiVAD insertion   123
  complications   119
  current VAD and TAH
    technologies   113–119
  decision algorithm for
    treatment of hypotension
    and hypertension
    123, 124
  indications   113
  induction of anesthesia
    and pre-bypass
    management   120
  post-VAD placement
    management   120–123
  relative
    contraindications   113
ventricular compliance   7
ventricular end-systolic
  pressure–volume
  points   132, *134*
ventricular failure   186
ventricular fibrillation
  186, 253
ventricular function
  assessment   101
ventricular hypertrophy   22
ventricular output   10
ventricular pacing   198
ventricular septal defects
  (VSDs)   11, 39, 94, 100,
  153, 161, 167, 171, 177,
  183, 193, 213, 225, 229,
  233, 249, 285. *See also*
  atrial septal defects (ASDs)
  anatomy   167
  anesthetic management
    169–170

ventricular septal defects
(VSDs) (*cont'd*)
   apical four-chamber view
      with anterior
      angulation   *168*
   catheterization laboratory
      intervention   169
   induction and maintenance
      169–170
   locations   *168*
   noncardiac surgery   170
   physiology   167–169
   post-CPB management
      170
   surgical therapy   169
ventricular size and identity
   98–99
ventricular tachyarrhythmias
   139
ventriculoarterial
   connections   330

ventriculoarterial
   relationship   99
ventriculoatrial septum
   (VAS)   161
ventriculography   51–53
ventriculotomy   169, 222,
   226, 244
verapamil   305
video-assisted thoracoscopic
   surgery (VATS)   145
von Willebrand factor
   (vWF)   41
V wave   49

W
Warden procedure   164
waterfall coagulation model.
   See classic cascade
Waterston and Potts
   shunts   217
wheezing   23, 281

Williams–Beurin
   syndrome   22, 193, 195
Windkessel effect   195
Withdrawal Assessment
   Tool-1   131
Wolff–Parkinson–White type
   of accessory
   pathway   333
Wood units   18, 59, 263

X
X descent   49

Y
Yasui procedure
   181, 278
Y descent   49

Z
Zellweger syndrome   **25**